METHODS IN MOLECULAR BIOLOGY

Series Editor
John M. Walker
School of Life and Medical Sciences
University of Hertfordshire
Hatfield, Hertfordshire, AL10 9AB, UK

For further volumes:
http://www.springer.com/series/7651

Chromosome Architecture

Methods and Protocols

Edited by

Mark C. Leake

Biological Physical Sciences Institute, University of York, Heslington, York, UK

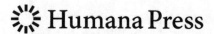 Humana Press

Editor
Mark C. Leake
Biological Physical Sciences Institute
University of York
Heslington, York, UK

ISSN 1064-3745   ISSN 1940-6029   (electronic)
Methods in Molecular Biology
ISBN 978-1-4939-8100-7   ISBN 978-1-4939-3631-1   (eBook)
DOI 10.1007/978-1-4939-3631-1

Printed on acid-free paper

This Humana Press imprint is published by Springer Nature
The registered company is Springer Science+Business Media LLC New York

Preface

Traditional insight into the composition, and functional properties, of chromosomes has stemmed largely either from conventional bulk ensemble average techniques in vitro or from optical microscopy methods on either fixed cell samples or living cells, but restricted to standard optical resolution limits. However, over the past few years several cutting-edge interdisciplinary methods have emerged which now enable us to understand the architecture of chromosomes with exceptionally enhanced resolution, both in terms of space and time; in other words, to probe the *dynamic* architecture of chromosomes, and at a *molecular length scale* of precision. These emerging interdisciplinary tools have grown in particular from biophysics, including several single-molecule methods and super-resolution techniques. This volume of *Chromosome Architecture* includes a valuable new collection of protocols and reviews of such emerging experimental and theoretical approaches, which have resulted in a substantial improvement to our understanding of chromosome architecture.

Biological Physical Sciences Institute (BPSI),   *Mark C. Leake*
University of York, UK

Contents

Contributors

JOHN ATKINSON • *School of Medical Sciences, Institute of Medical Sciences, University of Aberdeen, Foresterhill, Aberdeen, UK*

ANJANA BADRINARAYANAN • *Department of Biology, Massachusetts Institute of Technology, Cambridge, MA, USA*

SRINJAN BASU • *Department of Biochemistry, University of Cambridge, Cambridge, UK*

CHRISTOPH G. BAUMANN • *Department of Biology, University of York, Heslington, York, UK*

CLAIRE E. BROWN • *Department of Biology, University of York, Heslington, York, UK*

PIETRO CICUTA • *Cavendish Laboratory, University of Cambridge, Cambridge, UK*

STEPHEN J. CROSS • *Department of Biology, University of York, Heslington, York, UK*

NELLY DUABRRY • *MMSB - Molecular Microbiology and Structural Biochemistry, Université Lyon 1, Lyon Cedex, France*

TOMAS FESSL • *Astbury Centre for Structural Molecular Biology, University of Leeds, Leeds, UK*

SARAH HARRIS • *School of Physics and Astronomy, University of Leeds, Leeds, UK; Astbury Centre for Structural and Molecular Biology, University of Leeds, Leeds, UK*

MICHELLE HAWKINS • *Department of Biology, University of York, Wentworth Way, York, UK*

SOPHIA HEYDE • *Micron Advanced Bioimaging Unit, Department of Biochemistry, University of Oxford, Oxford, UK*

BART W. HOOGENBOOM • *London Centre for Nanotechnology and Department of Physics and Astronomy, University College London, London, UK*

ALESSIO V. INCHINGOLO • *School of Biosciences, University of Kent, Canterbury, UK*

CASSANDRAVICTORIA INNOCENT • *Micron Advanced Bioimaging Unit, Department of Biochemistry, University of Oxford, Oxford, UK*

AVELINO JAVER • *Cavendish Laboratory, University of Cambridge, Cambridge, UK*

GRACE JEREMY • *Structural & Molecular Biology, University College London, London, UK*

NEIL M. KAD • *School of Biosciences, University of Kent, Canterbury, UK*

ALAN KOH • *Centre for Bacterial Cell Biology, Institute for Cell & Molecular Biosciences, Newcastle University, Newcastle Upon Tyne, UK*

MARCO COSENTINO LAGOMARSINO • *Cavendish Laboratory, University of Cambridge, Cambridge, UK*

ERNEST D. LAUE • *Department of Biochemistry, University of Cambridge, Cambridge, UK*

MARK C. LEAKE • *Biological Physical Sciences Institute (BPSI), University of York, Heslington, York, UK*

STEVEN F. LEE • *Department of Chemistry, University of Cambridge, Cambridge, UK*

CHRISTIAN LESTERLIN • *MMSB - Molecular Microbiology and Structural Biochemistry, Université Lyon 1, Lyon Cedex, France*

KAREN LIPKOW • *Babraham Institute, Nuclear Dynamics Programme, Cambridge, UK; Cambridge Systems Biology Centre, University of Cambridge, Cambridge, UK*

CAMBRIDGE SYSTEMS BIOLOGY CENTRE UNIVERSITY OF CAMBRIDGE, CAMBRIDGE, UK

PAULA MONTERO LLOPIS • *Department of Microbiology & Immunobiology, Harvard Medical School, Boston, MA, USA*

ALAN R. LOWE • *Structural & Molecular Biology, University College London, London, UK; Department of Biological Sciences, Birkbeck College, University of London, London, UK; London Centre for Nanotechnology, London, UK*

ERIKA J. MANCINI • *School of Life Sciences, University of Sussex, Brighton, UK*

PETER MCGLYNN • *Department of Biology, University of York, Wentworth Way, York, UK*

EZEQUIEL MIRON • *Micron Advanced Bioimaging Unit, Department of Biochemistry, University of Oxford, Oxford, UK*

ROSA MORRA • *Faculty of Life Sciences, Manchester Institute of Biotechnology, University of Manchester, Manchester, UK*

HEATH MURRAY • *Centre for Bacterial Cell Biology, Institute for Cell & Molecular Biosciences, Newcastle University, Newcastle Upon Tyne, UK*

AGNES NOY • *School of Physics and Astronomy, University of Leeds, Leeds, UK*

ALICE L.B. PYNE • *London Centre for Nanotechnology and Department of Physics and Astronomy, University College London, London, UK*

VINCENT RÉCAMIER • *Laboratory Imaging, Praha, Czech Republic*

LOTHAR SCHERMELLEH • *Micron Advanced Bioimaging Unit, Department of Biochemistry, University of Oxford, Oxford, UK*

SVEN SEWITZ • *Babraham Institute, Nuclear Dynamics Programme, Cambridge, UK*

LUKE SPRINGALL • *School of Biosciences, University of Kent, Canterbury, UK*

JAMES STEVENS • *Department of Biological Sciences, Birkbeck College, University of London, London, UK*

THANA SUTTHIBUTPONG • *Theoretical and Computational Science Center (TaCS), Science Laboratory Building, Faculty of Science, King Mongkut University of Technology Thonburi, Thung Khru, Bangkok, Thailand*

YI LEI TAN • *Department of Biochemistry, University of Cambridge, Cambridge, UK*

EDWARD J.R. TAYLOR • *Department of Biochemistry, University of Cambridge, Cambridge, UK*

ROMAN TUMA • *Astbury Centre for Structural Molecular Biology, University of Leeds, Leeds, UK*

STEPHAN UPHOFF • *Department of Biochemistry, University of Oxford, Oxford, UK*

YUCHONG WANG • *Astbury Centre for Structural Molecular Biology, University of Leeds, Leeds, UK*

XINDAN WANG • *Department of Microbiology & Immunobiology, Harvard Medical School, Boston, MA, USA*

ADAM J.M. WOLLMAN • *Biological Physical Sciences Institute (BPSI), University of York, Heslington, York, UK*

Chapter 1

New Advances in Chromosome Architecture

Mark C. Leake

Abstract

Our knowledge of the "architecture" of chromosomes has grown enormously in the past decade. This new insight has been enabled largely through advances in interdisciplinary research methods at the cutting-edge interface of the life and physical sciences. Importantly this has involved several state-of-the-art biophysical tools used in conjunction with molecular biology approaches which enable investigation of chromosome structure and function in living cells. Also, there are new and emerging interfacial science tools which enable significant improvements to the spatial and temporal resolution of quantitative measurements, such as in vivo super-resolution and powerful new single-molecule biophysics methods, which facilitate probing of dynamic chromosome processes hitherto impossible. And there are also important advances in the methods of theoretical biophysics which have enabled advances in predictive modeling of this high quality experimental data from molecular and physical biology to generate new understanding of the modes of operation of chromosomes, both in eukaryotic and prokaryotic cells. Here, I discuss these advances, and take stock on the current state of our knowledge of chromosome architecture and speculate where future advances may lead.

Key words Single-molecule biophysics, Super-resolution, DNA, Nucleus

1 Introduction

This volume of Springer's Methods in Molecular Biology series consists of a collection of truly cutting-edge laboratory protocols, techniques and applications in use today by some of the leading international experts in the broad field of "Chromosome Architecture." A key difference, compared with previous collections of review articles published in this area over the past 5 years, is the emphasis on the development and application of complex techniques and protocols which increase the physiological relevance of chromosome architecture investigation compared to methods utilized previously—these developments are manifest both through application of far more complex bottom-up assays in vitro, as well as in striving to maintain the native physiological context through investigation of living, functional cells [1]. In particular, experimental methods which have used advances in light

Mark C. Leake (ed.), *Chromosome Architecture: Methods and Protocols*, Methods in Molecular Biology, vol. 1431,
DOI 10.1007/978-1-4939-3631-1_1, © Springer Science+Business Media New York 2016

microscopy [2], especially the use of fluorescence microscopy methods to probe functional, living cells, especially so using prokaryotic systems as model organisms [3–12]. The length scale of precision of experimental protocols in this area has improved dramatically over recent years and many cutting-edge methods now utilize state-of-the-art single-molecule approaches [13], both for imaging the DNA content of chromosome and proteins that bind to DNA, as well as using methods that can controllably manipulate single DNA molecules and can image its structure to a precision better the standard optical resolution limit.[14] This volume also includes more complex, physiologically representative methods to investigate chromosome architecture through the use of advanced computational methods and mathematical analysis.

What is clear is that the combination of pioneering molecular biology, biochemistry and genetics methods with emerging, exciting tools from biophysics, bioengineering, computer science, and biomathematics are transforming our knowledge of functional chromosome architecture. Improvements in these fields are likely to add yet more insight over the next few years into the complex interactions between multiple key molecular players inside chromosomes.

Acknowledgments

M.C.L. was assisted by a Royal Society URF and research funds from the Biological Physical Sciences Institute (BPSI) of the University of York, UK.

References

1. Wollman AJM, Miller H, Zhou Z et al (2015) Probing DNA interactions with proteins using a single-molecule toolbox: inside the cell, in a test tube and in a computer. Biochem Soc Trans 43:139–145

2. Wollman AJM, Nudd R, Hedlund EG et al (2015) From animaculum to single molecules: 300 years of the light microscope. Open Biol 5:150019

3. Lenn T, Leake MC, Mullineaux CW (2008) Are Escherichia coli OXPHOS complexes concentrated in specialized zones within the plasma membrane? Biochem Soc Trans 36:1032–1036

4. Plank M, Wadhams GH, Leake MC (2009) Millisecond timescale slimfield imaging and automated quantification of single fluorescent protein molecules for use in probing complex biological processes. Integr Biol 1: 602–612

5. Chiu S-W, Leake MC (2011) Functioning nanomachines seen in real-time in living bacteria using single-molecule and super-resolution fluorescence imaging. Int J Mol Sci 12: 2518–2542

6. Robson A, Burrage K, Leake MC (2013) Inferring diffusion in single live cells at the single-molecule level. Philos Trans R Soc Lond B Biol Sci 368:20120029

7. Bryan SJ, Burroughs NJ, Shevela D et al (2014) Localisation and interactions of the Vipp1 protein in cyanobacteria. Mol Microbiol 94(5):1179–1195

8. Llorente-Garcia I, Lenn T, Erhardt H et al (2014) Single-molecule in vivo imaging of bacterial respiratory complexes indicates delocalized oxidative phosphorylation. Biochim Biophys Acta 1837:811–824

9. Reyes-Lamothe R, Sherratt DJ, Leake MC (2010) Stoichiometry and architecture of

active DNA replication machinery in Escherichia coli. Science 328:498–501

10. Badrinarayanan A, Reyes-Lamothe R, Uphoff S et al (2012) In vivo architecture and action of bacterial structural maintenance of chromosome proteins. Science 338:528–531

11. Wollman AJM, Leake MC (2015) Millisecond single-molecule localization microscopy combined with convolution analysis and automated image segmentation to determine protein concentrations in complexly structured, functional cells, one cell at a time. Faraday Discuss 184:401–424.

12. Lenn T, Leake MC (2016) Single-molecule studies of the dynamics and interactions of bacterial OXPHOS complexes. Biochim Biophys Acta 1857(3):224–231

13. Leake MC (2013) The physics of life: one molecule at a time. Philos Trans R Soc Lond B Biol Sci 368(1611):20120248

14. Miller H, Zhaokun Z, Wollman AJM et al (2015) Superresolution imaging of single DNA molecules using stochastic photoblinking of minor groove and intercalating dyes. Methods 88:81–88

Chapter 2

Single-Molecule Narrow-Field Microscopy of Protein–DNA Binding Dynamics in Glucose Signal Transduction of Live Yeast Cells

Adam J.M. Wollman and Mark C. Leake

Abstract

Single-molecule narrow-field microscopy is a versatile tool to investigate a diverse range of protein dynamics in live cells and has been extensively used in bacteria. Here, we describe how these methods can be extended to larger eukaryotic, yeast cells, which contain subcellular compartments. We describe how to obtain single-molecule microscopy data but also how to analyze these data to track and obtain the stoichiometry of molecular complexes diffusing in the cell. We chose glucose mediated signal transduction of live yeast cells as the system to demonstrate these single-molecule techniques as transcriptional regulation is fundamentally a single-molecule problem—a single repressor protein binding a single binding site in the genome can dramatically alter behavior at the whole cell and population level.

Key words Single-molecule biophysics, Signal transduction, Yeast

1 Introduction

Bulk biochemical methods can only measure mean ensemble properties while single-molecule techniques allow the heterogeneity in molecular biology to be explored which often leads to a new understanding of the biological system involved [1]. The use of fluorescent protein fusions to act as reporters can provide significant insight into a wide range of biological processes and molecular machines, for enabling insight into stoichiometry and architecture as well as details of molecular mobility inside living, functional cells with their native physiological context intact [2–7]. Single-molecule narrow-field microscopy, and its similar counterpart Slimfield microscopy, is a versatile tool to investigate a diverse range of protein dynamics in live cells which can be used in conjunction with fluorescent protein fusion strains to generate enormous insight into biological processes at the single-molecule level. In bacteria, it has been used to investigate the components of the replisome [8] and the structural maintenance of chromosomes [9].

Mark C. Leake (ed.), *Chromosome Architecture: Methods and Protocols*, Methods in Molecular Biology, vol. 1431, DOI 10.1007/978-1-4939-3631-1_2, © Springer Science+Business Media New York 2016

In narrow-field microscopy, the normal fluorescence excitation field is reduced to encompass only a single cell. This produces a Gaussian excitation field ($\sim$30 μm^2) with 100–1000 times the laser excitation intensity of standard epifluorescence microscopy. This intense illumination causes fluorophores to emit many more photons, generating much greater signal intensity relative to normal camera-imaging noise and, hence, facilitates millisecond time-scale imaging of single fluorescently labeled proteins. The millisecond time scale is fast enough to keep up with the diffusional motion present in the cytoplasm of cells and can also sample the fast molecular transitions that occur, particularly during signal transduction. Single fluorescent proteins or complexes of proteins can be considered point sources of light and so appear as spatially extended spots in a fluorescence image due to diffraction by the microscope optics [10]. Narrow-field microscopy data consists of a time-series of images of spots which require a significant amount of in silico analysis. Spots must be identified by software, the intensity of these spots quantified to calculate their stoichiometry and their position tracked over time to produce a trajectory.

We have applied narrow-field microscopy to glucose signal transduction in budding yeast, *Saccharomyces cerevisiae*. All cells dynamically sense their environment through signal transduction mechanisms. The majority of these mechanisms rely on gene regulation through cascades of protein–protein interactions which transmit signals from sensory elements to responsive elements within each cell. The Mig1 protein is an essential transcription factor in this mechanism in yeast. Mig1 is a Cys2-His2 zinc finger DNA binding protein [11] which binds several glucose-repressed promoters [12–15]. In the presence of extracellular glucose it is poorly phosphorylated and predominantly located in the nucleus [16, 17] where it recruits a repression complex to the DNA [18]. If extracellular glucose concentration levels are depleted, Mig1 is phosphorylated by the sucrose non-fermenting protein (Snf1) [19–21], resulting in a redistribution of mean localization of Mig1 into the cytoplasm [16, 22, 23]. Thus, Mig1 concentration levels in the cell nucleus and cytoplasm serve as a readout of glucose signal transduction in budding yeast [24]. Mig1 has been labeled with the green fluorescent protein, GFP, and in the same strain, a ribosome component, Nrd1, almost completely localized to the nucleus, has been labeled with the mCherry fluorescent protein [17]. We have used narrow-field microscopy to track single Mig1-GFP complexes as they diffuse in the nucleus and cytoplasm in the presence and absence of extracellular glucose.

Here we describe in detail how to obtain single-molecule data of fluorescently labeled transcription factors in live yeast but also methods used to analyze the data obtained. We describe ADEMS code [25], the custom Matlab software we have created to track fluorescent molecules and quantify their stoichiometry. We also show how fluorescence images of Mig1-GFP and Nrd1-mcherry can be segmented to identify the boundary of the cell and nucleus respectively and thus how trajectories can be categorized by their different subcellular compartments.

2 Materials

2.1 Fluorescently Labeled Yeast Strains

1. MATa MIG1-GFPHIS3 NRD1-mCherry- hphNT1METLYS *S. cerevisiae* strain in the BY4741 background [17] stored at −80 °C in YNB media supplemented with 20% glycerol.

2. YNB media pH 6.

2.2 Sample Preparation

1. Standard microscope slides (Fisher).

2. Coverslips (Menzel-Gläser).

3. Gene frames (17 mm×28 mm) and spreaders (Thermo Scientific).

4. 2% agarose solution.

5. Plasma cleaner (Harrick Plasmas PDC-32G).

6. Desktop centrifuge (Sigma 1-14).

2.3 Narrow-Field Microscope

For narrow-field microscopy, ~6 W/cm² excitation light must be delivered to the sample centered at 488 nm for millisecond imaging of GFP. This must be combined with a high speed (kHz) camera capable of detecting single fluorescent proteins. Our microscope is constructed from:

1. A Zeiss microscope body with a 100× TIRF 1.49 numerical aperture (NA) Olympus oil immersion objective lens and an xyz nano positioning stage (Nanodrive, Mad City Labs).

2. 50 mW Obis 488 nm and 561 nm lasers for fluorescence excitation.

3. A dual pass GFP/mCherry dichroic with 25 nm transmission windows centered on 525 and 625 nm was used underneath the objective lens turret.

4. A high speed camera (iXon DV860-BI, Andor Technology, UK) was used to image at typically 5 ms/frame with the magnification set at ~80 nm per pixel.

5. The camera CCD was split between a GFP and mCherry channel using a bespoke color splitter consisting of a dichroic centered at pass wavelength 560 nm and emission filters with 25 nm bandwidths centered at 525 and 594 nm.

6. The microscope was controlled using our in-house bespoke LabVIEW (National Instruments) software.

2.4 Computational Analysis	1. We use MATLAB 2014b, which has the advantage that many functions are built in such as curve fitting etc. but these methods could be implemented in other packages such as IDL, LabVIEW or Python, C++, or Java.

3   Methods

3.1 Growing Yeast Strains	1. Prepare 5 ml YNB supplemented with 4% glucose in 15 ml Falcon tube.
	2. Scrape a small quantity of frozen yeast culture from the cryovial using a pipette tip without defrosting the vial.
	3. Swirl pipette tip in prepared media and leave the culture to grow overnight at 30 °C, shaking at 200 rpm.

3.2 Plasma Cleaning Coverslips

Glass coverslips must be plasma cleaned before use to remove any material left on the glass from manufacture. We have found this material to be fluorescent under the intense excitation light of narrow-field microscopy. This produces a fluorescent background in an image or false positive spots.

1. Place coverslips into the plasma cleaner.

2. Seal with the valve door and turn on the vacuum pump, pressing the edges of the door to insure a good seal.

3. Turn the radio frequency (RF) generator to high. If the vacuum pressure is low enough, a pink-violet glow will emanate from the chamber, but if the pressure is not yet low enough, continue to press on the seal until more air is evacuated by the pump.

4. Once plasma is generated, slightly open the valve to allow a small amount of air into the chamber. The plasma will change color to violet indicating oxygen plasma.

5. After coverslips have been exposed to oxygen plasma for ~1 min, turn off the RF and vacuum pump and slowly open the valve.

6. Once atmospheric pressure is restored, remove the coverslips and store in a clean petri dish.

3.3 Preparing Cell Samples

1. For glucose conditions, the overnight culture can be used as the cell sample.

2. For absence of glucose conditions, prepare 1 ml of YNB.

3. Pellet 1 ml of cell culture by spinning in a desktop centrifuge for 2 min at 3000 rpm ($660 \times g$) and discard the supernatant.

4. Resuspend in 500 μl YNB and pellet again.

5. Discard the supernatant and resuspend in 100 μl YNB or more depending on cell density.

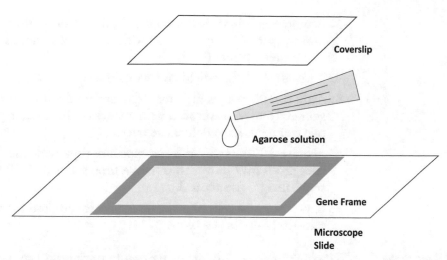

Fig. 1 Schematic of agarose pad assembly

3.4 Agarose Pad Preparation

Cells were imaged on agarose pads suffused with media. This ensures cells remain healthy during imaging but also immobilizes them. Figure 1 illustrates agarose pad assembly.

1. Prepare 500 μl 2× YNB, supplemented with 8% glucose to image cells in high glucose conditions.

2. Remove the larger of the two clear plastic covers from the gene frame and apply the frame to a glass slide to create a rectangular well.

3. Melt 2% agarose solution in a microwave.

4. Pipette 500 μl of hot agarose into the 2× YNB and quickly mix before removing 500 μl and pipetting into the well on the slide.

5. Quickly apply a plastic spreader (included with Gene Frames) to the well to remove excess agarose and leave a thin even layer in the well.

6. Slide the spreader off the pad carefully and remove the second plastic cover from the gene frame.

7. Pipette 5 μl of cell sample onto the pad in ~10 droplets and leave to dry for ~5 min before covering with a plasma cleaned coverslip.

3.5 Obtaining Single-Molecule Data

1. Place the sample on the microscope and locate a cell by imaging in bright field.

2. Focus on the mid body of the cell by adjusting the focus to the point of minimum contrast.

3. Acquire ten bright-field frames at 50 ms exposure time with no camera gain. All images saved with raw pixel values as stacked Tag Image Format (TIF) files.

4. Turn off the bright-field and set gain to maximum.

5. Acquire 100 frames at 5 ms exposure time with the 561 nm laser at 15 mW power to obtain images of the mCherry signal, this will be used to define the nucleus.

6. Acquire 1000 frames at 5 ms exposure time with the 488 nm laser at 30 mW power to obtain a time series of GFP fluorescence images (*see* **Note 1**).

7. Repeat for ~30 cells or however many are required for a robust statistical sample (*see* **Note 2**).

3.6 Tracking Single Molecules

Bespoke Matlab code has been written to track bright spots in fluorescence image time series. The steps performed by the code are outlined here.

Load TIF file containing single-molecule tracks, in this case the 1000 frame 488 nm exposure, into MATLAB as an $m \times n \times p$ array, m pixels by n pixels by p frames.

1. Apply a top hat transformation to each frame to even the background and threshold the resulting image using Otsu's method.

2. Dilate the resulting binary image with a disk shaped structural element and then erode with the same element to remove bright noise pixels.

3. Perform an ultimate erosion to leave only non-zero pixels at potential spot locations (*see* **Note 3**).

4. At each of these potential spot locations, define a square 16 pixel region of interest (ROI) and a 5 pixel radius circular ROI centered on the intensity centroid of the potential spot.

5. Convolve the circular ROI with a 2D Gaussian function with 3 pixel width centered on the current intensity centroid and use this to determine a new intensity centroid

6. Repeat **step 6** until the centroid position converges on the final sub-pixel spot center coordinates. Figure 2 illustrates one iteration of a Mig1-GFP spot.

7. Define the spot's total intensity as the sum of the pixel values inside the circular ROI corrected for background by subtracting the mean pixel value of the remaining pixels in the square ROI.

8. Define the spots signal to noise ratio (SNR) as the spot's total intensity divided by the standard deviation of the remaining pixels in the square ROI and discard spots with SNR < 0.4.

9. The center of the mask gives the sub-pixel centroid coordinates of the spot.

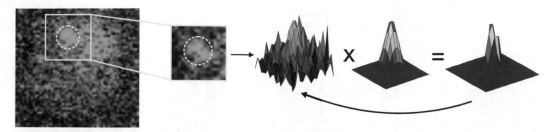

Fig. 2 Schematic of iterative Gaussian masking to determine spot centroid. *Left*: a fluorescence image of Mig1-GFP in a yeast cell with a spot identifiable. *Right*: schematic illustration of iterative Gaussian masking to find the spot centroid. The spot pixels are shown as a 3D surface and convolved with a 2D Gaussian centered on the centroid estimate. The resulting image is used to find a new centroid estimate and the process iterated until convergence

10. Determine the width of each spot by constrained fitting of a 2D Gaussian function inside the square ROI, with the width and central intensity the only variables.

11. Once all spots are found and characterized in at least two consecutive frames, they can be linked together into trajectories.

12. Calculate the pairwise distance between all pairs of spots in consecutive frames and keep any which are below 5 pixels.

13. Link closest pairs as long as their intensities or widths do not differ by >2× and assign a new trajectory number or continue an existing one if a spot is already part of a trajectory. Thus a complete set of trajectories for the time series is acquired.

3.7 Analyzing Single-Molecule Trajectories

Once trajectories are obtained, they are analyzed to determine the number of fluorophores present in each spot. The intensity of a single fluorophore is first found from the distribution of all spot intensities over the whole time series. The most common intensity value is that of a single fluorophore as all traces bleach to this value. The number of fluorophores present in each spot can be determined by dividing the initial value by the single fluorophore value. The initial intensity is determined by fitting an exponential decay function to each trace.

1. Generate histogram or kernel density estimation (KDE) of all the intensity values of all the spots found in trajectories. Figure 3 left shows the KDE of mig1-GFP intensity values obtained in a single cell.

2. As every complex of fluorophores is bleaching, the most common intensity value in the intensity distribution is the characteristic single fluorophore intensity and the peak value in the distribution. Figure 3 right shows spot intensity as a function of time with the single GFP value marked with a line (*see* **Note 4**).

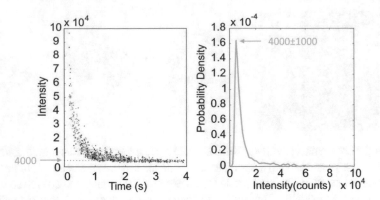

Fig. 3 *Left* spot intensity as a function of time with the single GFP intensity value marked as a *dotted line. Right* distribution of spot intensities with the single GFP value marked

3. Fit an exponential to all the spot intensity values as a function of time.

4. Use the time constant from the global fit, to fit exponentials to each trajectory, provided it is >3 points, within the first 200 frames and its initial intensity is >2× the single fluorophore intensity.

5. The number of fluorophores present in each spot is the initial intensity in each trajectory's fit divided by the characteristic single fluorophore intensity (*see* **Note 5**).

3.8 Categorizing Tracks by Cell Compartment

Trajectories are analyzed in terms of their location in the cell. The cell and nuclear boundaries are determined by segmenting GFP and mCherry fluorescence frame averaged images. This allows trajectories to be defined as nuclear, cytoplasmic, and transnuclear. Figure 4 shows example frame averages and segmentation and categorized trajectories overlaid on a bright-field image of a yeast cell.

1. Generate frame averages over first five frames of the Nrd1-mCherry and Mig1-GFP acquisitions. These will be used to determine the nucleus and cell boundary.

2. Threshold these images above the full width half maximum (FWHM) of the background peak in the pixel intensity distribution to obtain a binary image.

3. Erode this image with a 4 pixel disk shaped structural element to remove any bright single pixels and create a smoother edge around the object. These masks define the nucleus and cell pixels.

4. Divide the tracks into those which are always in the nucleus, always in the cytoplasm or are in both at different times—*trans*nuclear tracks.

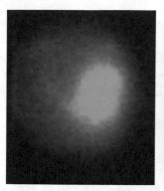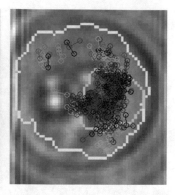

Fig. 4 *Left fluorescence image* of Mig1-GFP, *middle fluorescence image* of Nrd1-mCherry, *Right bright-field image* with cell and nucleus outlines (*yellow* and *cyan*, respectively) and nuclear, cytoplasmic, and transnuclear tracks (*red, green,* and *blue*, respectively) overlayed

4   Notes

1. During fluorescence acquisitions, the camera must begin acquiring frames just before the laser illuminates the sample. This allows all of the emitted light from the sample to be captured by the camera which is crucial for analysis.

2. When moving through the sample during imaging, care must be taken to move in a set direction through the sample. This ensures that every cell that is imaged has not had any prior exposure to the laser and thus no photobleaching has occurred.

3. **Steps 2–4** in Subheading 3.6 identify candidate spots in fluorescence images. This process is not strictly necessary as spots are evaluated using iterative Gaussian masking which could be performed at every pixel location in an image. This would be very computationally intensive but by identifying candidates, the number of possible spot locations is reduced along with the processing time.

4. The intensity of a single fluorophore can be independently verified in an in vitro assay by imaging antibody immobilized fluorophores on a coverslip. This intensity will vary from that observed in vivo due to the different conditions inside a cell, particularly the differing pH.

5. Any fluorophores which are within the diffraction limited spot width of each other (~250 nm for GFP) will appear to be a single spot in a narrow-field image. This distance is large compared to the size of proteins such as Mig1 of a few nanometres and so it is possible that some spots in a frame are not molecular complexes but separate molecules within 250 nm of each other. These events are short-lived for diffusing molecules and so the stoichiometry of complexes is obtained from the fits to the intensity vs time traces.

Acknowledgments

We thank Sviatlana Shashkova and Stefan Hohmann (University of Gothenburg, Sweden) for donation of yeast cell strains and assistance with yeast cell culturing. M.C.L. was assisted by a Royal Society URF and research funds from the Biological Physical Sciences Institute (BPSI) of the University of York, UK.

References

1. Wollman AJM, Miller H, Zhou Z et al (2015) Probing DNA interactions with proteins using a single-molecule toolbox: inside the cell, in a test tube and in a computer. Biochem Soc Trans 43:139–145

2. Lenn T, Leake MC, Mullineaux CW (2008) Are Escherichia coli OXPHOS complexes concentrated in specialized zones within the plasma membrane? Biochem Soc Trans 36:1032–1036

3. Plank M, Wadhams GH, Leake MC (2009) Millisecond timescale slimfield imaging and automated quantification of single fluorescent protein molecules for use in probing complex biological processes. Integr Biol 1:602–612

4. Chiu S-W, Leake MC (2011) Functioning nanomachines seen in real-time in living bacteria using single-molecule and super-resolution fluorescence imaging. Int J Mol Sci 12: 2518–2542

5. Robson A, Burrage K, Leake MC (2013) Inferring diffusion in single live cells at the single-molecule level. Philos Trans R Soc Lond B Biol Sci 368:20120029

6. Bryan SJ, Burroughs NJ, Shevela D et al (2014) Localisation and interactions of the Vipp1 protein in cyanobacteria. Mol Microbiol 94(5):1179–1195

7. Llorente-Garcia I, Lenn T, Erhardt H et al (2014) Single-molecule in vivo imaging of bacterial respiratory complexes indicates delocalized oxidative phosphorylation. Biochim Biophys Acta 1837:811–824

8. Reyes-Lamothe R, Sherratt DJ, Leake MC (2010) Stoichiometry and architecture of active DNA replication machinery in Escherichia coli. Science 328:498–501

9. Badrinarayanan A, Reyes-Lamothe R, Uphoff S et al (2012) In vivo architecture and action of bacterial structural maintenance of chromosome proteins. Science 338:528–531

10. Wollman AJM, Nudd R, Hedlund EG et al (2015) From animaculum to single molecules: 300 years of the light microscope. Open Biol 5:150019–150019

11. Lundin M, Nehlin JO, Ronne H (1994) Importance of a flanking AT-rich region in target site recognition by the GC box-binding zinc finger protein MIG1. Mol Cell Biol 14:1979–1985

12. Nehlin JO, Carlberg M, Ronne H (1991) Control of yeast GAL genes by MIG1 repressor: a transcriptional cascade in the glucose response. EMBO J 10:3373–3377

13. Klein CJL, Olsson L, Nielsen J (1998) Glucose control in Saccharomyces cerevisiae: the role of MIG1 in metabolic functions. Microbiology 144:13–24

14. Ghillebert R, Swinnen E, Wen J et al (2011) The AMPK/SNF1/SnRK1 fuel gauge and energy regulator: structure, function and regulation. FEBS J 278:3978–3990

15. Broach JR (2012) Nutritional control of growth and development in yeast. Genetics 192:73–105

16. De Vit MJ, Waddle J, Johnston M (1997) Regulated nuclear translocation of the Mig1 glucose repressor. Mol Biol Cell 8:1603–1618

17. Bendrioua L, Smedh M, Almquist J et al (2014) Yeast AMP-activated protein kinase monitors glucose concentration changes and absolute glucose levels. J Biol Chem 289: 12863–12875

18. Treitel MA, Carlson M (1995) Repression by SSN6-TUP1 is directed by MIG1, a repressor/activator protein. Proc Natl Acad Sci U S A 92:3132–3136

19. Smith FC, Davies SP, Wilson WA et al (1999) The SNF1 kinase complex from Saccharomyces cerevisiae phosphorylates the transcriptional repressor protein Mig1p in vitro at four sites within or near regulatory domain 1. FEBS Lett 453:219–223

20. Ostling J, Carlberg M, Ronne H (1996) Functional domains in the Mig1 repressor. Mol Cell Biol 16:753–761

21. Ostling J, Ronne H (1998) Negative control of the Mig1p repressor by Snf1p-dependent phosphorylation in the absence of glucose. Eur J Biochem 252:162–168

22. Frolova E (1999) Binding of the glucose-dependent Mig1p repressor to the GAL1 and GAL4 promoters in vivo: regulation by glucose and chromatin structure. Nucleic Acids Res 27:1350–1358

23. DeVit MJ, Johnston M (1999) The nuclear exportin Msn5 is required for nuclear export of the Mig1 glucose repressor of Saccharomyces cerevisiae. Curr Biol 9:1231–1241

24. Wollman A, Leake MC (2015) Single molecule microscopy: millisecond single-molecule localization microscopy combined with convolution analysis and automated image segmentation to determine protein concentrations in complexly structured, functional cells, one cell at a time. Farad Discuss 184:401–424

25. Miller H, Zhaokun Z, Wollman AJM et al (2015) Superresolution imaging of single DNA molecules using stochastic photoblinking of minor groove and intercalating dyes. Methods 88:81–88

Chapter 3

Single-Molecule Imaging to Characterize the Transport Mechanism of the Nuclear Pore Complex

Grace Jeremy, James Stevens, and Alan R. Lowe

Abstract

In the eukaryotic cell, a large macromolecular channel, known as the Nuclear Pore Complex (NPC), mediates all molecular transport between the nucleus and cytoplasm. In recent years, single-molecule fluorescence (SMF) imaging has emerged as a powerful tool to study the molecular mechanism of transport through the NPC. More recently, techniques such as single-molecule localization microscopy (SMLM) have enabled the spatial and temporal distribution of cargos, transport receptors and even structural components of the NPC to be determined with nanometre accuracy. In this protocol, we describe a method to study the position and/or motion of individual molecules transiting through the NPC with high spatial and temporal precision.

Key words Nucleus, Nuclear pore complex, Single-molecule tracking, Super-resolution microscopy

1 Introduction

1.1 The Nuclear Pore Complex

The eukaryotic cell contains an envelope bound nucleus, a structure facilitating the spatial and temporal partitioning of the genetic material and molecules critical to normal function. The movement of molecules, termed cargos, across the envelope is called nucleo-cytoplasmic transport. This process is key for regulating nuclear composition and gene expression. The Nuclear Pore Complex (NPC) is the major channel of passage between the nucleus and cytoplasm, facilitating passive transport of small cargo and the regulated transport of larger molecules. NPCs are formed from many copies of ~30 nucleoporin proteins (Nups), with a total of 500–1000 Nups forming a single NPC. "Barrier Nups" are found throughout the NPC channel structure and are composed of phenylalanine glycine rich repeat (FG) motifs [1]. These FG-Nups control the selective transport of large cargoes through the central channel of the NPC [2]. The FG motifs protrude into the central channel, generating a permeability barrier which permits the unhindered passage of small, nonpolar molecules (ions,

Mark C. Leake (ed.), *Chromosome Architecture: Methods and Protocols*, Methods in Molecular Biology, vol. 1431, DOI 10.1007/978-1-4939-3631-1_3, © Springer Science+Business Media New York 2016

metabolites) whilst occluding larger cargoes (macromolecules, proteins >40 kDa) [3].

Large cargoes destined for transport possess specific amino acid sequences or patches called nuclear localization (NLS) signals [4]. These bind (via adaptor proteins) to Nuclear Transport Receptors (NTRs), such as Importin-beta (Impβ) [5]: proteins that facilitate transport by forming multiple interactions with the barrier Nups. Transport of Nup-interacting proteins is very efficient and greatly exceeds that of non-interacting proteins, with a translocation rate of $\sim10^3$ s^{-1} NPC^{-1} [6]. The directionality of Impβ-dependant transport is controlled by a sharp spatial gradient of the GTPase Ran in either its GDP- or GTP-bound state [7, 8]. RanGTP dominates the nuclear side whereas RanGDP is the prevalent cytoplasmic form. A typical import complex comprises Impβ, Impα, and cargo. Upon reaching the nuclear face of the NPC, the Impβ binds RanGTP, promoting the release of cargo into the nucleus [9].

Many models of transport, with varying functional arrangements of the FG-nups, have been proposed. The permeability of the NPC could result from a physical barrier as proposed in the "selective phase" model, with barrier Nups interacting to form a size-selective mesh preventing the movement of larger cargoes [6]. Alternatively it could be energetic as in the "virtual-gate" model, occluding molecules that do not interact with the FG-repeats as they cannot overcome the entropic barrier formed by the dense FG-lining of the central channel [10]. Other studies suggest the FG-nups form a hydrogel through cross-linking interactions, and that this acts as a sieve permitting passage of NTR complexes [11, 12]. Recent studies also suggest that a FG-nup meshwork is only partially stable, and that NTRs may influence inter-Nup interactions to permit the active movement of cargo [13, 14]. However, despite the many theories, and a wealth of experimental data, the mechanism of translocation is still largely unresolved.

1.2 Single-Molecule Imaging of the NPC

In recent years, single-molecule fluorescence (SMF) imaging has emerged as a complimentary technique for studying the mechanism of the NPC. SMF microscopy is a highly specific and noninvasive imaging method, capable of visualizing individual fluorophores conjugated to biological molecules of interest. As such it has been utilized, to great effect, to study individual transport reactions in cells in real-time. Several different experimental geometries have been established to enable quantitative measurements of either the transport reaction, or of the structural arrangement of components of the NPC (Fig. 1). Typically, these experiments use *Digitonin* permeabilized mammalian cells [15] and a reconstituted recombinant import system, including a fluorescently labeled molecule of interest (e.g., NTR, cargo, or component of the NPC itself).

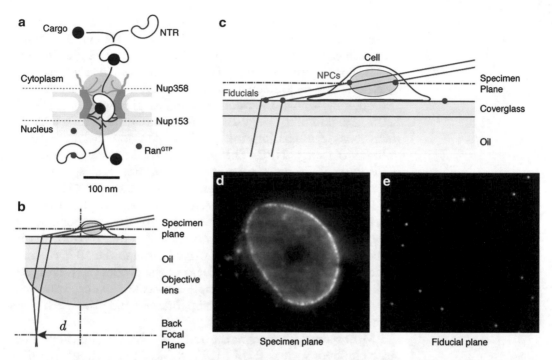

Fig. 1 Schematic describing simplified NPC transport mechanism and imaging assay to probe cargo–NTR interactions. (**a**) A simplified schematic describing active import of cargos into the nucleus. A cargo bearing a Nuclear Localization Signal (NLS), must bind to cognate Nuclear Transport Receptors (NTRs) enabling the cargo to enter into the NPC. A sharp spatial gradient of the GTP form of Ran GTPase provides the directionality to active transport. The scale bar refers to the NPC structure rather than the soluble components (Cargo, NTRs, and Ran). (**b**) Illumination setup to increase imaging signal-to-noise. Rather than standard epifluorescence illumination the laser can be inclined through the sample, by introducing an offset, *d*, in the position of the imaging laser at the BFP of the objective. Additionally, adding a slit in the conjugate plane to the specimen plane (HILO) can improve S/N further. (**c**) Schematic showing the two focal planes which must be imaged, the specimen plane containing the NPCs, and the fiducial plane where fluorescent beads can be utilized to correct lateral drift. (**d**) Example of a HILO image of labeled NTRs interacting with the NPC. Individual NPCs can be identified as discrete puncta. (**e**) Example wide-field image of fluorescent beads localized to the surface of the glass coverslip

Total Internal Reflection Fluorescence (TIRF) microscopy is often used to perform SMF imaging experiments due to the enhanced signal-to-noise ratio (S/N), but this limits the illumination volume to only ~100 nm above the cover glass surface. In most cases, the nucleus, and hence the NPCs are located above this illumination volume, therefore many alternative strategies have been developed to directly visualize the basal and equatorial planes of the nucleus.

For example, wide-field and narrow-field (enhancing the S/N) epifluorescence have been used to measure NTR transport times and the localization of NTR–NPC interaction sites within single NPCs [16], as well as the effect of NTR concentration on transport kinetics [17]. These NTR dwell time and binding site distribution measurements have aided determination of likely transport models and lead to the suggestion that multiple transport pathways are present in a single NPC [18, 19]. Highly inclined and laminated optical sheet (HILO) microscopy further increases S/N, enabling measurement of cargo–NTR dissociation constants and quantification of the number of NTRs present at single NPCs [20]. Single-Point Edge-Excitation subDiffraction (SPEED) microscopy can also improve S/N, by limiting the illumination volume to a single NPC. This has been used to observe transient NTR–cargo–Nup interactions [21] suggesting that spatially distinct routes exist for facilitated and passive transport [22].

In addition, alternative fluorescent probes have been utilized to measure different aspects of the transport reaction. For example cargo tracking experiments utilizing semiconductor nanoparticles have visualized transport of large cargos through the NPC channel, exploiting the photostability and size of the probes [23]. Dye pairs have been used to perform single-molecule Förster Resonance Energy Transfer (smFRET) experiments, revealing the mechanism of impα–cargo dissociation [24].

Most recently, "super-resolution" SMLM imaging (in particular, techniques such as PALM [25], STORM [26], and dSTORM [27]) has been used to precisely localize many molecules within NPCs. For example HILO-dSTORM has enabled precise visualization of the spatial distribution of NTRs, and inter-NPC variability under different conditions [13]. dSTORM has also been utilized independently [28] and combined with correlative electron microscopy [29] to assess the organization of structural domains within the NPC [30].

In this protocol, we will describe, in detail, our most current workflow for imaging the location and/or motion of cargos and NTRs using SMLM imaging and single-particle tracking (SPT). The same basic protocol can be used to perform either type of experiment, with the major experimental difference being whether the sample is fixed (SMLM, dSTORM) or live (SPT), and how the data are processed.

Our workflow comprises several steps:

1. Expression and purification of recombinant transport receptors and cargos.

2. Chemical labeling of the NTRs or cargo with fluorescent moieties.

3. Digitonin permeabilization of cells and addition of recombinant transport system.

4. Single-molecule imaging using highly inclined illumination (HILO).

5. Single particle tracking or localization microscopy (e.g., dSTORM).

6. Data analysis to generate composite maps of the NPC.

2 Materials

2.1 Protein Expression and Purification

1. *Escherichia coli* cells (OneShot BL21 (DE3), Life Technologies).
2. Expression plasmid for His$_6$-tagged cargo, NTRs, or Ran.
3. 2 l LB medium with appropriate antibiotics.
4. 1 M IPTG.
5. 5 ml HisTrap column (GE Healthcare).
6. Elution buffer containing imidazole: 3 mM imidazole, 2 mM DTT in PBS, pH 7.4.

2.2 Labeling of the NTRs or Cargo with Fluorescent Moieties

1. Gene encoding photoactivatable fluorescent protein (such as mEOS3).
2. Chemical dye such as the *N*-hydroxysuccinimidyl ester of Alexa Fluor 647 (Life Technologies A-20006).
3. Nanoparticles such as Amino (PEG) Quantum Dots (Life Technologies Q21501MP).

2.3 Preparation of Cells for Imaging

1. HeLa cells.
2. 75 cm^2 tissue culture flasks.
3. 10 ml of growth media: 1:1 solution of Dulbecco's Modified Eagle Medium and F12 (Gibco), 10% fetal calf serum (FCS) (Gibco), and 1% penicillin–streptomycin (Gibco).
4. Incubator (37 °C, 5% (v/v) CO$_2$).
5. HBSS (Gibco).
6. 0.05% EDTA–trypsin (Gibco).
7. Glass bottom dishes (Ibidi, μ-Dish 35 mm, high).

2.4 Recombinant Transport Assay

1. Phosphate buffered saline (PBS): 50 mM, pH 7.4.
2. Permeabilization buffer (PB): 50 mM HEPES pH 7.3, 50 mM KOAc, 8 mM MgCl$_2$.
3. Digitonin-permeabilization buffer (DPB): PB plus 0.1 mM digitonin in DMSO, 80 μM ATP, 80 μM GTP, 3.2 mM creatine phosphate, and 40 Units creatine kinase in PBS.
4. Transport buffer (TB): 20 mM HEPES pH 7.3, 110 mM KOAc, 5 mM NaOAc, 2 mM Mg(OAC)$_2$, 4 mM DTT, pH 7.3.
5. Import Mix (IMx): 1.5 μM Impβ, 8 μM ATP, 8 μM GTP, 320 μM creatine phosphate, 4 Units creatine kinase in PBS, 2 μM DTT, 1× TB, in dH$_2$O.
6. Ran Mix (RMx): 0.03 μM RanGAP, 4 nM RanBP, 10.3 μM GDP, 0.06 μM NTF2.
7. Energy Mix (EMx): 0.75 mM ATP, 0.75 mM GTP, 15 mM creatine phosphate, 0.075 mg/ml creatine kinase in HEPES, 0.075 mM DTT, 0.075 mM Mg(OAC)$_2$, pH 7.5.

8. Fluorescent beads (0.1 μm TetraSpeck Fluospheres, Life Technologies) as fiducial markers for drift correction.

9. Imaging buffer 100 mM mercaptoethylamine, 0.5 mg/ml glucose oxidase, 0.2 % vol/vol catalase, and 10 % wt/vol d-glucose in PBS pH 7.4.

10. Nail varnish and cover glass, to seal the chamber for SMLM.

2.5 Single-Molecule Imaging Instrumentation

We perform single-molecule using a custom-built microscope, based on an Olympus IX81 base (Fig. 2). The system is set-up to allow epifluorescence, TIRF or inclined illumination of the sample. Inclined illumination schemes (including HILO) can be used to improve the S/N ratio of the imaging, by reducing the illumination of molecules above and below the focal plane of interest. TIRF illumination cannot be employed since the NPCs are typically located above the shallow (~100 nm) evanescent field of illumination. The system comprises the following features:

1. Four lasers (100 mW 405 nm Coherent Obis, 100 mW 488 nm Coherent Sapphire, 150 mW 561 nm Coherent Sapphire and a 150 mW Toptica iBeam Smart, *see* **Note 1**), each with their own shutter control, are expanded to the same diameter and combined using a series of dichroic mirrors (Semrock LaserMUX) into a single free-space beam. Half-wave plates were used to adjust the polarization before passing the beams

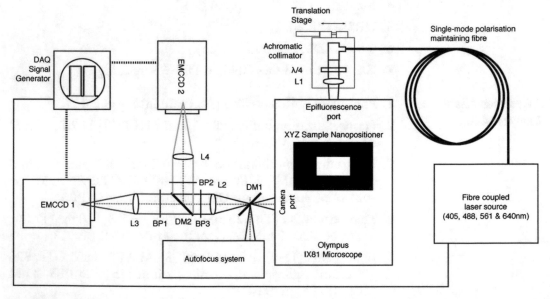

Fig. 2 Schematic of single-molecule localization microscope optical layout. An Olympus IX81 base with high NA objective is used as the body of the microscope. Laser illumination is coupled into the system using a single-mode fiber. Two EMCCD cameras are attached to the camera port via a relay, enabling simultaneous two-color imaging. Cameras and lasers are synchronized using an external signal generator. An infrared laser autofocus system is coupled via the camera port to maintain a focus lock during image acquisition

through an Acousto-Optical Tunable Filter (AOTF, AA Optoelectronics, France) to quickly modulate laser power. The combined beams are again expanded and launched into a single-mode optical fiber (Thorlabs PM-S405-XP) using an inexpensive Olympus 10X (0.1 N.A. air) objective lens.

2. The output of the optical fiber is collimated using an achromatic parabolic mirror collimator and passed through a quarter-wave plate to circularly polarize the beam to prevent orientation specific excitation of fluorophores. The free beam is then passed through a "TIRF lens" (Thorlabs AC254-200-A-ML), focussing the expanded beam, via a multi-edge dichroic filter (Semrock Di01-R405/488/561/635-25x36), directly onto the back focal plane of an apochromatic Olympus 100× 1.49 N.A. objective lens. This entire subsystem can be mounted on a translation stage to adjust the translation of the beam across the back focal plane of the objective, and therefore adjust the inclination of the beam at the sample plane (*see* **Note 2**).

3. Actively cooled EMCCD cameras (Andor iXon Ultra DU-897U-CS0-#BV) are coupled to the camera port of the microscope via an additional 1.5× magnifying relay. The magnifying relay ensures that optimal Shannon–Nyquist sampling is achieved in the final image. An additional dichroic mirror in the Fourier plane of the relay can be used to simultaneously image a second color on the second camera. Full frame camera acquisition is performed at 33 Hz (corresponding to an exposure time of 30 ms).

4. Appropriate bandpass filters (e.g., Semrock FF01-520/35-25 for GFP) are mounted in the Fourier space before of each camera, in order to select the emission of the fluorescent molecule used.

5. The laser shutters, AOTF and camera firing are synchronized using the external clock of a Data Translation DT9834 data acquisition module.

6. Sample positioning is controlled via a manual micrometer stage coupled with a 200 μm range three-axis nanopositioning stage (Physik Instrumente P-545.3R7).

Focal drift can be minimized using a focus-locking system (*see* **Note 3**). Here we present a design for a simple, low-cost, home-built focus-locking system based on total internal reflection of a near-IR laser off of the cover glass, with the return beam monitored by a linear two-axis position sensitive detector (Fig. 3). A simple low-noise bipolar power supply (modified from: http://tangent-soft.net/elec/vgrounds.html) can be created for powering the lateral effect sensor, which can then be read out using an Arduino or high-resolution A/D converter. A PID (Proportional, Integral, Differential) control loop drives the nanopositioner to correct and

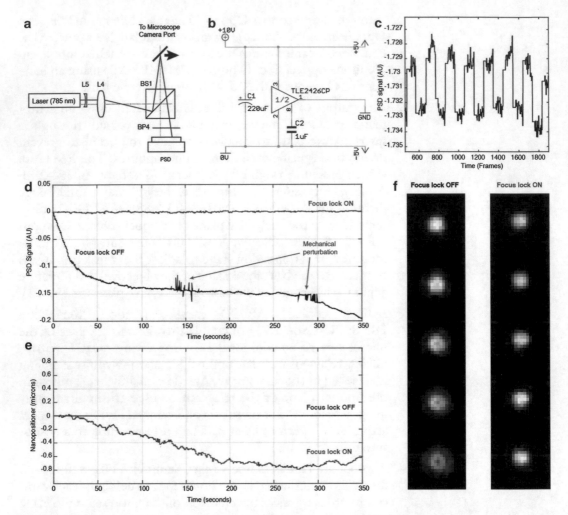

Fig. 3 Real-time focus locking system employed to maintain the imaging plane in focus. (**a**) Optical layout of total internal reflection of a near IR laser onto a position sensitive detector via the camera port of the microscope. (**b**) Low cost bipolar power supply design for the PSD. (**c**) Readout of PSD with 1 Hz, 50 nm square-wave applied to the nanopositioner. (**d**) PSD signal of sample with the focus-locking device either on or off. With the focus-lock off, the PSD signal rapidly decreases, corresponding to the mechanical drift of the objective turret. With the focus-lock engaged, the PSD signal stays constant. (**e**) Output of the PID control loop to the nanopositioner with the focus lock engaged, shows the corrections applied to the system to maintain focus. (**f**) Images of 100 nm fluorescent fiducial markers as a function of time with the focus lock off and on, demonstrating maintenance of the focus

maintain the sample position and account for focus drift. Translational drift is corrected post acquisition. The components required for the focus lock system are:

1. Data Translation DT9834 analog-to-digital converter.

2. Thorlabs PDP90A lateral effect sensor.

3. Thorlabs 785 nm laser (CPS780S).

4. 10 V power supply (we used an Isotech IPS303DD DC power supply).

5. Texas Instruments TLE2426IP rail virtual ground with noise reduction.

6. Hirose HR10A-7R-6S(73) 6-pin circular connector.

7. Panasonic EEU-FC1V221L 220uF aluminum electrolytic capacitor.

8. Panasonic ECQ-V1H105JL 1uF film capacitor.

9. IR Dichroic mirror and IR notch filter (Semrock FF750-SDi02-25x36).

Pins 4, 5, and 6 of the PDP90A are connected to the +5v, Ground, and –5v of the bipolar supply respectively. Pins 1, 2, and 3 (X-position, Δx, Y-position, Δx, and Sum voltage, S) are connected to the analog inputs of either the DAQ or an Arduino (via an additional circuit). The return beam position is calculated using the sensor size ($Lx = Ly = 10$ mm) as:

$$x = \frac{L_x \cdot \Delta x}{2S}, y = \frac{L_y \cdot \Delta y}{2S}$$

This return beam directly reports on the distance (separation) between the objective lens and the glass/water interface of the sample and can be used to correct/maintain the focus in real time.

2.6 Software

Software is required to localize (track, if live), and align the single-molecule trajectories from the camera acquisition data. In practice many software packages are available to localize molecules and perform drift correction (e.g., QuickPALM [31], ThunderSTORM [32], MLE [33]) using a Gaussian approximation of the Point Spread Function (PSF). Tracking can be performed using open source software such as the Crocker and Grier particle tracking code (http://physics.nyu.edu/grierlab/software.html) [34] or TrackMate (http://fiji.sc/TrackMate) [35].

In practice, we use a mixed C++/Python software library, ImPy, developed in-house, to localize, drift-correct, and track molecules, and a simple MATLAB interface to perform subsequent single-particle data analysis. The latest version of the source code for the image analysis tools can be downloaded from *github*:

```
git clone https://github.com/quantumjot/impy-tools
git    clone    https://github.com/quantumjot/NPC-local-
isation-tools
```

3   Methods

3.1   Protein Expression and Purification

Escherichia coli cells can be transformed with the appropriate plasmid for a His$_6$-tagged cargo, NTRs, or Ran, grown up in 1–2 l cultures induced with of 1 M IPTG overnight at 37 °C. Lyse cells with a cell homogenizer, and purify the protein using a 5 ml HisTrap column, eluting with a gradient of elution buffer containing imidazole (300 mM imidazole, 2 mM DTT in PBS, pH 7.4).

3.2   Labeling of Proteins

Proteins can either be expressed as fusion proteins containing a photo-convertible fluorescent protein (e.g., mEOS3) or chemically labeled using fluorescent dyes such as an *N*-hydroxysuccinimidyl ester of Alexa Fluor 647 as per the manufacturers instructions (*see* **Note 4**).

3.3   Preparation of Cells for Imaging

1. Grow HeLa cells in 75 cm^2 tissue culture flasks containing 10 ml of growth media in an incubator (37 °C, 5 % (v/v) CO$_2$).

2. Once grown to approximately 80 % confluence, aspirate the media from the flasks and wash cells with 5 ml HBSS prior to incubation with 2 ml 0.05 % EDTA/trypsin (5 min, 37 °C, 5 % (v/v) CO$_2$).

3. After detachment, add 7 ml HBSS/10 % FCS and transfer to a 15 ml falcon tube for centrifugation (1200×*g*, 4 °C, 5 min).

4. Aspirate the resulting supernatant before resuspending the cell precipitate in 5 ml HBSS/10 % FCS. Seed the cells in 10 ml growth media at 2×10^6 cells per flask.

5. Wash glass bottom dishes (Ibidi, μ-Dish 35 mm, high) with 2 ml HBSS.

6. Seed dishes with HeLa cells (incubate in 2 ml growth media at 37 °C (5 % (v/v) CO$_2$, for 24 h) to allow attachment.

3.4   Cell Permeabilization and Transport Assay

At ~50 % confluence, remove dishes containing cells from the incubator and aspirate the growth media. Permeabilization of the cell membrane is performed by the following washes, adding the appropriate buffer, waiting for the specified time and then aspirating:

1. Three × 2 ml PBS, 5 min each.

2. One × 2 ml Permeabilization buffer (PB), 2 min.

3. One × 2.5 ml Digitonin-Permeabilization buffer (DPB), 10 min.

4. Three × 3 ml Transport buffer (TB), 5 min each.

5. Following permeabilization the excess buffer can be wicked away using a folded lint-free tissue, before adding the transport reaction mix.

6. Initiate the transport reaction by gently adding 200 μl of import mix onto the cells in the glass bottom dish. If using a labeled cargo, add it here (typical concentrations are 10–50 pM). Wrap the dish in aluminum foil to prevent any photo-conversion or photo-bleaching.

7. If imaging active transport add 1.0 μM RanGDP, alongside Ran Mix and Energy Mix (*see* **Note 5**).

8. A 1:1000 dilution of 0.1 μm fluorescent beads can be added to the import mix.

9. If fixing the sample, allow the reaction to proceed for 10–20 min, then apply 2 ml of a 4% paraformaldehyde (PFA in PBS pH 7.4) solution for 15 min, before washing off and replacing with imaging buffer (*see* **Note 6**).

10. Image acquisition should start immediately.

3.5 Image Acquisition and Processing

3.5.1 General Imaging Scheme

Since the equatorial plane of the nucleus of HeLa cells can be 3–7 μm above the cover glass (and hence the fiducial markers used for image registration are out of focus), image acquisition is performed as a sequence (as shown schematically in Fig. 4), alternating the focus between the imaging plane at equator of the nucleus and the fiducial markers at the surface of the coverslip. This acquisition scheme utilizes the laser focus-lock to maintain the focus at each plane to within ±5 nm, and uses the fiducial marker trajectories to perform drift correction post acquisition. EMCCD cameras are used in kinetic frame transfer mode, with cooling (−80 °C), EM "real" gain (typically 500–750) and short exposure times (10–30 ms). Imaging is performed as follows:

1. Wear protective eyewear while operating the microscope.

2. Put a drop of oil on the objective and mount the sample on the stage (*see* **Note 7**).

3. Verify that the imaging laser is collimated out of the objective by looking at the projection on the ceiling. Adjust the translation of the imaging laser to achieve highly inclined illumination.

4. Focus on the fluorescent beads adsorbed onto the cover glass surface.

5. Determine the relative z-displacement (ΔZ) of the equatorial imaging plane of the nucleus to the surface beads by measuring the laser return beam offset on the PSD, and nanopositioner z-offset at the two focal planes. Note that the focus lock system uses the stored PSD offset values to lock the focus.

6. Bleach down the sample if necessary by setting the imaging laser to full power (*see* **Note 8**).

7. Return the focus to the fiducial marker plane.

8. Start the image acquisition Python script:

   (a) Engage the focus lock, image for 10–30 s using a low laser power (1–5 mW 488 nm). Disengage the focus lock.

   (b) Move up to the equatorial plane (+ΔZ), engage the focus lock, and turn on the imaging laser (e.g., ~150 mW 640 nm for SMLM, <20 mW for tracking) and image for 30–120 s. The length of this acquisition, and the laser power can be optimized to account for the duration of events to be imaged. Note that lateral drift correction is worse for longer imaging periods (*see* **Note 9**). Disengage the focus-lock.

   (c) Move back down to the fiducial plane (−ΔZ).

   (d) Return to (a) unless >20 min of imaging data has been acquired.

9. Stop the acquisition.

3.5.2 Localization of Molecules

Under the conditions described, individual fluorophores should be visible (Fig. 4). Each spot represents the true position of the molecule convolved with the Point Spread Function (PSF) of the microscope, and additive noise. The PSF is equivalent to a probability distribution that defines the coordinates of the molecule, where fitting a two-dimensional Gaussian function can approximate the centroid. In practice, the localization precision of each molecule refers to how precisely we can define the center of the PSF, given the magnification and S/N of the image. Since we use a symmetrical Gaussian function to model the PSF, the mean-squared positional error is given by:

$$\sigma^2_{x,y} \approx \frac{s^2 + \dfrac{a^2}{12}}{N_\mathrm{m}} + \frac{4\sqrt{\pi}s^3 b^2_\mathrm{m}}{aN^2_\mathrm{m}}$$

where s is the standard deviation of the PSF, a is the pixel size in the image, N_m is the total number of photons measured from the molecule m, and b_m is the number of background photons measured in the localization window [36]. We calculate the photon conversion factor for our camera by measuring the mean and variance of the camera response counts as a function of illumination intensity. In general, the greater the number of photons, the more precise the fit is, so good localization can depend on using fluorescent molecules that emit many photons (*see* **Note 2**).

3.5.3 Drift Correction

Thermal and mechanical drift is a major problem in long timescale (>min), single-molecule imaging experiments. During acquisition, drift arising from movement of the stage (lateral) or objective

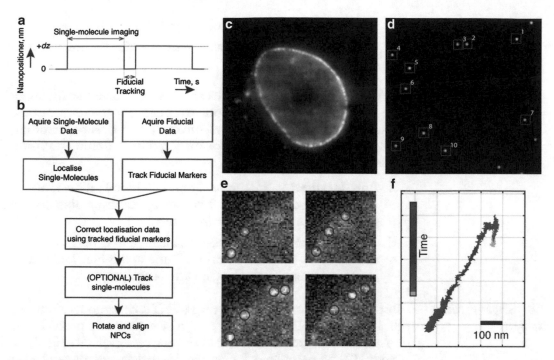

Fig. 4 Data acquisition and processing workflow. (**a**) Scheme for sequentially imaging two planes within the sample, the specimen plane and the fiducial plane. The nanopositioner (using feedback from the focus lock) maintains the position at either of the two planes. (**b**) Generalized method workflow describing the data acquisition and processing steps. (**c**) An example HILO image of a nucleus labeled with NTRs. Individual puncta are evident at the nuclear envelope. (**d**) Widefield image of fiducial markers at the cover glass surface. Software is used to identify the particles. (**e**) Raw frames from a live single-molecule tracking experiment showing individual molecules. Each molecule is localized in each frame. (**f**) Example fiducial marker trajectory from a long imaging acquisition showing an example of translational drift during acquisition

turret or sample (axial/focus drift) can lead to blurry or incorrectly aligned images. Focus drift is corrected using the focus-locking mechanism described earlier, typically to within ±5 nm. Translational drift of the sample is corrected post acquisition using the image data taken from the cover glass immobilized fiducial markers. The protocol for drift correction is as follows:

1. Use the software to identify at least three fiducial markers close to the cell of interest.

2. Track these particles over time, and interpolate the trajectory where necessary.

3. Overlay all of the trajectories and create a mean trajectory (drift vector).

4. Assess the width of the distribution of the each fiducial trajectory minus the drift vector.

5. Discard those with few time points or where there is significant deviation from the drift vector.

6. Iteratively refine by repeating **steps 1–5**.

7. Correct the localization data by subtracting the time dependent drift vector.

3.5.4 Image Creation

A final diffraction-limited image can be reconstructed by summing
the images from the acquisition. Generating a two-dimensional
histogram of the localization data can create a final, super-resolved,
image. Typically a bin size approximating the localization precision
is used.

1. Run **localisation_image.m** from NPC-localisation-tools to
bin-sort the data, using a bin size *h*, corresponding to the
localization precision of the instrument.

2. The bin-sorting algorithm also maintains a hash map that maps
the bin to the set of localizations found in this bin. This can be
used for fast look-up in single-particle analysis.

*3.6 Single-Particle
Analysis*

In order to create a composite map of NTR or cargo localizations
in a canonical NPC structure, we first extract the positions of
putative NPC complexes found at the nuclear envelope (Fig. 5, *see*
Note 10). All parameters for the single-particle analysis can be set
using the **options.m** file.

1. First, define the nuclear envelope (NE) as a series of vectors, in
the 2-dimensional plane of our image, describing a closed
curve, arranged in a clockwise direction. The directionality of
the curve is important as this allows one to calculate the orientation of the surface normal vector according to the right hand
rule. This orientation directly relates to the nucleocytoplasmic
axis vector of the NPC.

2. The software passes a scanning window, corresponding to a
rotated rectangle whose long axis is aligned with the surface
normal vector, along the envelope curve in order to calculate
the number of localizations as a function of position on the
envelope curve. Let **X** be the set of *n* single-molecule localizations $x_1,...,xn$. Let *P* be a rectangle with four vertices,
width *w* and length *l*, centered at point p_0, rotated by some
angle relative to the origin, θ and found on the envelope
curve. Polygon P is defined in terms of the unit tangent, **t**
and normal, **n** vectors (Fig. 5d). The width and length parameters are chosen such that the width is approximately that of
the feature we are interested in, and the length to be several
times that of the feature, to allow refinement of the axial centroid later. We can define a subset **Y** of all localizations, falling
within this window. In practice, we can dramatically increase
the speed of this calculation by not testing every member of
X and restricting the set of localizations used to calculate

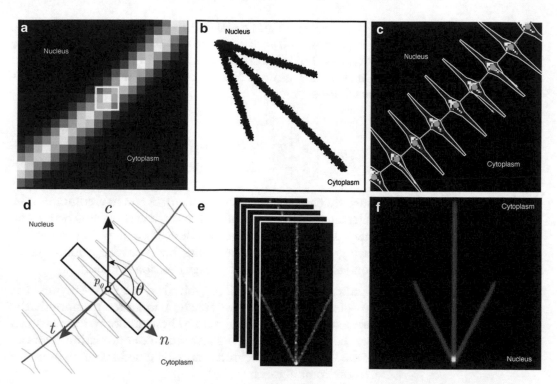

Fig. 5 Single-particle analysis of SMLM microscopy data. This figure uses simulated data where NPCs are represented as directional *arrows* arranged along an envelope structure. (**a**) Simulated diffraction limited image of *arrow* structures arranged at an envelope. (**b**) Example of the underlying localizations representing the arrow structure highlighted in (**a**). (**c**) After having drawn (or fit) the envelope vector (*blue line*), the software generates an envelope histogram with putative NPC structures marked with *green dots*. (**d**) Geometry of the alignment transformation. Three vectors are shown, *c* the unit alignment vector, *t*, the envelope tangent vector and *n*, the orientation vector of the putative NPC centered at point *p0*. The structure is extracted and rotated by the angle θ to bring all structures into register. (**e**) Examples of individual structures to be aligned. (**f**) Mean image of aligned structures, following cross-correlation or ICP based alignment from (**e**)

window occupancy to those within a reasonable distance from point p_0, using a hash map.

3. Utilizing the hash-map and the scanning window, calculate a linearized histogram of localizations along the NE vector by calculating the cardinality of the subset $|\mathbf{Y}|$ (i.e., the number of localizations within the scanning window). The software will identify peaks within this distribution (utilizing peak height, width and separation as control parameters), which correspond to candidate complexes.

Once we have identified the centroids of candidate NPCs along the envelope vector, we can extract and rotationally align the point clouds. This rotational alignment assures that each candidate NPC structure maintains its cytoplasm-to-nucleus orientation vector, but assumes that the NPC is orientated normally to the envelope vector.

1. Using a common axis $\mathbf{c} = [0, 1]^T$ to determine the angle of the rotated box as $\theta = \arccos(\mathbf{n} \times \mathbf{c})$, the software will rotate the point cloud of localizations found within the box into the new common axis using a Euclidean transform in homogeneous coordinates:

$$\begin{bmatrix} x' \\ y' \\ 1 \end{bmatrix} = \begin{bmatrix} \cos\theta & -\sin\theta & -p_x \\ \sin\theta & \cos\theta & -p_x \\ 0 & 0 & 1 \end{bmatrix} \begin{bmatrix} x \\ y \\ 1 \end{bmatrix}$$

2. Once we have rotationally aligned data sets to a common axis, we create small images of each pore, again by bin-sorting the data with an appropriate coarseness, h. At all points in the following procedure, the mapping between the original point cloud and the discretized (image) version is maintained.

3. Next, each small image is convolved with a radially symmetric two-dimensional Gaussian function in order to smooth the image and facilitate alignment. These smoothed images can then be aligned using a normalized cross-correlation method, or the original point clouds can be aligned using an Iterative Closest Point algorithm (ICP).

4. Specify a suitable template image, and calculate the translational offset of each image in the set relative to the template. Use this offset to align the original point cloud of each structure.

5. Once all of the structures have been aligned, remove those with very large displacements or poor correlation with the remaining data set.

6. Assemble a mean image from the aligned structures.

7. The performance of the alignment procedure can be assessed utilizing synthetic images. Run **demo.m** from NPC-localisation-tools.

4   Notes

1. Different lasers can be utilized for different experimental geometries. For example the 640 nm laser is often used for *d*STORM type experiments using Alexa 647 as a reporter, while the 561 nm laser for PALM experiments, using mEOS as a reporter. In both cases, the 405 nm laser can be used to photo-convert/activate depending on the fluorophore used. By tuning the 405 nm laser power, the amount of photoactivation/conversion can be tightly controlled. The 488 nm laser is often used for semiconductor nanocrystal tracking experiments (SPT) or for visualizing GFP constructs.

2. Additionally, by inserting an aperture in a conjugate plane to the specimen plane (with the appropriate relay lenses), the system can be also used for true HILO illumination.

3. Several commercial focus-lock systems are available from major microscope manufacturers. There are also several open source solutions such as PGFocus (http://big.umassmed.edu/wiki/index.php/PgFocus). Here we utilize our own, since it is cheap and highly customizable for the acquisition protocol.

4. For SMLM, dyes such as Alexa 647 show ideal photo-physical properties (blinking, quantum yield, etc.). Semiconductor nanocrystals such as Quantum Dots can be utilized to create synthetic cargos capable of being tracked for minutes. However, these particles are larger in size than synthetic moieties or fluorescent proteins. In some cases this precludes them from use for particular types of SPT experiments.

5. Once the cells have been permeabilized and the cytoplasm washed out, the RanGTP gradient has been abolished. The Ran and Energy Mixes therefore contain all of the components required to reinitialize and maintain the RanGTP gradient within the permeabilized cells, and therefore permit active transport. This should be tested using model cargos.

6. The imaging buffer is an oxygen scavenging system to remove oxygen and thus preventing photobleaching. The buffer also contains an appropriate amount of reducing agent (typically β-mercaptoethanol or β-mercaptoethylamine) that promotes the blinking required for SMLM or indeed can reduce blinking in nanocrystal tracking experiments. Care needs to be taken over the pH of the buffer, as it will decay over time. Also, some commercially available buffers have a high refractive index that may interfere with the use of the focus-lock system.

7. Sample drift is often most pronounced at the beginning of the experiment, and generally immediately after the sample is mounted on the microscope. To minimize the amount of drift observed in the experiment, let the sample settle for a period of minutes before beginning the acquisition.

8. For SMLM it can be advisable to "bleach down" the sample, using a high-laser power, prior to acquisition to ensure that single fluorophores are visible and sparse. Many localization algorithms can generate artifacts if the data are not sparse.

9. There exists a trade-off between observing longer interactions and the accuracy of registration using the drift correction. Longer interactions require a longer period of imaging, during which the fiducial markers cannot easily be tracked.

10. Labeling a second component of the NPC, such as POM-121 or Nup358, with a second dye, can be used to verify the identity and orientation of putative NPCs.

Acknowledgements

Grace Jeremy is supported by a Wellcome Trust studentship. We thank Anthony Roberts for criticial reading of the manuscript. We also thank the Hayward, Waksman and Fassati labs for contributions of reagents, equipment, and expertise. The Lowe lab acknowledges support from the Medical Research Council award MR/K015826/1 Super Resolution Imaging for Cell Biology and Neuroscience at UCL.

References

1. Devos D, Dokudovskaya S, Williams R, Alber F, Eswar N, Chait BT, Rout MP, Sali A (2006) Simple fold composition and modular architecture of the nuclear pore complex. Proc Natl Acad Sci U S A 103(7):2172–2177. doi:10.1073/pnas.0506345103

2. Grossman E, Medalia O, Zwerger M (2012) Functional architecture of the nuclear pore complex. Annu Rev Biophys 41:557–584. doi:10.1146/annurev-biophys-050511-102328

3. Terry LJ, Shows EB, Wente SR (2007) Crossing the nuclear envelope: hierarchical regulation of nucleocytoplasmic transport. Science 318(5855):1412–1416. doi:10.1126/science.1142204

4. Kalderon D, Roberts BL, Richardson WD, Smith AE (1984) A short amino acid sequence able to specify nuclear location. Cell 39(3 Pt 2):499–509

5. Cingolani G, Petosa C, Weis K, Müller CW (1999) Structure of importin-beta bound to the IBB domain of importin-alpha. Nature 399(6733):221–229. doi:10.1038/20367

6. Ribbeck K, Görlich D (2001) Kinetic analysis of translocation through nuclear pore complexes. EMBO J 20(6):1320–1330. doi:10.1093/emboj/20.6.1320

7. Izaurralde E, Kutay U, von Kobbe C, Mattaj IW, Gorlich D (1997) The asymmetric distribution of the constituents of the Ran system is essential for transport into and out of the nucleus. EMBO J 16(21):6535–6547. doi:10.1093/emboj/16.21.6535

8. Kalab P, Weis K, Heald R (2002) Visualization of a Ran-GTP gradient in interphase and mitotic Xenopus egg extracts. Science 295(5564):2452–2456. doi:10.1126/science.1068798

9. Görlich D, Panté N, Kutay U, Aebi U, Bischoff FR (1996) Identification of different roles for RanGDP and RanGTP in nuclear protein import. EMBO J 15(20):5584–5594

10. Rout MP, Aitchison JD, Magnasco MO, Chait BT (2003) Virtual gating and nuclear transport: the hole picture. Trends Cell Biol 13(12):622–628

11. Frey S, Richter RP, Görlich D (2006) FG-rich repeats of nuclear pore proteins form a three-dimensional meshwork with hydrogel-like properties. Science 314(5800):815–817. doi:10.1126/science.1132516

12. Frey S, Görlich D (2007) A saturated FG-repeat hydrogel can reproduce the permeability properties of nuclear pore complexes. Cell 130(3):512–523. doi:10.1016/j.cell.2007.06.024

13. Lowe AR, Tang JH, Yassif J, Graf M, Huang WY, Groves JT, Weis K, Liphardt JT (2015) Importin-β modulates the permeability of the nuclear pore complex in a Ran-dependent manner. eLife 4:doi:10.7554/eLife.04052

14. Bestembayeva A, Kramer A, Labokha AA, Osmanović D, Liashkovich I, Orlova EV, Ford IJ, Charras G, Fassati A, Hoogenboom BW (2015) Nanoscale stiffness topography reveals structure and mechanics of the transport barrier in intact nuclear pore complexes. Nat Nanotechnol 10(1):60–64. doi:10.1038/nnano.2014.262

15. Adam SA, Marr RS, Gerace L (1990) Nuclear protein import in permeabilized mammalian cells requires soluble cytoplasmic factors. J Cell Biol 111(3):807–816

16. Dange T, Grünwald D, Grünwald A, Peters R, Kubitscheck U (2008) Autonomy and robustness of translocation through the nuclear pore complex: a single-molecule study. J Cell Biol 183(1):77–86. doi:10.1083/jcb.200806173

17. Yang W, Musser SM (2006) Nuclear import time and transport efficiency depend on importin beta concentration. J Cell Biol 174(7):951–961. doi:10.1083/jcb.200605053

18. Kubitscheck U, Grünwald D, Hoekstra A, Rohleder D, Kues T, Siebrasse JP, Peters R

(2005) Nuclear transport of single molecules: dwell times at the nuclear pore complex. J Cell Biol 168(2):233–243. doi:10.1083/jcb.200411005

19. Kahms M, Lehrich P, Hüve J, Sanetra N, Peters R (2009) Binding site distribution of nuclear transport receptors and transport complexes in single nuclear pore complexes. Traffic 10(9):1228–1242. doi:10.1111/j.1600-0854.2009.00947.x

20. Tokunaga M, Imamoto N, Sakata-Sogawa K (2008) Highly inclined thin illumination enables clear single-molecule imaging in cells. Nat Methods 5(2):159–161. doi:10.1038/nmeth1171

21. Ma J, Yang W (2010) Three-dimensional distribution of transient interactions in the nuclear pore complex obtained from single-molecule snapshots. Proc Natl Acad Sci U S A 107(16):7305–7310. doi:10.1073/pnas.0908269107

22. Yang W (2013) Distinct, but not completely separate spatial transport routes in the nuclear pore complex. Nucleus 4(3):166–175. doi:10.4161/nucl.24874

23. Lowe AR, Siegel JJ, Kalab P, Siu M, Weis K, Liphardt JT (2010) Selectivity mechanism of the nuclear pore complex characterized by single cargo tracking. Nature 467(7315):600–603. doi:10.1038/nature09285

24. Sun C, Yang W, Tu LC, Musser SM (2008) Single-molecule measurements of importin alpha/cargo complex dissociation at the nuclear pore. Proc Natl Acad Sci U S A 105(25):8613–8618. doi:10.1073/pnas.0710867105

25. Betzig E, Patterson GH, Sougrat R, Lindwasser OW, Olenych S, Bonifacino JS, Davidson MW, Lippincott-Schwartz J, Hess HF (2006) Imaging intracellular fluorescent proteins at nanometer resolution. Science (NY) 313(5793):1642–1645. doi:10.1126/science.1127344

26. Rust M, Bates M, Zhuang X (2006) Sub-diffraction-limit imaging by stochastic optical reconstruction microscopy (STORM). Nat Methods 3(10):793–796

27. Heilemann M, van de Linde S, Mukherjee A, Sauer M (2009) Super-resolution imaging with small organic fluorophores. Angew Chem Int Ed Engl 48(37):6903–6908. doi:10.1002/anie.200902073

28. Löschberger A, van de Linde S, Dabauvalle MC, Rieger B, Heilemann M, Krohne G, Sauer M (2012) Super-resolution imaging visualizes the eightfold symmetry of gp210 proteins around the nuclear pore complex and resolves the central channel with nanometer resolution. J Cell Sci 125(Pt 3):570–575. doi:10.1242/jcs.098822

29. Löschberger A, Franke C, Krohne G, van de Linde S, Sauer M (2014) Correlative super-resolution fluorescence and electron microscopy of the nuclear pore complex with molecular resolution. J Cell Sci 127(Pt 20):4351–4355. doi:10.1242/jcs.156620

30. Szymborska A, de Marco A, Daigle N, Cordes VC, Briggs JA, Ellenberg J (2013) Nuclear pore scaffold structure analyzed by super-resolution microscopy and particle averaging. Science 341(6146):655–658. doi:10.1126/science.1240672

31. Henriques R, Lelek M, Fornasiero EF, Valtorta F, Zimmer C, Mhlanga MM (2010) QuickPALM: 3D real-time photoactivation nanoscopy image processing in ImageJ. Nat Methods 7(5):339–340. doi:10.1038/nmeth0510-339

32. Ovesny M, Krizek P, Borkovec J, Svindrych Z, Hagen GM (2014) ThunderSTORM: a comprehensive ImageJ plug-in for PALM and STORM data analysis and super-resolution imaging. Bioinformatics 30(16):2389–2390. doi:10.1093/bioinformatics/btu202

33. Starr R, Stahlheber S, Small A (2012) Fast maximum likelihood algorithm for localization of fluorescent molecules. Opt Lett 37(3):413–415

34. Crocker J, Grier D (1996) Methods of digital video microscopy for colloidal studies. J Colloid Interface Sci 179(1):298–310

35. Jaqaman K, Loerke D, Mettlen M, Kuwata H, Grinstein S, Schmid SL, Danuser G (2008) Robust single-particle tracking in live-cell time lapse sequences. Nat Methods 5(8):695–702. doi:10.1038/nmeth.1237

36. Thompson R, Larson D, Webb W (2002) Precise nanometer localization analysis for individual fluorescent probes. Biophys J 82(5):2775–2783

Chapter 4

Using Fluorescence Recovery After Photobleaching (FRAP) to Study Dynamics of the Structural Maintenance of Chromosome (SMC) Complex In Vivo

Anjana Badrinarayanan and Mark C. Leake

Abstract

The SMC complex, MukBEF, is important for chromosome organization and segregation in *Escherichia coli*. Fluorescently tagged MukBEF forms distinct spots (or "foci") in the cell, where it is thought to carry out most of its chromosome associated activities. This chapter outlines the technique of Fluorescence Recovery After Photobleaching (FRAP) as a method to study the properties of YFP-tagged MukB in fluorescent foci. This method can provide important insight into the dynamics of MukB on DNA and be used to study its biochemical properties in vivo.

Key words Chromosome organization, MukBEF, *E. coli*, Fluorescence microscopy, FRAP

1 Introduction

The bacterial chromosome is compacted nearly a 1000-fold into a cell where it is faithfully replicated, transcribed, and segregated. Not only is it highly compacted, but it is also spatially organized with chromosomal regions occupying specific positions inside the cell [1, 2]. The highly conserved Structural Maintenance of Chromosome (SMC) complex, MukBEF, plays a central role in *E. coli* to maintain chromosome organization and ensure faithful chromosome segregation [3, 4]. The MukBEF complex consists of three proteins: The SMC-like MukB and two accessory proteins MukE and MukF. Deletion of any of these components results in a Δ*muk* phenotype that includes temperature sensitivity, production of anucleate cells and loss of wild-type chromosome organization. Functional fluorescent fusions of MukB, E, or F all form foci in cells (Fig. 1), with two foci on average around the origin of replication [3, 5]. Recent studies using an array of microscopy-based approaches and genetic tools have provided insight into the properties of Muk foci and have supported the idea that foci are the

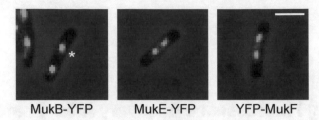

MukB-YFP   MukE-YFP   YFP-MukF

Fig. 1 Fluorescent fusions of MukBEF form foci in cells. YFP-tagged MukB, MukE, and MukF form foci in cells. Representative cells are shown in this figure. Fluorescent focus is highlighted with *asterisk*

centers of activity of the MukBEF complex [3–7]. The techniques used in these studies are widely applicable to understanding the functions of other proteins/protein complexes in vivo.

In general, advances in live-cell imaging in combination with the use of Green Fluorescent Protein (GFP) and its variants have facilitated the ability to study the composition and dynamics of protein complexes in a cellular context [8–19]. In this chapter we describe the techniques of Fluorescence Recovery After Photobleaching (FRAP) [20] and Fluorescence Loss In Photobleaching (FLIP) to study the dynamics of YFP-tagged MukB, E, or F in foci [6]. During FRAP, a subset of fluorescent molecules (typically, molecules in one of the two Muk foci) are irreversibly photobleached using a laser beam with high intensity of illumination. After the brief pulse of bleaching, images are recorded for subsequent time-frames at lower laser intensities to observe the recovery of fluorescence at the bleached spot either by diffusion of the non-bleached molecules or by active exchange of bleached molecules in the focus with unbleached ones. Since MukBEF forms two fluorescent foci, we can also record the loss in fluorescence of the unbleached focus (FLIP) during the photobleaching experiment. In an ideal scenario, the rate of recovery after photobleaching should be comparable to the loss in intensity of the unbleached focus.

This chapter briefly describes the method to grow cells and prepare slides, similar to that described previously [21] and outlines a typical FRAP experiment as well as a simple method of data analysis. As states earlier, the method can be modified to study other protein complexes as well. For these experiments, *E. coli* cells are grown under conditions that result in non–overlapping replication cycles, so each cell has two Muk foci on average.

2   Materials

Instructions for the construction of YFP-tagged MukBEF components are beyond the scope of this chapter. However, a note is included on strain construction that might be useful (*see* **Note 1**).

2.1 Growth Media

1. Luria Broth: 10 g Yeast Extract, 5 g NaCl and 5 g Tryptone in 1 L of water. pH is adjusted to 7 and LB is sterilized by autoclaving.

2. 10× M9 salt solution: 63 g Na_2HPO_4, 30 g KH_2PO_4, 5 g NaCl, and 10 g NH_4Cl in 1 L of water. Sterilize by autoclaving.

3. 1× M9–glycerol: 1× M9 salts, 0.5 mg/mL of thiamine, 0.1% 1 M $MgSO_4$, 0.1% 100 mM $CaCl_2$, and 0.2% of glycerol as carbon source in water. Make 100 mL of this solution.

4. 2× M9–glycerol: Same as 1× M9–glycerol but in half the quantity of water. Make 50 mL of this solution.

5. 2% agarose: Invitrogen ultrapure agarose can be used for this. For 50 mL, add 1 g of agarose to 50 mL of water.

6. 1% agarose + M9–glycerol (this mixture is used for microscope slide preparation): Mix melted 2% agarose with 2× M9–glycerol in a 1:1 ratio. We usually mix 500 μL of each solution by pipetting in an eppendorf and immediately use this to prepare the microscopy slide.

2.2 Slides and Microscope

1. Microscope slides: VistaVision microscope slides (VWR).

2. Coverslips: Micro cover glasses, Thickness 1.5, 24×50 mm (VWR).

3. Gene Frame Seals. (Thermo Scientific Catalog number AB0578).

4. Microscope: UltraView PerkinElmer spinning disk confocal microscope with FRAP module, 100× 1.35NA oil immersion objective, Electron-multiplying charge-coupled device (ImagEM, Hamamatsu Photonics) and UltraView PK Bleaching Device for photobleaching. Assuming that you will be imaging YFP-tagged MukBEF, the microscope should have laser lines for 514 nm (*see* **Note 2** for alternative laser lines).

5. Immersion oil: Immersol W oil NA 1.339 (Zeiss).

6. Software: Volocity imaging software (PerkinElmer) for image acquisition and ImageJ for image analysis.

3 Methods

3.1 Preparation of Bacterial Cultures for Microscopy

1. Streak bacterial cells from a frozen stock on LB agar plates with appropriate antibiotic at 37 °C. As far as possible, use fresh cells no more than 2 weeks old. All cultures are grown by shaking to provide sufficient aeration. Most cells can grow at 37 °C. (*See* **Note 3** about growing Δ*mukBEF* cells). The steps listed below are for a strain carrying an YFP-tagged version of MukB. The same procedure can be followed for other tagged components of the complex.

2. Pick a single colony from the plate prepared in **step 1** and resuspend it in 5 mL of LB. Allow the culture to grow until stationary phase (5–6 h).

3. Make a 1 in 5000 dilution of the above into 5 mL of 1× M9–glycerol and allow this culture to grow overnight.

4. The following day, subculture the cells in fresh 1× M9–glycerol (~1 in 1000 dilution) and allow the cells to grow till OD 0.1–0.2 (measured using a spectrophotometer). This should take 2–3 h (*see* **Note 4** for details about generation time of *E. coli* cells grown in M9–glycerol)

5. Spin down 500 μL of culture from **step 4** at 8000 rpm (~6000 rcf) for 1 min. Remove the supernatant and resuspend the pellet in 50 μL of 1× M9–glycerol. Cells are now ready to be spotted on the microscope slide and imaged.

3.2 Preparation of Microscopy Slide

The procedure described here has been previously outlined in detail in another volume of this series [21]. A condensed version of this protocol is provided below.

1. The Gene Frame is first stuck on a clean glass slide by removing its clear plastic cover. Make sure to stick the frame smoothly on all side without leaving wrinkles (*see* **Note 5** on why Gene Frames are used).

2. Take 500 μL of 1% agarose + M9–glycerol and immediately transfer it to the center of the gene frame prepared in the above step (*see* **Note 6**).

3. Place a coverslip on top of this and press it down to remove excess agarose and flatten the solution evenly in the frame. Let this stand for a few minutes, until the agarose has dried and solidified.

4. Once the agarose has solidified, slide the coverslip off and let the agarose dry for a couple of extra minutes.

5. Take 5 μL of culture prepared earlier (**step 5**, Subheading 3.1) and spot it on the agarose. Try to evenly distribute it across the slide by applying multiple spots and tilting the slide to allow spreading. Allow the slide to dry for a couple of more minutes. It is essential to do so as excess water will hamper **step 6** of this section.

6. Remove the top plastic cover of the gene frame. On the sticky side of the frame carefully place a coverslip. Make sure that the coverslip is placed evenly and avoid the formation of air pockets. Once the coverslip has made contact with all four sides of the frame, you can press it down gently to even out its adhesion.

3.3 Microscopy

1. Turn on the lasers, microscope, and computer. Then turn on Volocity (the acquisition software).

2. Add a drop of immersion oil to the objective and place the slide on top of the lens.

3. Cells should be focused using bright field or DIC. Avoid focusing using fluorescence to prevent photobleaching. An ideal field of view for imaging should have cells evenly distributed and in focus. A typical field can have up to 50 cells.

4. Open the settings for YFP (514 nm laser) on Volocity and reduce laser power to 4–6% (*see* **Note 7**). Under camera settings, set the frame rate to 300 ms for image capture. Focus and take a picture.

5. In the picture, you will be able to see typically two distinct MukB-YFP foci per cell. The aim of the experiment is to bleach one of the two foci and record fluorescence recovery after bleaching (*see* **Note 8** on use of cephalexin to elongate cells).

6. Open the FRAP module to set up bleaching conditions (*see* **Note 9** on FRAP calibration). Pulse bleach is ideally done with 6–15% laser intensity for 15 ms. The number of cycles of bleaching is limited to 1. A region of interest (ROI) is drawn around the focus to be bleached. This is usually a diffraction limited region of ~300 nm (*see* **Note 10** on size of ROI).

7. Using the PhotoKinesis menu, choose up to six ROIs (one ROI per cell) in one field of view. ROIs can be chosen by drawing a region around a MukB-YFP focus. Then set the conditions for acquisition. Typically, take 2–3 pre-bleach images and after pulse-bleaching (**step 6**), record recovery of fluorescence every 15 s for 3 min or every 30 s for 5 min. Again, image capture should be done at lower laser intensity (4–6%) at a 300 ms capture rate. The entire module is automated. Once the settings have been applied and acquisition has started, images will be acquired in the sequence desired: two pre-bleached images, followed by pulse-photobleaching of the ROIs selected, followed by image capture with low laser intensities for 3 or 5 min. Movies are saved as stack files that can be opened in ImageJ.

8. Repeat the above procedure after moving to a new field of view that is distinct from the field previously imaged (*see* **Note 11**).

3.4 Image Analysis

1. Open images (saved as a stack) in ImageJ. It is important to remove background fluorescence prior to extracting information on focus intensity. This is done using the background subtraction module in ImageJ. Apply subtraction to the entire stack.

2. For FRAP measurements draw a region of interest around the spot that was bleached in the experiments in Subheading 3.3. Also draw a second ROI around the entire cell to calculate

total cellular fluorescence intensity for the cell undergoing pulse-bleaching. Use ImageJ's "Measure Intensity" tool to extract mean and total intensity values for each ROI through the entire stack.

3. For FLIP measurements, the same procedure (**step 2**) should be repeated for an ROI drawn around the unbleached focus in the cell undergoing pulse-bleaching.

4. FRAP, FLIP, and total cellular fluorescence intensities for a cell in a movie can now be copied and pasted into Excel. To compare recovery across cells, intensity of ROIs should be normalized to highest pre-bleach intensities.

5. Before calculating recovery times, it is important to correct for photobleaching during imaging. This is done by normalizing total cellular intensity at each time point to the total cellular intensity soon after photobleaching.

6. Now the intensity of a bleached focus at a given time point can be calculated using the following equation, which corrects measured intensity values for any photobleaching which may have occurred:

$$I(t) = (\mathrm{Ib}(t) \,/\, \mathrm{Ib}_{max}) \,/\, (\mathrm{Ic}(t) \,/\, \mathrm{Ic}_{max})$$

Where:

$\mathrm{Ib}(t)$ = intensity of ROI at time t (post bleach).

Ib_{max} = maximum intensity of ROI (pre bleach).

$\mathrm{Ic}(t)$ = intensity of whole cell at time t.

Ic_{max} = intensity of whole cell soon after bleach.

7. By plotting the $I(t)$ values for a bleached or unbleached focus over the time of imaging, you can get an estimate of FRAP or FLIP respectively (*see* **Note 12** on expected outcomes and controls) (Fig. 2).

4   Notes

1. It is ideal to construct fluorescent fusions of proteins in the chromosome at the endogenous locus of the gene. One efficient way of strain construction in *E. coli* is using the λ-Red recombination system [22]. MukBEF genes are arranged in an operon (in the order *mukF–mukE–mukB*). While C-terminal fusions to MukB and MukE are fully functional, MukF needs to be tagged in its N-terminus for function to be maintained. A short linker of about 8–10 amino acids (glycine, serine, and alanine rich) is typically inserted between MukB, E, or F and the fluorescent protein (monomeric form of YFP, mYPet, has been used to image MukBEF in previous experiments [6]).

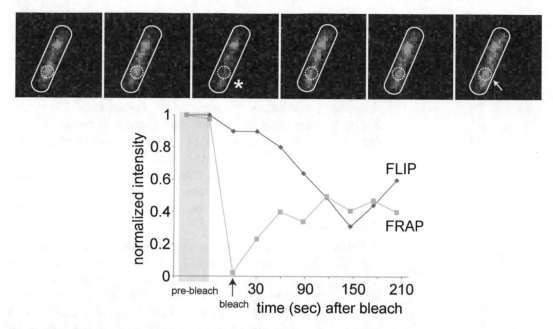

Fig. 2 Using FRAP to study dynamics of MukB-YFP in foci. *Above*: Representative time-lapse of a cell with MukB-YFP foci during a FRAP experiment is shown. The region of interest (ROI) that is pulse-bleached is high-lighted with a *circle*, pulse-bleaching is indicated with *asterisk* and recovery after bleaching is indicated by the *arrow. Below*: Quantification of FRAP experiment is shown. Two pre-bleach images were taken prior to pulse-bleaching of fluorescence in the ROI. Images were taken every 30 s after bleaching to record fluorescence recovery after bleaching. Normalized intensity in plotted for the bleached focus (FRAP) and for the control, unbleached focus (FLIP) in the same cell

2. Typically pulse-bleaching should be carried out using the same wavelength as used for imaging. In the case of YFP this is the peak excitation wavelength of 514 nm. In the event that the YFP laser is not powerful enough for pulse-bleaching, a 488 nm laser can be used for this step of the experiment.

3. Wild type *E. coli* cells can be grown at 37 °C in rich or minimal media. However, *ΔmukB, E*, or *F* strains or strains with mutants of MukB are temperature sensitive and ideally grow at room temperature (~22 °C). When doing an experiment that involves *ΔmukB* (or mutant MukB) and wild type cells, you should grow both cultures at 22 °C so that the conditions are comparable during imaging as well.

4. The generation time for *E. coli* in M9–glycerol is ~100 min. Cells grown in these conditions have non-overlapping replication cycles and are simpler to study processes such as chromosome organization, replication and segregation using microscopy. When growing cells in M9–glycerol, it is important to ensure that cells do not go into late stationary phase ($OD_{600} \sim 1$) as the recovery time (lag phase) to return to exponential growth will be prolonged.

5. Agarose pads can dry out or dessicate when kept for a long period during imaging (especially at high temperatures such as 37 °C). In order to prevent this, gene frames are used.

6. As stated earlier, M9–glycerol provides ideal growth conditions for microscopy-based experiments in *E. coli*. Another important advantage of using M9–glycerol over LB is the lower autofluorescence in M9. Background fluorescence can pose a problem during imaging and in particular, during analysis of fluorescence intensity in the cell. It is always advisable to use media with low levels of autofluorescence for this reason. Autofluorescence can be further reduced using low fluorescence agarose, for example the Nusieve GTG Agarose from Lonza Biosciences.

7. Ideal laser intensity settings will vary between microscope setups. It is recommended to use low laser intensities during imaging in order to reduce photobleaching or phototoxicity effects. The same applies for laser intensity used for pulse-bleaching. It is recommended to use an intensity that is high enough to completely bleach fluorescence in the region of interest, but not too high that other regions of the cell are bleached as well.

8. Since *E. coli* cells are small in size, FRAP experiments can sometimes cause bleaching across the entire cell, which can complicate analysis of fluorescence recovery. One way of circumventing this problem is to treat *E. coli* cells with the cell division inhibitor cephalexin (100 mg/mL) for 2–3 generations prior to imaging. This will result in the production of elongated cells with multiple, segregated chromosomes. If cephalexin is used, it should also be added to the agarose pad to prevent cells from dividing during imaging.

9. Before you start a FRAP experiment it is important to ascertain that the pulse-bleach is centered on the region of interest chosen in the cell. This can be done using the "FRAP Calibration Wizard" in Volocity. For this, you will need a slide with GFP fluorescence (We use a fluorescence marker to make this).

10. Since bacterial cells are small, try to use a small ROI for pulse-bleaching to avoid bleaching a large area of the cell.

11. While imaging, it is important to ensure that cells are still actively growing on the agarose pad. I recommend FRAP imaging of cells on an agarose pad for no longer than 2 h. More traditional time-lapse movies can be carried out for longer time (as long as the cells continue to grow).

12. There are, broadly, two typical outcomes of a FRAP experiment: (a) there is no recovery after photobleaching and the slight increase in fluorescence intensity in the ROI after pulse-bleaching is due to diffusion of free fluorescent molecules into

the area. (b) There is active recovery of fluorescence as assessed by a significant increase in intensity in the ROI after pulse-bleaching. You should be able to see the return of a MukB focus in this case. In order to test for the physiological relevance of this recovery, you can use MukB mutants that should not show recovery after photobleaching [6].

Acknowledgements

A.B. is supported by a Human Frontier Science Program Postdoctoral Fellowship.

References

1. Le TB, Laub MT (2014) New approaches to understanding the spatial organization of bacterial genomes. Curr Opin Microbiol 22C:15–21

2. Wang X, Llopis PM, Rudner DZ (2013) Organization and segregation of bacterial chromosomes. Nat Rev Genet 14:191–203

3. Danilova O, Reyes-Lamothe R, Pinskaya M et al (2007) MukB colocalizes with the oriC region and is required for organization of the two Escherichia coli chromosome arms into separate cell halves. Mol Microbiol 65:1485–1492

4. Nolivos S, Sherratt D (2014) The bacterial chromosome: architecture and action of bacterial SMC and SMC-like complexes. FEMS Microbiol Rev 38:380–392

5. Badrinarayanan A, Lesterlin C, Reyes-Lamothe R et al (2012) The Escherichia coli SMC complex. MukBEF, shapes nucleoid organization independently of DNA replication. J Bacteriol 194:4669–4676

6. Badrinarayanan A, Reyes-Lamothe R, Uphoff S et al (2012) In vivo architecture and action of bacterial structural maintenance of chromosome proteins. Science 338:528–531

7. Nicolas E, Upton AL, Uphoff S et al (2014) The SMC complex MukBEF recruits topoisomerase IV to the origin of replication region in live Escherichia coli. mBio 5:e01001–e01013

8. Shaner NC, Steinbach PA, Tsien RY (2005) A guide to choosing fluorescent proteins. Nat Methods 2:905–909

9. Schermelleh L, Heintzmann R, Leonhardt H (2010) A guide to super-resolution fluorescence microscopy. J Cell Biol 190:165–175

10. Wollman AJM, Miller H, Zhou Z et al (2015) Probing DNA interactions with proteins using a single-molecule toolbox: inside the cell, in a test tube and in a computer. Biochem Soc Trans 43:139–145

11. Plank M, Wadhams GH, Leake MC (2009) Millisecond timescale slimfield imaging and automated quantification of single fluorescent protein molecules for use in probing complex biological processes. Integr Biol 1:602–612

12. Robson A, Burrage K, Leake MC (2013) Inferring diffusion in single live cells at the single-molecule level. Philos Trans R Soc Lond B Biol Sci 368:20120029

13. Llorente-Garcia I, Lenn T, Erhardt H et al (2014) Single-molecule in vivo imaging of bacterial respiratory complexes indicates delocalized oxidative phosphorylation. Biochim Biophys Acta 1837:811–824

14. Lenn T, Leake MC (2012) Experimental approaches for addressing fundamental biological questions in living, functioning cells with single molecule precision. Open Biol 2:120090

15. Chiu S-W, Leake MC (2011) Functioning nanomachines seen in real-time in living bacteria using single-molecule and super-resolution fluorescence imaging. Int J Mol Sci 12:2518–2542

16. Leake MC (2010) Shining the spotlight on functional molecular complexes: the new science of single-molecule cell biology. Commun Integr Biol 3:415–418

17. Bryan SJ, Burroughs NJ, Shevela D et al (2014) Localisation and interactions of the Vipp1 protein in cyanobacteria. Mol Microbiol 94(5):1179–1195

18. Chiu S-W, Roberts MAJ, Leake MC et al (2013) Positioning of chemosensory proteins and FtsZ through the Rhodobacter sphaeroides cell cycle. Mol Microbiol 90:322–337

19. Lenn T, Leake MC, Mullineaux CW (2008) Are Escherichia coli OXPHOS complexes concentrated in specialized zones within the plasma membrane? Biochem Soc Trans 36:1032–1036

20. Sprague BL, McNally JG (2005) FRAP analysis of binding: proper and fitting. Trends Cell Biol 15:84–91

21. Reyes-Lamothe R (2012) Use of fluorescently tagged SSB proteins in in vivo localization experiments. Meth Mol Biol (Clifton, NJ) 922:245–253

22. Datsenko KA, Wanner BL (2000) One-step inactivation of chromosomal genes in Escherichia coli K-12 using PCR products. Proc Natl Acad Sci U S A 97:6640–6645

Chapter 5

Imaging DNA Structure by Atomic Force Microscopy

Alice L.B. Pyne and Bart W. Hoogenboom

Abstract

Atomic force microscopy (AFM) is a microscopy technique that uses a sharp probe to trace a sample surface at nanometre resolution. For biological applications, one of its key advantages is its ability to visualize substructure of single molecules and molecular complexes in an aqueous environment. Here, we describe the application of AFM to determine superstructure and secondary structure of surface-bound DNA. The method is also readily applicable to probe DNA–DNA interactions and DNA–protein complexes.

Key words Atomic force microscopy, AFM, DNA, Supercoiling, Double helix, DNA–protein binding

1 Introduction

Atomic force microscopy (AFM, *see* Fig. 1) is a unique tool to obtain structural information of single biomolecules at ~1 nm spatial resolution. In addition, it allows for characterization of these molecules adsorbed on a planar substrate in aqueous solution, i.e., without the need for chemical fixation, staining, or vitrifying. AFM can be performed in fluid or in air. In-air AFM is more straightforward in operation and can provide static snapshots of reactions that involve DNA in solution (i.e. taking place while the DNA was free in solution and not bound to the planar substrate) by drying the sample before imaging. However, AFM in liquid has both yielded the highest spatial resolution on DNA [2–4], and can also be used to observe biomolecules at work [5–7]. AFM has been extensively used to visualize DNA supercoiling [8–11] and DNA–protein complexes [12–16], with the additional advantage that binding events and conformational changes can be monitored in real time [6, 7, 16]. In terms of spatial resolution, AFM can discern the helical pitch of DNA [17–20], and under appropriate imaging conditions, resolve the two strands of the DNA double helix [2–4].

For high-resolution AFM imaging, the sample must be adsorbed onto an atomically flat substrate, such that observed topographic features can be attributed to the biological sample

Mark C. Leake (ed.), *Chromosome Architecture: Methods and Protocols*, Methods in Molecular Biology, vol. 1431,
DOI 10.1007/978-1-4939-3631-1_5, © Springer Science+Business Media New York 2016

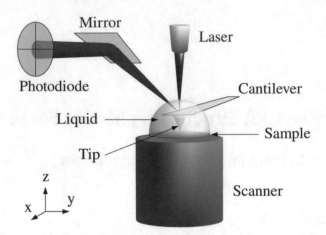

Fig. 1 Schematic of AFM in aqueous solution. A sharp tip is scanned line-by-line across the sample surface to build up an image of the surface topography. The topography at each scanned point is a function of the tip–sample interaction which is monitored via measuring the bending of the cantilever to which the tip is attached. The bending of the cantilever is usually detected via a laser beam deflected on a position-sensitive detector (4-quadrant photodiode). The sample is mounted on a (usually piezoelectric) scanner for three-dimensional positioning with sub-nanometer accuracy. The sample, the tip and the cantilever are immersed in liquid. Reproduced from [1]

and not to the substrate. Muscovite mica is often used as a substrate for AFM imaging, since its structure consists of many weakly interacting planes. These planes can be cleaved using sticky tape, resulting in an atomically flat surface. The disadvantage of mica as a substrate for DNA imaging is that both mica and DNA are negatively charged at neutral pH in aqueous solution, impeding the adsorption of DNA to the mica. Various methods that modify the surface charge of mica have been developed to facilitate DNA adsorption. These include: functionalizing the mica with aminopropyltriethoxy silane (APTES) or aminopropyl silatrane (APS) to create a positively charged surface [21]; using monovalent and divalent cations to bridge the charge repulsion [22]; adsorbing a positively charged lipid bilayer to the mica to facilitate electrostatically driven adsorption [18]; and the use of basic peptide solutions (e.g., poly-L-lysine) to create a positively charged monolayer on the surface [10]. Here we cover the divalent cation method and the use of poly-L-lysine.

In typical AFM experiments, the sample preparation is a compromise between the need to immobilize the DNA for high spatial resolution and, for real-time imaging of binding events and conformational changes, the need to allow DNA sufficient freedom for structural rearrangements. In addition, when using salts to facilitate DNA adsorption on a substrate, there is—in particular for the commonly used $NiCl_2$—the possibility of salt accumulation on the substrate, which may compromise the resolution and interpretation of the resulting AFM images [2–4].

In addition to the sample preparation, a critical element for high resolution AFM imaging is force sensitivity and control [2–4]. Generally, the AFM probe needs to exert a force on the sample to be able to record the surface topography. However if this force is too large, it can cause sample deformation or contamination of the probe, both of which can reduce the resolution of the resulting image. To minimise the force exerted on the sample, a wide range of operational modes have been developed.

Here, we describe two methods for in-liquid AFM imaging of DNA that have been successfully employed to visualize the DNA double helix: the widely implemented amplitude modulation mode (also called tapping, intermittent contact, or AC mode); and the rapid force-distance imaging mode (also called PeakForce tapping or Quantitative Imaging mode, depending on the AFM manufacturer). Our description presumes some knowledge about elementary AFM operation, such as can be found in instrument manuals.

2 Materials

2.1 General Materials and Equipment

1. Glass beakers and bottles.
2. Eppendorf tubes, 0.5 or 2 mL.
3. Falcon tubes, 15 mL.
4. Scalpel.
5. 2, 20, and 200 μL Gilson pipettes with 2–20 and 20–200 μL plastic tips.
6. Stainless steel tweezers.
7. 1.2 cm magnetic steel pucks.
8. Thin and flexible Teflon sheet.
9. 0.99 cm mica disks.
10. Bondloc B2030 primer.
11. Loctite 406 superglue.
12. Scotch tape.
13. 0.01% poly-L-lysine solution (Molecular weight 70,000–150,000).

2.2 Buffer Solutions (See Note 1)

1. Ultrapure water (MilliQ, resistivity > 18.2 MΩ).
2. Nickel adsorption buffer: 10 mM $NiCl_2$, 20 mM HEPES pH 7.4 (store at 4 °C (*see* **Note 2**). To Prepare 1 L weigh out 4.76 g HEPES (molecular weight: 238.30 g/mol) and 2.38 g $NiCl_2$ (molecular weight: 237.69 g/mol). Dissolve in 100 mL ultrapure water (>18.2 mΩ) in a glass beaker, using a thoroughly cleaner magnetic stirrer to aid the dissolution process if required. Once fully dissolved, add ultrapure water

to a final volume of 1 L. Check the pH of the solution using a well-calibrated and cleaned pH meter, and adjust the pH to 7.4 using small amounts of concentrated (~1 M) HCl or NaOH (*see* **Note 3**).

3. Nickel imaging buffer: 2 mM NiCl$_2$, 20 mM HEPES pH 7.4, store at 4 °C (*see* **Note 2**). Prepare 1 L as descibed above using 0.475 g NiCl$_2$ and 4.76 g HEPES.

4. Poly-L-lysine imaging buffer (*see* **Note 4**): 10 mM Tris–HCl, 150 mM NaCl (*see* **Note 5**), pH 7.4 (store at 4 °C) (*see* **Note 2**). Prepare 1 L as described above, using 1.214 g TRIS (molecular weight 121.14 g/mol) and 8.8 g NaCl (molecular weight: 58.44 g/mol).

2.3 DNA

1. 3486 base-pair plasmid DNA (store at 4 °C) (*see* **Note 2**) in 10 mM Tris–HCl pH 8.0, at a concentration of ~10 ng/μL (*see* **Note 6**).

2. 339 base-pair DNA minicircles (store at 4 °C) (*see* **Note 2**) in 10 mM Tris–HCl pH 8.0 at a concentration of ~10 ng/μL (*see* **Note 6**).

3 Methods

3.1 Preparation of Mica Substrate

Mica substrates can be bought as disks of 0.99 cm diameter, which can be attached to a steel puck to be mounted on magnetic sample holders as common in AFM instruments (*see* **Note 7**).

1. Lay a Teflon sheet out on the bench, if you have a 1.2 cm punch you can pre-form the teflon circles for attachment to the steel disks (*see* **Note 8**).

2. Apply the Bondloc primer to the Teflon surface, over a surface equivalent to that of the steel puck.

3. Use a small amount of Loctite 406 to glue the steel puck to the primer coated Teflon.

4. Cut the Teflon around the puck using a scalpel, such that the Teflon does not exceed the puck area.

5. Apply the Bondloc primer to the center of the bare Teflon surface.

6. Use a small amount of Loctite 406 to glue a mica disk to the primer coated Teflon.

7. Once the glue has dried, the mica can be cleaved using Scotch tape to reveal an atomically flat clean substrate (*see* **Note 9**).

3.2 Two Methods for DNA Adsorption on a Mica Substrate for AFM Imaging in Fluid

Mica and DNA are both negatively charged at a neutral pH in aqueous solution, which complicates the adsorption of DNA to the mica. The following sections describe two methods to facilitate DNA adsorption on mica, which are appropriate for imaging DNA in liquid (*see* **Note 10**).

3.2.1 DNA Adsorption Using Divalent Cations

Divalent cations (in this case Ni^{2+}) can be used to overcome the electrostatic repulsion between DNA and mica, thus facilitating DNA adhesion to the mica, which can also be tuned via the cationic concentration in the solution as outlined below.

1. Immediately before DNA adsorption, cleave a mica disk that has been prepared as described in Subheading 3.1.

2. Cover the freshly cleaved mica with 48 μL of nickel adsorption buffer (*see* **Note 11**).

3. Add 2 μL (*see* **Note 12**) DNA (10 ng/μL) and distribute evenly in the meniscus by gently purging.

4. Adsorb for 5 minutes. Then gently exchange the buffer to the nickel imaging buffer to remove any unbound DNA and reduce the nickel concentration, thereby minimizing the formation of salt aggregates on the surface (which otherwise compromise the image quality).

5. Add sufficient nickel imaging buffer on the sample and in the AFM fluid cell (dependent on the AFM system).

6. Mount sample on AFM.

7. Allow to equilibrate for 30 min.

3.2.2 DNA Adsorption Using poly-L-lysine

DNA adsorption on mica can also be assisted by surface modification of mica. Poly-L-lysine creates a cationic monolayer on the mica surface due to its protonated amino groups. DNA can then bind to the positively charged groups. The procedure for this is outlined below.

1. Immediately before exposure to poly-L-lysine, cleave a mica disk that has been prepared as described in Subheading 3.1.

2. Cover the mica with 25 μL 0.01 % poly-L-lysine solution.

3. Incubate for 5 min.

4. Wash 5× with ultrapure water.

5. Add 50 μL poly-L-lysine imaging buffer.

6. Add 5 μL (*see* **Notes 12** and **13**) DNA (10 ng/μL) and distribute evenly in the meniscus by gently purging.

7. Absorb for 5 minutes. Then gently exchange the buffer to the poly-L-lysine imaging buffer, to remove any unbound DNA (*see* **Note 14**).

8. Add sufficient poly-L-lysine imaging buffer on the sample and in the AFM fluid cell (dependent on the AFM system).

9. Mount sample on AFM.

10. Allow to equilibrate for 30 min (*see* **Note 15**).

Figure 2 shows DNA minicircles adsorbed on a mica substrate by both the divalent cation (Fig. 2a) and poly-L-lysine (Fig. 2b) methods. Both methods yield a stable DNA adsorption on the substrate for imaging by AFM.

3.3 AFM Setup for High Resolution Imaging in Fluid

Several variables need to be optimized to record high-resolution images by AFM. These variables include sample preparation, cantilever characteristics and AFM operation. The sample preparations above should yield DNA that is sufficiently bound to the mica substrate to facilitate high-resolution imaging.

1. Prepare a DNA sample as described in Subheadings 3.1 and 3.2.1 or 3.2.2 (*see* **Note 10**).

2. Select an appropriate cantilever for imaging DNA.

    (a) Cantilevers with spring constants ≤0.3 N/m are preferable for achieving the highest resolution when using the AFM imaging modes described here—allowing imaging of DNA at forces <100 pN.

    (b) To perform high resolution imaging, a sharp tip is required to probe the surface, such that tip-convolution does not dominate small corrugations of the sample surface. A tip radius of ~1 nm can yield images of the secondary structure of DNA, while with tip radii larger than 2 nm, secondary structure is harder to resolve. The apparent width of the DNA results from a convolution of the DNA and the AFM tip.

    (c) It would follow that the smaller the tip radius, the higher resolution that can be achieved, but this is not always the case. For smaller tip radii the same tip–sample force is exerted on a smaller area of the sample, applying a larger pressure, and correspondingly a larger risk of sample distortion.

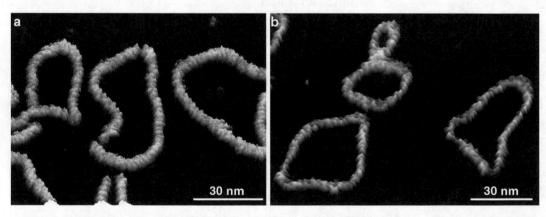

Fig. 2 AFM topographic images of 339 bp DNA minicircles captured in rapid force-distance mode in buffer solution using the divalent cation method (**a**) and poly-L-lysine method (**b**). The banded corrugation along the molecule corresponds to the strands of the DNA double helix, separated by major and minor grooves [2–4]. Sample courtesy: Michael Piperakis and Tony Maxwell (John Innes Centre, Norwich, UK)

3. Approach the cantilever manually to within a few hundred micrometers of the sample using the motors, ensuring that the cantilever does not crash on the surface.

4. Once the cantilever is immersed in fluid, align the laser on the cantilever for a maximum sum signal on the split photodetector, and zero the deflections by centering the laser spot on the detector.

5. Set the image size to a minimum (i.e. 0–10 nm) to avoid large tip motions over the sample at the start of the measurement. This allows for correction of any parameters which were suboptimal during approach. These parameters can then be adjusted after the approach prior to larger-scale imaging, to avoid damaging the tip.

6. Set the approach parameters to achieve a setpoint that corresponds to a force of ~60 pN, as can be easily determined in rapid-force distance mode (*see* **Note 16**). For imaging in amplitude modulation mode, drive the cantilever close to the resonant frequency, at an amplitude of ~4 nm, and select a setpoint that is ~70% of the free amplitude of the oscillation for the approach.

7. Approach the cantilever to the sample (*see* **Note 17**).

3.4 Optimizing AFM Imaging for High Resolution AFM Imaging on DNA

The best high-resolution AFM images in the literature appear highly similar. This illustrates that there is more than one route to high-resolution imaging given that all required parameters are optimized. However, these modes may vary in the ease by which the imaging is achieved. AFM builds an image by raster scanning the surface, which exerts lateral drag forces on the sample. To minimize these forces, amplitude modulation AFM and rapid force-distance AFM (*see* **Note 18**) modulate the vertical tip–sample distance whilst scanning. Here, these two methods are described, focusing on their application for imaging DNA on mica in aqueous solution.

3.4.1 High Resolution Imaging of DNA by Rapid Force-Distance AFM

Rapid force-distance AFM measures the force applied by the tip to the sample during imaging. It does so by taking repeated force curves across the sample whereby the tip is approached to and retracted from the surface. As the tip interacts with the surface the applied force is measured with respect to the baseline away from the surface, for each force curve. By measuring the height at which the force reaches a predefined setpoint, we can determine the sample topography at each interaction point. The height and level of detail of the topography can change as a function of the applied force (*see* Fig. 3), which is a key factor for high resolution imaging.

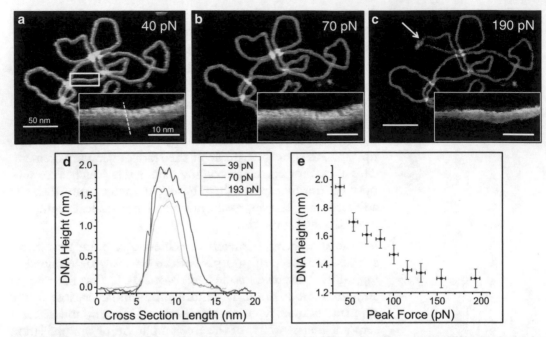

Fig. 3 Double-helix, corrugation and height of a DNA plasmid in AFM topography, with the DNA adsorbed using Ni^{2+} ions (Subheading 3.2.1) and the data acquired by rapid force-distance imaging (Subheading 3.4.1). (**a–c**) A plasmid imaged at maximum forces of 39, 70, and 193 pN, respectively, with the major and minor grooves of the DNA double helix visualized at higher magnification (*insets*). Color scales: 3 nm (for low magnification); 2 nm (for the *insets*). (**d**) Height profiles, measured across the DNA, as marked on the *inset* of **b** by a *dashed line*, for different applied forces. (**e**) Measured height along the same section across the molecule (as **d**), as a function of maximum (peak) force. Adapted from ref. 4, with permission

1. Once the tip has reached the surface, minimize the setpoint to the point at which the maximum force barely exceeds the force noise (~30 pN).

2. Reduce the total length of the force curve (z length or ramp) to ≤10 nm, thus ensuring that the tip spends most of the time in the immediate vicinity of the surface.

3. Begin scanning an area of ~500 × 500 nm^2.

4. Locate a DNA molecule of interest.

5. Increase the feedback gains (if appropriate) to ensure the molecule is tracked and traced properly.

6. If the molecule cannot be tracked (*see* **Note 19**), increase the force to allow tracking of the molecule.

7. Ensure that the molecule being tracked is stable under imaging (correctly adsorbed) by verifying that it does not significantly shift between subsequent scan lines.

8. Reduce the scan size to ~120 nm to image at high resolution, by zooming in on the DNA molecule of interest.

9. Increase the number of pixels per line to obtain ~0.5 nm per pixel (e.g., 256 pixels per line for a 120 nm scan).

10. Reduce the applied force if required (*see* **Note 20**).

11. Increase the gains to just below the point at which the noise in the surface topography begins to significantly increase.

12. Lateral drift or creep may be visible as the objects appearing to move across the image between subsequent scans (*see* **Note 21**). Under such conditions, higher scan speeds may improve resolution.

13. Align the molecule to the direction along which the scan lines are recorded (the so-called fast scan direction) for highest resolution (*see* **Note 22**).

14. Optimize the applied force and gains by increasing and decreasing the force in the range where the DNA molecule is not overly compressed (i.e., the measured height of the DNA should be ~20% of its known 2 nm diameter, *see* Fig. 3) to maximize resolution.

Figure 3 shows the effect of altering the applied force on a DNA plasmid imaged in rapid force-distance mode. The DNA was immobilized using the divalent cation method and gains were optimized at each force. At low force, the molecule cannot be adequately tracked (Fig. 3a), whereas at high force, the plasmid is significantly compressed, and the DNA starts to be moved laterally by the AFM tip (Fig. 3c). At optimum force, the banded or stranded DNA structure is clearly resolved along the plasmid (Fig. 3b, inset) whilst compression accounts for a ~20% reduction in the expected height of the molecule. The effect of the applied force can be seen as a reduction in the height of the molecule in Fig 3d. This follows a trend, shown in Fig 3e.

3.4.2 High Resolution Imaging of DNA by Amplitude Modulation AFM

In amplitude modulation AFM the tip is oscillated at its resonant frequency (or just below it), causing a "tap" or intermittent contact on the surface at the bottom of each oscillation cycle. The amplitude of oscillation when scanning is set to a predefined setpoint, usually about 70% of the free amplitude of oscillation (*see* **Note 23**). The amplitude of oscillation of the probe is influenced by the topography, reducing as the probe detects protrusions from the surface. In amplitude modulation AFM the tip–sample distance is adjusted as the probe scans over the sample, to maintain a constant amplitude of oscillation. The sample topography is then reconstructed from the changes in tip height.

1. Once the tip is approached to the surface, *increase* the amplitude setpoint, thus *reducing* the applied force on the molecule, until the tip begins to lift off the sample.

2. Begin scanning an area of ~500×500 nm².

3. Carefully reduce the setpoint until the tip is in contact with the surface.

4. Locate a DNA molecule of interest.

5. Increase the gains to just below the point where the noise in the surface topography (ringing) begins to significantly increase.

6. If the molecule cannot be tracked (*see* **Note 19**) further decrease the setpoint to better trace the molecule.

7. Ensure that the molecule being tracked is stable under imaging (correctly adsorbed), by verifying that it does not significantly shift between subsequent scan lines.

8. Reduce the scan size to ~120 nm to image at high resolution, by zooming in on the DNA molecule of interest.

9. Increase the number of pixels per line to a minimum of ~0.5 nm per pixel (e.g., 256 pixels per line for a 120 nm scan).

10. Reduce the applied force if required (*see* **Note 20**).

11. Increase the gains to just below the point at which they begin to ring.

12. If the DNA appears distorted or to move between scans, increasing the scan speed may improve resolution. The higher scan speeds act to mitigate the effects of lateral drift or creep which may cause these effects (*see* **Note 21**).

13. Adjust the scan orientation such that the molecule (or area of interest on the molecule) is aligned to the direction along which the scan lines are recorded (the so-called fast-scan direction), to achieve the highest resolution (*see* **Note 22**).

14. Optimize the applied force and gains by increasing and decreasing the setpoint, aiming to enhance contrast, while ensuring that the molecule is not overly compressed (~20%) to maximize resolution.

When using sufficiently sharp AFM tips, both rapid-force distance and amplitude modulation AFM can be used for high resolution imaging of the double helix of DNA. Figure 4 shows two high resolution scans of DNA plasmids, showing the secondary structure of DNA.

4   Notes

1. Ensure all buffers are clean and free of contamination from chemicals. Any contamination in flasks, beakers, buffer solutions or DI water will contaminate the image and reduce resolution. Clean glassware with detergent and rinse with copious amounts of Ultrapure water, and ensure chemicals are stored

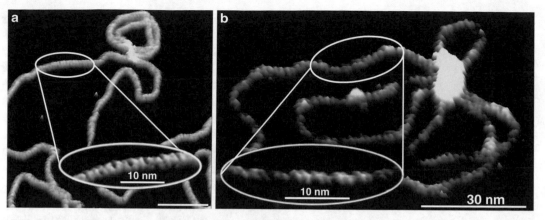

Fig. 4 AFM topographic images of DNA plasmids adsorbed on mica by the divalent cation method taken in both rapid force-distance mode (**a**, adapted from ref. 1, with permission) and amplitude modulation mode (**b**). Both images show corrugation along the plasmid which corresponds to the major and minor grooves of the DNA double helix. (**a**) *Inset:* (both) a higher resolution image showing the major and minor grooves of the DNA plasmid more clearly. Color scale (*see* Fig. 3 of Chapter 4 for scale bar): 2 nm (main), 1.1 nm (*inset*)

correctly. It is good practice to verify buffer cleanliness by imaging a freshly cleaved mica surface in the buffer: The mica should appear atomically flat and not show any noticeable contamination.

2. DNA and buffers should be stored in a fridge for continual use, and can be frozen if not needed for a long period of time.

3. HCl is used to reduce the pH of the solution, however if the pH is adjusted to values that are too acidic, small amounts of a ~1 M NaOH solution can be used to increase the pH to the required value.

4. NiCl$_2$ or other divalent ions are not required if the mica is chemically functionalized to make its surface positively charged.

5. NaCl is used to screen the electrostatic repulsion between the tip and the DNA which are both negatively charged in solution at physiological pH. This allows for better resolution as the tip can follow the contours of the DNA more easily.

6. Stocks may be stored at any concentration and diluted in the buffer to the final concentration shown.

7. Alternatively and depending on the AFM instrument, the mica disk can be glued to a glass slide, and the surrounding glass treated with a hydrophobic pen.

8. A layer of (hydrophobic) Teflon is placed below the mica to confine the liquid solution to the mica disk and avoid contamination and spillage when imaging in fluid.

9. If liquid is placed on the mica before the superglue is dry, the glue may contaminate it.

10. The divalent-cation preparation is most straightforward for imaging in air. For imaging in liquid, Ni^{2+} ions may be preferred because they provide stronger binding of DNA to the mica substrate than, e.g., Mg^{2+}. The disadvantage of using $NiCl_2$, however, is that it tends to precipitate on the mica surface, with increased risk of contaminating the AFM probe. The poly-L-lysine preparation has the advantage of not requiring particular salts in the solution, but because of its affinity to typical AFM tips, it can compromise amplitude modulation imaging with soft AFM probes.

11. The strength of DNA adsorption can be tuned by altering the $NiCl_2$ concentration in the buffer. Typically, higher Ni^{2+} concentrations lead to a stronger binding of adsorbed DNA molecules to the mica, which facilitates AFM imaging, but also result in an increased surface contamination by precipitating $NiCl_2$.

12. The exact quantity of DNA required can vary depending on the nature of the sample.

13. The amount of DNA required to adsorb DNA with good coverage using the poly-L-lysine preparation is slightly higher than that required when using the divalent cation method.

14. The buffer may be exchanged for any imaging buffer to remove DNA that is not adsorbed. This step can be missed out if the user requires.

15. The DNA and buffers may need to equilibrate to the temperature of the AFM, to minimize the effect of drift in the measurements.

16. Setpoints are often measured in Volts as directly read via the detector readout of the cantilever deflection. To convert these into forces, the Setpoint value in Volts can be multiplied by the sensitivity of the deflection detection and the spring constant of the cantilever.

17. At low approach setpoints, using soft cantilevers, the cantilever may finish its approach before having made contact with the surface. In this case approach the cantilever again. If the approach fails repeatedly, you may need to increase the approach setpoint.

18. Other imaging modes exist. In particular, early DNA double helix imaging was carried out using phase and frequency modulation techniques, which typically achieve high sensitivity using stiffer cantilevers [2, 3].

19. At low applied forces, the tip may not be able to track the molecule well. Even with the feedback gains high, this may result in an effect known as parachuting, where the tip fails to quickly move back towards the surface after having moved up

on contact with a protrusion such as adsorbed DNA. This can lead to streaky features extending from the molecule in the direction of scanning.

20. On reducing the scan size, the imaging setpoint may need to be reduced and the gains should be readjusted, as the tip now spends more time interacting with the same sample area, which can imply an increased risk of damage to the DNA molecule(s).

21. Such drift or creep may be reduced by operating the AFM with a so-called closed-loop scanner, but may also depend on the microscope design.

22. Aligning the molecule in the fast scan direction is particularly helpful when drift or creep reduced the position accuracy between scan lines.

23. The free amplitude is the amplitude of oscillation of the tip when it is not interacting with the sample. This will be the amplitude obtained during tuning of the cantilever, which must be done away from the surface. Because of hydrodynamic interactions, the tip amplitude typically decreases closer to the surface even without making direct contact. When defining the free amplitude as the amplitude at ≤ 1 μm from the surface, the setpoint can be significantly higher than 70%.

References

1. Hoogenboom BW (2015) AFM in liquids. In: Bhushan B (ed) Encyclopedia of nanotechnology, 2nd edn. Springer, Amsterdam, pp 83–89. doi:10.1007/978-90-481-9751-4

2. Leung C, Bestembayeva A, Thorogate R, Stinson J, Pyne A, Marcovich C, Yang JL, Drechsler U, Despont M, Jankowski T (2012) Atomic force microscopy with nanoscale cantilevers resolves different structural conformations of the DNA double helix. Nano Lett 12(7):3846–3850. doi:10.1021/nl301857p

3. Ido S, Kimura K, Oyabu N, Kobayashi K, Tsukada M, Matsushige K, Yamada H (2013) Beyond the helix pitch: direct visualization of native DNA in aqueous solution. ACS Nano 7(2):1817–1822. doi:10.1021/nn400071n

4. Pyne A, Thompson R, Leung C, Roy D, Hoogenboom BW (2014) Single-molecule reconstruction of oligonucleotide secondary structure by atomic force microscopy. Small 10(16):3257–3261. doi:10.1002/smll.201400265

5. Crampton N, Yokokawa M, Dryden DTF, Edwardson JM, Rao DN, Takeyasu K, Yoshimura SH, Henderson RM (2007) Fast-scan atomic force microscopy reveals that the type III restriction enzyme EcoP15I Is capable of DNA translocation and looping. Proc Natl Acad Sci U S A 104(31):12755–12760. doi:10.1073/pnas.0700483104

6. Lyubchenko YL (2014) Nanoscale nucleosome dynamics assessed with time-lapse AFM. Biophys Rev 6(2):181–190. doi:10.1007/s12551-013-0121-3

7. Miyagi A, Ando T, Lyubchenko YL (2011) Dynamics of nucleosomes assessed with time-lapse high-speed atomic force microscopy. Biochemistry 50(37):7901–7908. doi:10.1021/bi200946z

8. Adamcik J, Jeon J-H, Karczewski KJ, Metzler R, Dietler G (2012) Quantifying supercoiling-induced denaturation bubbles in DNA. Soft Matter 8(33):8651–8658. doi:10.1039/C2SM26089A

9. Fogg JM, Kolmakova N, Rees I, Magonov S, Hansma H, Perona JJ, Zechiedrich EL (2006) Exploring writhe in supercoiled minicircle DNA. J Phys Condens Matter 18(14):S145–S159. doi:10.1088/0953-8984/18/14/S01

10. Bussiek M (2003) Polylysine-coated mica can be used to observe systematic changes in the supercoiled DNA conformation by scanning force microscopy in solution. Nucleic Acids Res 31(22):137. doi:10.1093/nar/gng137

11. Li D, Lv B, Zhang H, Lee JY, Li T (2014) Positive supercoiling affiliated with nucleosome formation repairs non-B DNA structures. Chem Commun 50(73):10641–10644. doi:10.1039/C4CC04789C

12. Osada E, Suzuki Y, Hidaka K, Ohno H, Sugiyama H, Endo M, Saito H (2014) Engineering RNA–protein complexes with different shapes for imaging and therapeutic applications. ACS Nano 8(8):8130–8140. doi:10.1021/nn502253c

13. Kundukad B, Cong P, van der Maarel JRC, Doyle PS (2013) Time-dependent bending rigidity and helical twist of DNA by rearrangement of bound HU protein. Nucleic Acids Res 41(17):8280–8288. doi:10.1093/nar/gkt593

14. Gaczynska M, Osmulski PA, Jiang Y, Lee J-K, Bermudez V, Hurwitz J (2004) Atomic force microscopic analysis of the binding of the Schizosaccharomyces pombe origin recognition complex and the spOrc4 protein with origin DNA. Proc Natl Acad Sci U S A 101(52):17952–17957. doi:10.2307/3374175

15. Heddle JG, Mitelheiser S, Maxwell A, Thomson NH (2004) Nucleotide binding to DNA gyrase causes loss of DNA wrap. J Mol Biol 337(3):597–610. doi:10.1016/j.jmb.2004.01.049

16. Katan AJ, Vlijm R, Lusser A, Dekker C (2015) Dynamics of nucleosomal structures measured by high-speed atomic force microscopy. Small 11(8):976–984. doi:10.1002/smll.201401318

17. Hansma HG (2001) Surface biology of DNA by atomic force microscopy. Annu Rev Phys Chem 52(1):71–92. doi:10.1146/annurev.physchem.52.1.71

18. Mou J, Czajkowsky DM, Zhang Y, Shao Z (1995) High-resolution atomic-force microscopy of DNA: the pitch of the double helix. FEBS Lett 371(3):279–282. doi:10.1016/0014-5793(95)00906-P

19. Maaloum M, Beker A-F, Muller P (2011) Secondary structure of double-stranded DNA under stretching: elucidation of the stretched form. Phys Rev E 83(3):031903. doi:10.1103/PhysRevE.83.031903

20. Santos S, Barcons V, Christenson HK, Billingsley DJ, Bonass WA, Font J, Thomson NH (2013) Stability, resolution, and ultra-low wear amplitude modulation atomic force microscopy of DNA: small amplitude small set-point imaging. Appl Phys Lett 103(6):063702. doi:10.1063/1.4817906

21. Lyubchenko YL, Shlyakhtenko LS (2009) AFM for analysis of structure and dynamics of DNA and protein–DNA complexes. Methods 47(3):206–213. doi:10.1016/j.ymeth.2008.09.002

22. Hansma HG, Laney DE (1996) DNA binding to mica correlates with cationic radius: assay by atomic force microscopy. Biophys J 70(4):1933–1939. doi:10.1016/S0006-3495(96)79757-6

Chapter 6

Investigating Bacterial Chromosome Architecture

Christian Lesterlin and Nelly Duabrry

Abstract

How is the bacterial chromosome organized within the bacterial cell? Over the last 60 years, a variety of approaches have been used to investigate this question. More recently, the parallel development of epifluorescence microscopy and genetic tools has enabled the direct visualization of the intracellular positioning of DNA sequences in live cells and has consequently revolutionized our view of the architecture of the nucleoid *in vivo*. In this chapter I present a comprehensive methodology designed to characterize the architecture of the nucleoid DNA and the positioning of specific DNA sequences in live *Escherichia coli* cells. DNA localization systems, preparation of stable agarose-mounted microscopy slides, and basic image analysis tools are mentioned.

Key words Bacterial chromosome, DNA architecture and dynamics, Live cell imaging, Epifluorescence microscopy

1 Introduction

Within the bacterial cell, the chromosome DNA is highly organized into a compact structure, the nucleoid, which occupies most of the cell volume. For a long time, the small size of bacteria and the lack of nuclear envelop or X-shaped chromosomes made the study of the architecture of the bacterial nucleoid quite challenging. Early direct observations of the bacterial chromosome in live cells have been produced using light microscopy imaging of cells mounted on a gelatine-containing surface [1]. Despite the lack of resolution, this pioneer technic revealed the complex dynamics of the chromosome during unperturbed growth. In the seventies, Electron-Microscopy has provided numbers of high-resolution images of the chromosome DNA in fixed cells, which appeared highly organized and compacted [2–6]. In parallel to these direct visualization approaches, a wide range of studies used molecular biology or genetic recombination assays to indirectly investigate the local and global DNA organization, DNA topology and sequence interaction ability in vivo [7–13]. All together, these works contributed to the establishment of early fundamental models describing the

Mark C. Leake (ed.), *Chromosome Architecture: Methods and Protocols*, Methods in Molecular Biology, vol. 1431,
DOI 10.1007/978-1-4939-3631-1_6, © Springer Science+Business Media New York 2016

intracellular architecture of the bulk of the DNA *in vivo*. However, it is only since the early 2000s that the combination of fluorescence microscopy and DNA localization systems has provided new means to visualize the position and dynamics of the DNA in live cells [14–21]. First, the shape and movement of the whole nucleoid DNA can be characterized using fluorescent DNA-staining molecules or fluorescently labeled versions of proteins associated with the chromosome (NAPs) [22, 23]. Second, genetic DNA localization systems enable monitoring the position of specific sequences of interest. This revealed that the positioning of the chromosome DNA is nonrandom during cell growth, but rather follows a predetermined choreography reliably reproduced over generations. Each chromosome part occupies a specific intracellular volume and migrates to the future daughter cells according to a segregation program, which is strictly correlated to the progression of DNA replication and cell division.

Here, I describe a combination of DNA localization tools, light microscopy imaging, and basic image analysis tools, which has proven to be a fruitful method to gain insights into the intracellular architecture and dynamics of the chromosome in the live bacterial cell.

2   Materials

2.1   Minimal Medium for Cell Culture and Staining Solutions

1. M9 salts 10× solution (1 L): Prepare 70 g of $Na_2HPO_4 \cdot 7H_2O$; 30 g of KH_2PO_4; 5 g of NaCl, and 10 g of NH_4Cl and add MilliQ water to a volume of 1 L. Mix well until complete dissolution of crystals and autoclave.

2. Minimal medium supplemented with 0.2% glucose for liquid culture: For 1 L, add 100 mL of M9 solution 10× to 800 mL of water in a 1 L graduated cylinder. Add 10 mL of sterile glucose 20%, 1 mL of 1 M $MgSO_4$, 400 μL of thiamine (B1 vitamin). Finally add MilliQ water to a volume of 1 L and 80 μL of 1 M $CaCl_2$ (*see* **Note 1**). Mix well and filter with a 0.2 μm membrane to sterilize the freshly prepared ready to use minimal medium supplemented with 0.2% glucose. This medium should be complemented with relevant amino acids depending on the auxotrophy of the strain.

3. 4′,6-diamidino-2-phenylindole (DAPI) is diluted in water or DMF and mixed with cells at 4 μg/mL final concentration.

2.2   Agarose-Mounted Slides

1. 2× minimal medium supplemented with 0.2% glucose for agarose pads. For 100 mL, add 10 mL of M9 solution 10× to 80 mL of water in a 100 mL graduated cylinder. Add 1 mL of glucose 20%, 0.1 mL of 1 M $MgSO_4$, 40 μL of thiamine (B1 vitamin), and 8 μL of 1 M $CaCl_2$. Finally add water to a volume

of 100 mL. Mix well and filter with a 0.2 μm membrane to sterilize the freshly prepared ready to use minimal medium supplemented with 0.2 % glucose.

2. 2 % agarose for pad preparation: For 100 mL, weigh 2 g of low fluorescence agarose (Bio-Rad) and add water to a volume of 100 mL. Mix well and autoclave.

3. Gene frame 125 μL (17×28 mm) (Thermo scientific).

4. Glass slide (76×28 mm) and coverslip Slides and coverslips (24×50 mm; 1.5 μm thickness). Glass coverslips can be burned to remove any fluorescent background particles.

2.3 Visualization of the Entire Nucleoid DNA

1. DNA staining with 4′,6-diamidino-2-phenylindole (DAPI) is used for snapshot imaging of the bacterial nucleoid. Due to its brightness and photostability, DAPI produces a robust and strong fluorescent signal, which is suitable for conventional epifluorescence microscopy but also for three-dimensional SIM imaging. However, DAPI staining impedes cell growth and is then inappropriate for the study of DNA dynamics in live cells.

2. Genetically encoded systems have been developed to allow the time-lapse imaging of the nucleoid DNA in live cells. In bacteria, the chromosomal DNA is decorated with a number of small and abundant binding proteins, the NAPs (Nucleoid Associated Proteins), which are involved in a variety of cellular functions [24]. The localization of functional fluorescently labelled version of NAPs is used to reveal the intracellular position of the whole chromosomal DNA in live cells. *E. coli* nucleoids have been visualized using the fluorescently tagged HupA protein, which is a subunit of the abundant nucleoid-associated factor HU [23]. The heterologous *Anabaena* HU has also been used in *E. coli* and gave similar results than those obtained with a fluorescent protein fusion to Fis DNA binding protein [22].

2.4 Genetic Systems for Localization of Specific DNA Sequences

Several genetic tools have been developed to monitor the physical positions of DNA sequences in the living cell and their movement in the course of the cell cycle. These genetic localization systems require the insertion of a specific DNA sequence (binding site) into the DNA locus of interest and the production of the corresponding binding protein labelled with a fluorescent protein through translational fusion. The resulting chimera protein produced will form a discrete focus under the microscope that reveals the intracellular position of the DNA sequence carrying the insertion of the binding site. Note that binding sites are usually inserted in intergenic regions and preferentially in between convergent genes of the chromosome in order to limit the perturbation of the genetic context. Also, the level of expression of the fluorescently labelled binding proteins needs to be finely tuned in order to avoid perturbation of the dynamics of the DNA region. Appropriate promoters should be chosen to obtain the minimal level of protein production that allows satisfactory focus detection. These fusion proteins can be produced either form an plasmid or an ectopic chromosomal locus [16, 19, 25]. Such localization systems are used for snapshot and time-lapse imaging with any fluorescence microscope equipped with appropriate optics, light source and filters (*see* **Note 2**).

1. The ParB/*parS* systems enable the intracellular localization of specific chromosome loci. The *parS* site is inserted in the DNA region of interest and is bound by the fluorescent version of the corresponding ParB binding protein, which also binds the neighboring DNA [16]. The simultaneous use of two of these ParB/*parS* systems, one from P1 bacteriophage and one from pMT1 plasmid has been well characterized previously [19]. In theory, up to four different ParB/*parS* systems can be used simultaneously to characterize the localization of four different DNA sequences in a cell [26]. This requires the translational fusion of each four ParB binding proteins to compatible fluorescent proteins that can be visualized simultaneously.

2. Alternatively, FROS (Fluorescent Repressor Operator Systems) such as LacI/*lacO* or TetR/*tetO* operator systems can be used [14, 17, 27]. In these systems, fluorescently labelled LacI and TetR repressor proteins bind to *lacI* and *tetO* operator sites resulting in the formation a discrete focus that reveals the intracellular position of the chromosome locus carrying the operator insertions. In this case, the number of binding proteins is directly correlated to the number of binding sites inserted.

2.5 Semiautomated Image Analysis Suite

1. Quantitative image analysis MicrobeTracker [28] is used for cell segmentation, signal quantification, and basic analysis (download at http://microbetracker.org).

2. Custom routines programmed in Matlab (Mathworks) are designed to analyze the data previously generated by MicrobeTracker (*see* [29, 30]).

3. ImageJ/Fiji, Icy [31], and Imaris software (Bitplane) allow image analysis and 3D or 4D rendering.

---

3   Methods

Carry out all procedures at room temperature unless otherwise specified. Growth conditions (medium, temperature, agitation) should be determined depending on the organism studied and the wanted physiological state (*see* **Note 3**). Below, I describe the experimental procedure for characterization of chromosome archi-tecture of *E. coli* strains cultured in minimal medium at 30 °C, which allow moderate growth following a cell cycle without over-lapping replication periods (*see* **Note 4**).

3.1 Cell Culture

1. Streak the strain of interest onto LB agar plates containing appropriate antibiotic in order to obtain isolated colonies. Inoculate a single *colony* into 5 mL of minimal medium supple-mented with 0.2% glucose and with appropriate antibiotic. Incubate overnight at 30 °C with agitation.

2. Dilute the overnight culture 1/100 in 5 mL of fresh minimal medium supplemented with 0.2% glucose and with appropri-ate antibiotic and grow at 30 °C with agitation until exponen-tial phase, i.e., A600 ~ 0.1–0.2. Take a 1 mL sample of culture in a micro-tube. DAPI staining should be performed at this stage if required (*see* **Note 5**).

3. Centrifuge the cell culture sample at ~7000 × g for 2 min and resuspend gently with a pipette in 50 μL of fresh minimal medium supplemented with 0.2% glucose (*see* **Note 6**). Cells are now ready for immobilization on the agarose mounted slide and observation under the microscope.

3.2 Agarose Pad Preparation

The following method describes preparation of microscopy slides that enable the observation of bacterial cells growing on a smooth and flat surface composed of growth medium and agarose, in a sealed compartment to avoid desiccation (Fig. 1). The resulting standardized agarose-mounted slides are highly stable and can be used for a variety of high-resolution microscopy imaging technics: PALM and Live-PALM [32, 33] or Structured-Illumination Microscopy [30].

1. Remove the plastic film from the bottom of the blue frame, leaving the hollowed plastic film on the other side. Stick the blue frame on the glass slide (*see* **Note 7**).

2. Melt the H_2O 2% agarose solution in a boiling bath and mix with equivalent volume of 2× minimal medium solution to obtain a 1% agarose minimal medium solution (*see* **Note 8**).

3. Pipette 200 μL of the 1% agarose minimal medium solution and pour in the 125 μL compartment inside the blue frame (Fig. 1a). Rapidly cover with a clean coverslip (Fig. 1b). This will remove the excess of liquid and flatten the agarose surface (*see* **Note 9**). Wait a few minutes for the agarose to solidify at RT or 4 °C (*see* **Note 10**).

4. When the cell sample is ready, remove and discard the coverslip with your thumb. Wait a few minutes until the excess of liquid has disappeared and the surface of the agarose pad has become matt. Finally, remove the hollowed plastic film from the blue frame.

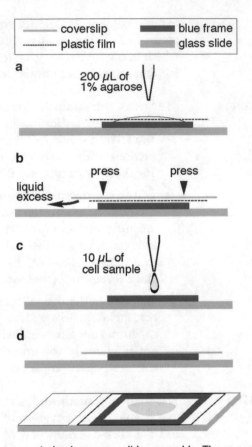

Fig. 1 Agarose-mounted microscopy slide assembly. The successive steps of slide preparation detailed in the text are shown. (**a**) Pour 200 μL of the 1 % agarose minimal medium solution in the 125 μL compartment formed by the blue frame. (**b**) Put a coverslip on the plastic film and press gently to remove the excess of liquid. (**c**) Pour 10 μL of prepared cell sample, tilt the glass slide to spread the droplet, and wait for the droplet to be adsorbed by the agarose pad. (**d**) Seal the sample by sticking a clean coverslip on the blue frame

5. Pour 10 μL of cell sample in the middle of the agarose pad and tilt the glass slide gently to spread the liquid droplet (Fig. 1c) (*see* **Note 11**). When all the liquid has been adsorbed, seal the sample by sticking a clean coverslip on the blue frame. It is important to avoid the formation of air bubble underneath the coverslip. The microscopy slide is now ready to use (Fig. 1d) (*see* **Note 12**).

3.3 Imaging Acquisition

Epifluorescence microscopes generally allow acquisition of large fields of view. Acquisition of large cell population samples (>1000 cells) will facilitate statistical treatment of the data and improve the statistical significance of the observations. There are no standard acquisition parameters, as a consequence optimum parameters have to be empirically determined by the user for each specific fluorescent constructs and experimental condition. The quality of the acquired image not only depends on the quality of the microscope components but also on numerous factors such as the brightness, the dynamics and the quantity of fluorescent molecules present in the cells. When the acquisition requires multiple exposures (as in the case of time-lapse or 3D imaging) the photostability of the fluorescent molecule will also become a critical parameter. It that case, the exposure time will have to be reduced to the minimum that allows satisfying fluorescent signal collection.

For 3D-SIM imaging, image stacks should be composed of at least 12 z-sections of 125 nm each (corresponding to a sample thickness of 1.375 μm) in order to acquire to whole cell. Optimized acquisition settings are DAPI, 20 ms exposure with 405 nm laser (100% transmission); FM4-64, 30 ms exposure with 593 nm laser (100% transmission). Other optimized parameters can be found in the literature [17, 19, 20, 30, 34, 35]. Remark that it might be preferable to acquire phase contrasts images to facilitate the cell segmentation by MicrobeTracker analysis software.

3.4   Image Analysis

1. Nucleoids observed either by fluorescently labelled NAPs or DAPI-staining can be analyzed using image processing software such as Fiji, Imaris (Bitplane), or the open informatics platform Icy [31]. Figure 2 presents the results obtained for basic intensity analysis of nucleoids observed using 3D-Widefield imaging of Hu-mCherry (Fig. 2a, b) and 3D-SIM imaging of DAPI-stained nucleoids (Fig. 2c–g). Indeed, variations in fluorescence signal intensity, which reflect variations in local DNA density, can be visualized using the Analyze/3D-surface plot function in Fiji (Fig. 2b, c, f). The resulting 2D-map reveals fluctuation in local DNA compaction within the nucleoid lobes and allow calculating the transition intensity value that defines the nucleoid boundaries. Subsequent 3D-surface renderings (Imaris) using the previously defined transition intensity value as a threshold reveals the shape of the nucleoid within the cell compartment (Fig. 2g). Both examples shown in Fig. 2 reveal the nucleoid as a highly structured object with a twisted shape, composed of several lobs separated by DNA free regions. The nucleoid DNA is not filling the whole cell compartment since DNA-free spaces are visible at the periphery of the cell and between the lobes.

2. The intracellular position of specific DNA sequences in the course of the cell cycle can be presented in a number of different graphs. Figure 3 shows a few examples of basic graphical outputs that are commonly used in DNA localization studies. The x-axis often shows the cell length, which directly reflects the cell age from birth to the next division. This enable to reconstruct the different stages of the cell cycle from popula-

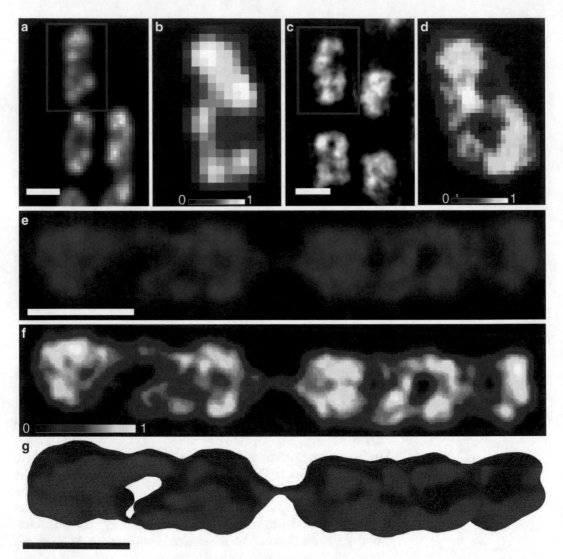

Fig. 2 Visualization of the nucleoid DNA in *Escherichia coli* cells. z-Projection of (**a**) 3D-Widefield imaging of HU-mCherry and (**c** and **e**) 3D-SIM imaging of DAPI-stained nucleoids in fast growing *E. coli* cells. The *red frame* shows the nucleoid that is analyzed in the following panel. (**b, d** and **f**) 3D-surface plot generated with Fiji, showing the variations in fluorescent intensities normalized to 1, from low-DNA density (value = 0, corresponding to *black*) and higher-DNA density (value = 1, corresponding to *white*) displayed by the nucleoids. (**g**) 3D-surface rendering generated by Imaris software (Bitplane) reveals the nucleoid shape within the cell compartment (thresholding set at intensity value = 0.15 corresponding to *blue* in the color scale). Scale bars are 1 μm

tion snapshot analysis. Cells are first segmented from phase contrast images using quantitative image analysis software MicrobeTracker [28]. The position of the spots is determined either manual using the spotfinderM function or automatically using spotfinderZ function. DNA locus intracellular position and number are revealed by focus number histograms,

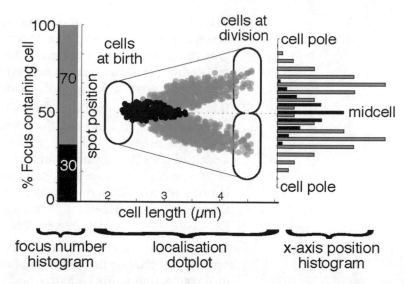

Fig. 3 Example of DNA locus localization basic analysis. One focus cells are shown in *black* and two foci cells are shown in *grey*. From *left* to *right*: histogram of the fraction of cells with one or two foci; dotplot of DNA locus position as a function of cell length, from cell birth to cell division; *histograms* of locus positioning along the cell length

2D-localization dot plots and long-axis position histograms (Fig. 3). More specific analysis can be performed depending on the localization feature that has to be addressed, such as focus size, brightness or Inter-Focal-Distance. For these I would recommend to refer to published works [17, 19, 20, 30, 34, 35]. Although not detailed here, snapshot analysis is nicely complemented by time-lapse imaging of DNA sequence localization systems, which allow to characterize the dynamics of the DNA sequence at short or longer time scales. This enable a range of analysis describing the movement of the DNA regions, such as the characterization of the speed and directionality of the movement, the mean square displacement (MSD) and the diffusion behavior. Protocols for particle tracking are referenced in several DNA locus localization studies [30, 34, 36].

4 Notes

1. It is required to add $CaCl_2$ solution after the water to avoid precipitation.

2. It is critical to carefully choose fluorescent protein or synthetic dyes that are compatible so that they can be visualized simultaneously. When possible, avoid using fluorescent proteins that requires excitation with short wave length light because of the greater phototoxicity.

3. The shape and compaction of the bacterial nucleoid varies depending on the growth rate, it is to say depending on the growth condition used and mainly the medium richness. In *E. coli* strains, the DNA content per cell and the DNA compaction are increased in fast growth conditions.

4. It is critical to use growth medium with reduced autofluorescence in order to limit the fluorescent background during image acquisition. For slow growth, the minimal media described here is convenient for imaging. The carbon source should be changed from glucose to glycerol or even succinate in order to slow down the growth rate. For fast growth, Rich Defined Medium (EZRDM, Teknova) should be preferred to LB medium since it exhibits very little autofluorescence.

5. DNA-staining with DAPI for should be performed at this stage by incubating the cell sample with DAPI at 4 μg/mL final concentration for 15 min.

6. As described in ref. 30. After staining with DAPI, this procedure 3 should be repeated twice to wash the excess of fluorescent dye.

7. Take care to position the blue frame in a way compatible with the position of the glass slide on the stage of your microscope.

8. The thiamine (B1 vitamin) contained in the minimal medium is thermolabile, consequently the melted H_2O 2% agarose has to be cooled down to ~55 °C before mixing with the 2× minimal medium solution. Fresh medium should be prepared for each experiment.

9. Remove the excess of liquid by pushing gently on the side of the coverslip, which upon the hollowed plastic film covering the blue frame. Do not press in the middle of the coverslip, this would generate and air bubble in the compartment.

10. At this stage, the agarose-mounted slide should be pre-incubated at the temperature that is going to be used during the microscopy experiment. This stabilizes the slide structure before the observation and thus limiting potential movements or drifting during imaging. This will also limits the temperature change for the cells. Alternatively, the agarose-mounted slide can be kept in the fridge for 2–3 days in a humid chamber. However, I would advise to prepare fresh agarose mounted slides before each microscopy experiment.

11. An appropriate cell density on the slide is a critical to the quality of the observation. It is useful to put the drop of cell sample on one side of the agarose pad, and spread it toward the other side by tilting the glass slide. Also, one should progress

unidirectional when putting the coverslip on the preparation. Doing so will generate a cell density gradient on the slide, which will facilitate the identification of a field of view that convenient for you image acquisition. It is best to avoid fields of view with conjunctives cells, which impede automated cell outline recognition by MicrobeTracker.

12. From the moment the sample is sealed, the oxygen level will start decreasing until it becomes limiting for the growth of aerobic bacteria. The duration of the observation has to be adapted accordingly.

Acknowledgments

Thanks to Nelly Dubarry for critical reading. This work was supported by ATIP-Avenir 2014 grant (CNRS and INSERM) and Finovi Funding to Christian Lesterlin.

References

1. Mason DJ, Powelson DM (1956) Nuclear division as observed in live bacteria by a new technique. J Bacteriol 71(4):474–479

2. Delius H, Worcel A (1974) Electron microscopic studies on the folded chromosome of Escherichia coli. Cold Spring Harb Symp Quant Biol 38:53–58

3. Delius H, Worcel A (1974) Letter: electron microscopic visualization of the folded chromosome of Escherichia coli. J Mol Biol 82(1):107–109

4. Hobot JA, Villiger W, Escaig J, Maeder M, Ryter A, Kellenberger E (1985) Shape and fine structure of nucleoids observed on sections of ultrarapidly frozen and cryosubstituted bacteria. J Bacteriol 162(3):960–971

5. Bohrmann B, Villiger W, Johansen R, Kellenberger E (1991) Coralline shape of the bacterial nucleoid after cryofixation. J Bacteriol 173(10):3149–3158

6. Bohrmann B, Haider M, Kellenberger E (1993) Concentration evaluation of chromatin in unstained resin-embedded sections by means of low-dose ratio-contrast imaging in STEM. Ultramicroscopy 49(1-4):235–251

7. Bliska JB, Cozzarelli NR (1987) Use of site-specific recombination as a probe of DNA structure and metabolism in vivo. J Mol Biol 194(2):205–218

8. Higgins NP, Yang X, Fu Q, Roth JR (1996) Surveying a supercoil domain by using the gamma delta resolution system in Salmonella typhimurium. J Bacteriol 178(10):2825–2835

9. Staczek P, Higgins NP (1998) Gyrase and Topo IV modulate chromosome domain size in vivo. Mol Microbiol 29(6):1435–1448

10. Postow L, Hardy CD, Arsuaga J, Cozzarelli NR (2004) Topological domain structure of the Escherichia coli chromosome. Genes Dev 18(14):1766–1779

11. Valens M, Penaud S, Rossignol M, Cornet F, Boccard F (2004) Macrodomain organization of the Escherichia coli chromosome. EMBO J 23(21):4330–4341

12. Stein RA, Deng S, Higgins NP (2005) Measuring chromosome dynamics on different time scales using resolvases with varying half-lives. Mol Microbiol 56(4):1049–1061

13. Lesterlin C, Gigant E, Boccard F, Espeli O (2012) Sister chromatid interactions in bacteria revealed by a site-specific recombination assay. EMBO J 31(16):3468–3479. doi:10.1038/emboj.2012.194, emboj2012194 [pii]

14. Webb CD, Teleman A, Gordon S, Straight A, Belmont A, Lin DC, Grossman AD, Wright A, Losick R (1997) Bipolar localization of the replication origin regions of chromosomes in vegetative and sporulating cells of B. subtilis. Cell 88(5):667–674

15. Gordon GS, Wright A (1998) DNA segregation: putting chromosomes in their place. Curr Biol 8(25):R925–R927

16. Li Y, Sergueev K, Austin S (2002) The segregation of the Escherichia coli origin and terminus of replication. Mol Microbiol 46(4):985–995

17. Lau IF, Filipe SR, Soballe B, Okstad OA, Barre FX, Sherratt DJ (2003) Spatial and temporal organization of replicating Escherichia coli chromosomes. Mol Microbiol 49(3):731–743

18. Wang X, Possoz C, Sherratt DJ (2005) Dancing around the divisome: asymmetric chromosome segregation in Escherichia coli. Genes Dev 19(19):2367–2377. doi:10.1101/gad.345305

19. Nielsen HJ, Ottesen JR, Youngren B, Austin SJ, Hansen FG (2006) The Escherichia coli chromosome is organized with the left and right chromosome arms in separate cell halves. Mol Microbiol 62(2):331–338. doi:10.1111/j.1365-2958.2006.05346.x

20. Lesterlin C, Pages C, Dubarry N, Dasgupta S, Cornet F (2008) Asymmetry of chromosome Replichores renders the DNA translocase activity of FtsK essential for cell division and cell shape maintenance in Escherichia coli. PLoS Genet 4(12), e1000288. doi:10.1371/journal.pgen.1000288

21. White MA, Eykelenboom JK, Lopez-Vernaza MA, Wilson E, Leach DR (2008) Non-random segregation of sister chromosomes in Escherichia coli. Nature 455(7217):1248–1250. doi:10.1038/nature07282

22. Hadizadeh Yazdi N, Guet CC, Johnson RC, Marko JF (2012) Variation of the folding and dynamics of the Escherichia coli chromosome with growth conditions. Mol Microbiol 86(6):1318–1333. doi:10.1111/mmi.12071

23. Fisher JK, Bourniquel A, Witz G, Weiner B, Prentiss M, Kleckner N (2013) Four-dimensional imaging of E. coli nucleoid organization and dynamics in living cells. Cell 153(4):882–895. doi:10.1016/j.cell.2013.04.006

24. Dame RT (2005) The role of nucleoid-associated proteins in the organization and compaction of bacterial chromatin. Mol Microbiol 56(4):858–870

25. Possoz C, Filipe SR, Grainge I, Sherratt DJ (2006) Tracking of controlled Escherichia coli replication fork stalling and restart at repressor-bound DNA in vivo. EMBO J 25(11):2596–2604. doi:10.1038/sj.emboj.7601155

26. Dubarry N, Pasta F, Lane D (2006) ParABS systems of the four replicons of Burkholderia cenocepacia: new chromosome centromeres confer partition specificity. J Bacteriol 188(4):1489–1496. doi:10.1128/JB.188.4.1489-1496.2006

27. Gordon GS, Sitnikov D, Webb CD, Teleman A, Straight A, Losick R, Murray AW, Wright A (1997) Chromosome and low copy plasmid segregation in E. coli: visual evidence for distinct mechanisms. Cell 90(6):1113–1121

28. Sliusarenko O, Heinritz J, Emonet T, Jacobs-Wagner C (2011) High-throughput, subpixel precision analysis of bacterial morphogenesis and intracellular spatio-temporal dynamics. Mol Microbiol 80(3):612–627. doi:10.1111/j.1365-2958.2011.07579.x

29. Fleurie A, Lesterlin C, Manuse S, Zhao C, Cluzel C, Lavergne JP, Franz-Wachtel M, Macek B, Combet C, Kuru E, VanNieuwenhze MS, Brun YV, Sherratt D, Grangeasse C (2014) MapZ marks the division sites and positions FtsZ rings in Streptococcus pneumoniae. Nature 516(7530):259–262. doi:10.1038/nature13966

30. Lesterlin C, Ball G, Schermelleh L, Sherratt DJ (2014) RecA bundles mediate homology pairing between distant sisters during DNA break repair. Nature 506(7487):249–253. doi:10.1038/nature12868

31. de Chaumont F, Dallongeville S, Chenouard N, Herve N, Pop S, Provoost T, Meas-Yedid V, Pankajakshan P, Lecomte T, Le Montagner Y, Lagache T, Dufour A, Olivo-Marin JC (2012) Icy: an open bioimage informatics platform for extended reproducible research. Nat Methods 9(7):690–696. doi:10.1038/nmeth.2075

32. Stracy M, Uphoff S, Garza de Leon F, Kapanidis AN (2014) In vivo single-molecule imaging of bacterial DNA replication, transcription, and repair. FEBS Lett 588(19):3585–3594. doi:10.1016/j.febslet.2014.05.026

33. Uphoff S, Sherratt DJ, Kapanidis AN (2014) Visualizing protein-DNA interactions in live bacterial cells using photoactivated single-molecule tracking. J Vis Exp 85:PMID:24638084. doi:10.3791/51177

34. Wang X, Lesterlin C, Reyes-Lamothe R, Ball G, Sherratt DJ (2011) Replication and segregation of an Escherichia coli chromosome with two replication origins. Proc Natl Acad Sci U S A 108(26):E243–E250. doi:10.1073/pnas.1100874108

35. Badrinarayanan A, Lesterlin C, Reyes-Lamothe R, Sherratt D (2012) The Escherichia coli SMC complex, MukBEF, shapes nucleoid organization independently of DNA replication. J Bacteriol 194(17):4669–4676. doi:10.1128/JB.00957-12

36. Uphoff S, Reyes-Lamothe R, Garza de Leon F, Sherratt DJ, Kapanidis AN (2013) Single-molecule DNA repair in live bacteria. Proc Natl Acad Sci U S A 110(20):8063–8068. doi:10.1073/pnas.1301804110

Chapter 7

Transverse Magnetic Tweezers Allowing Coincident Epifluorescence Microscopy on Horizontally Extended DNA

Stephen J. Cross, Claire E. Brown, and Christoph G. Baumann

Abstract

Longitudinal magnetic tweezers (L-MT) have seen wide-scale adoption as the tool-of-choice for stretching and twisting a single DNA molecule. They are also used to probe topological changes in DNA as a result of protein binding and enzymatic activity. However, in the longitudinal configuration, the DNA molecule is extended perpendicular to the imaging plane. As a result, it is only possible to infer biological activity from the motion of the tethered superparamagnetic microsphere. Described here is a "transverse" magnetic tweezers (T-MT) geometry featuring simultaneous control of DNA extension and spatially coincident video-rate epifluorescence imaging. Unlike in L-MT, DNA tethers in T-MT are extended parallel to the imaging plane between two micron-sized spheres, and importantly protein targets on the DNA can be localized using fluorescent nanoparticles. The T-MT can manipulate a long DNA construct at molecular extensions approaching the contour length defined by B-DNA helical geometry, and the measured entropic elasticity agrees with the worm-like chain model (force < 35 pN). By incorporating a torsionally constrained DNA tether, the T-MT would allow both the relative extension and twist of the tether to be manipulated, while viewing far-red emitting fluorophore-labeled targets. This T-MT design has the potential to enable the study of DNA binding and remodeling processes under conditions of constant force and defined torsional stress.

Key words Transverse magnetic tweezers, Coincident fluorescence microscopy, DNA micromanipulation, Single-molecule manipulation

1 Introduction

Magnetic tweezers (MT) have become a common single-molecule manipulation technique and are widely used to probe the elasticity of supercoiled DNA and the dynamics of DNA processing enzymes involved in modulating chromosome architecture [1]. Most MT instruments are designed to stretch out a single tethered DNA molecule orthogonal to the microscope coverslip surface ("longitudinal" configuration). Positioning of fixed pole magnets above the surface causes a superparamagnetic microsphere (SP-MS) attached at the untethered end of the DNA molecule to move away from the coverslip surface, thus stretching out the DNA

Mark C. Leake (ed.), *Chromosome Architecture: Methods and Protocols*, Methods in Molecular Biology, vol. 1431, DOI 10.1007/978-1-4939-3631-1_7, © Springer Science+Business Media New York 2016

molecule. The force acting on the DNA molecule is altered as the vertical position of the magnets is changed. In this longitudinal MT (L-MT) geometry it is possible to negatively and positively supercoil the tether by rotating the magnets, if the DNA molecule is attached to the SP-MS and coverslip surfaces via both DNA strands, i.e., torsionally constrained [2]. The dynamics of DNA processing enzymes can be studied using L-MT; however, in these experiments enzymatic activity is inferred from changes in DNA tether length and/or linking number [3]. This results in all information on the location of the enzymatic event on the DNA tether being lost. In addition, L-MT experiments necessitate a long-lived DNA–enzyme complex, thus it is not feasible to study enzymes or proteins that associate with DNA but do not alter its topology, e.g., proteins undergoing 1D sliding on DNA.

Although the majority of magnetic tweezers systems adopt the longitudinal configuration there are a few systems designed for use in a horizontal or "transverse" configuration, i.e., transverse magnetic tweezers (T-MT). These systems utilize the same basic principle as L-MT, whereby a single tether is extended between a stationary surface and a SP-MS moving in response to an applied magnetic field. However, unlike the longitudinal configuration, the tether is extended in the focal plane of the objective lens. This affords the notable advantage of permitting real-time observation of events on the tethered substrate, as with laminar flow extension and optical tweezers manipulation of DNA, while maintaining the ability to introduce positive or negative twist into the DNA molecule.

Currently, no standard configuration for a T-MT microscope exists, with relatively few systems having thus far been published. One of the first examples was reported by Danilowicz et al., where DNA tethers were formed between a SP-MS (2.8 μm diameter) and the antibody-functionalized surface of a cylindrical capillary (330 μm diameter) [4]. This assembly was placed inside a square micro-cell (600 μm cross-section), which permitted fluidic sample delivery and buffer exchange. Force was applied using a stack of five permanent magnets (each $6.4 \times 6.4 \times 2.5$ mm^3) placed to one side of the micro-cell and the corresponding SP-MS response observed using a 10× objective lens (NA = 0.25) placed underneath the sample. Although not explicitly stated, the low resolving power of the optics indicates a long working distance and was likely a compromise designed to permit both wide-field imaging and close proximity of the magnet stack and sample. While this allowed forces up to 30 pN to be measured simultaneously for dozens of tethers, the low magnification of the microscope limited its use to the reported multiplex application.

The compromise of low magnification in favor of a higher applied force was reversed in a similar design reported by Graham et al. [5]. In this system, tethers were formed directly onto the micro-cell surface (1 mm cross-section; VitroCells; VitroCom) and extended at an acute angle relative to this surface. Fluorescence imaging was done through the bottom surface of the micro-cell using a 60× magnification oil-immersion objective lens (NA = 1.25, PlanApo; Olympus) and epi-illumination. The SP-MS (Dynabeads M-280; Invitrogen) was manipulated using a stack of four cubic NdFeB magnets (12.7 mm cross section) held perpendicular to the objective lens optical axis on the end of a micromanipulator. With this configuration, forces up to 3 pN were tested; higher applied forces may have been possible but this was not reported.

Using an electron-multiplying CCD camera, Graham et al. were able to observe DNA-binding by the proteins Fis, HU and NHP6A with a high signal-to-noise ratio [5]; however, epi-illumination ultimately limits the contrast possible through significant bulk fluorescence excitation. This can be addressed via implementation of total internal reflection fluorescence (TIRF) microscopy as demonstrated by Schwarz et al. [6]. Fundamentally, the microscope configuration is nearly identical to that reported by Graham et al., but with tethers formed from the lower surface, permitting TIRF) illumination. This is only a partial solution, because the finite SP-MS diameter will result in non-horizontal tether inclination and limit the amount of DNA within the evanescent field. For typical 1 μm diameter SP-MS, only one-fifth of the tether will be within the 100 nm penetration depth of the evanescent field. While the exponential field decay will likely result in observation beyond this range, a significant decrease in fluorescence intensity would be observed. This would make molecular tracking and stoichiometry of DNA-associated protein complexes difficult to quantify. Similar to the epifluorescence system, this method also suffers from limited force generation, with the highest reported value being 1.5 pN when using a single cubic permanent magnet ($5 \times 5 \times 1$ mm³; Q-05-05-01-HN; Supermagnete).

A permanent magnet-based tweezers system has also been reported by van Loenhout et al. [7]. They used a standard longitudinal configuration to initially twist DNA, but with a second magnet to pull the coiled tether horizontally. This was used in conjunction with the fluorescent dye Cy3 to view plectoneme dynamics in DNA. While demonstrated using epifluorescence, such a configuration is not too dissimilar to that described by Schwarz et al. [6]. As with the methods of Graham et al. and Schwarz et al., lateral forces appear to be restricted, with magnitudes no greater than 3.2 pN reported.

An alternative approach to realization of a T-MT is to use electromagnets, whereby electromagnetic coils placed either side of the sample generate a relatively uniform magnetic field [8]. While this configuration was reported to yield forces of ~15 pN (using M280 SP-MS; Invitrogen), the use of a water-immersion objective necessitated a larger coil spacing, thus limiting forces to ~1.7

pN. Furthermore, resistive heating of the coils required implementation of an active water-cooling system; a problem characteristic of electromagnets [8, 9]. Through implementation of micro-fabricated electromagnets, Chiou et al. were able to achieve three-dimensional control of magnetic substrates [10]. This configuration was reported to benefit from reduced heat generation and produce applied forces exceeding 20 pN when acting on 2.8 μm diameter SP-MS, while maintaining compatibility with high numerical aperture light microscopy and epi-illumination [10]. The notable disadvantage of such electromagnetic approaches is a significant increase in implementation complexity relative to a permanent magnet-based tweezers system.

Several methods to manipulate individual DNA molecule extension while permitting simultaneous single-molecule fluorescence observation have been reported. Despite this, there is no easily applicable, standardized approach for manipulating twist in a horizontal DNA template. The emerging trend is to adapt the established L-MT technique, in which DNA is extended orthogonally from the tethering substrate, to permit extension within the observable plane of the microscope. However, the relatively few published techniques are limited in at least one of the following: maximum achievable applied force, optical spatial resolution and the capacity to generate truly horizontal tethers. Compromise between force and resolution is necessary since short sample-to-magnet separations are required to apply high force, yet such positioning is generally precluded by the large objective lenses used for high numerical aperture microscopy. Similarly, high spatial resolution and truly horizontal tethers have thus far been mutually exclusive, with inclined extension from the lower sample surface used in conjunction with TIRF microscopy.

There is a need for an easily implementable approach to allow single-molecule localization experiments to be conducted on torsionally constrained and characterizable DNA tethers. This can be realized through implementation of design alterations to the aforementioned horizontal magnetic tweezers configurations. Firstly, use of thin fluid cells (<10 μm) in which experiments are conducted limits bulk fluorescence excitation, thus facilitating use of epi-illumination, as opposed to spatially restricted TIRF illumination. As a result, tethers can be extended horizontally in the center of the sample chamber, rather than attached to the lower surface and extended at an acute angle. Secondly, use of a long-working distance objective lens to permit reduced sample-to-magnet separations increases the applicable force range dramatically. Finally, use of nanoscopic fluorescent probes (e.g., TransFluoSpheres; Invitrogen), rather than individual extrinsic organic dyes, reduces the deleterious effects sample photobleaching can have on the length of time over which DNA-associated events can be tracked. Additionally, the relatively large number of fluorophores present in a single TransFluoSphere further facilitates implementation of epifluorescence imaging, where reductions in signal-to-noise ratio relative to TIRF microscopy are inevitable.

In this chapter, a T-MT instrument is described which incorporates permanent magnets and a long-working distance microscope objective (Fig. 1). This enables the permanent magnet–superparamagnetic microsphere distance to be minimized, thus increasing the maximum force that can be applied to the DNA tether. This allows a single DNA tether to be manipulated at extensions equal to the molecular contour length determined by the B-form helix (=0.338 nm rise per base pair multiplied by number of base pairs in the DNA tether), where intramolecular interactions would occur with a very low probability (probability of loop formation in stretched polymer chain estimated in ref. 11) and protein-mediated DNA looping could be probed. This design enables the entire length of the tether to be imaged using wide-field epifluorescence microscopy at video rate (30 Hz) (Fig. 2) in

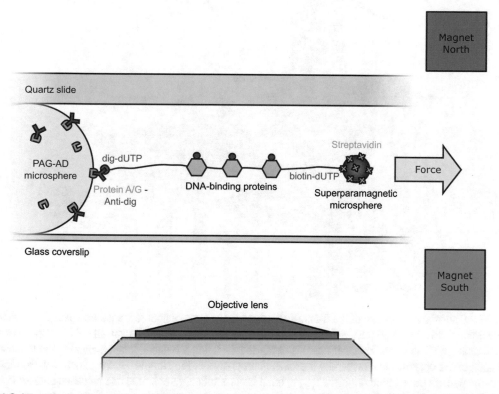

Fig. 1 Schematic diagram showing tethering configuration for generating horizontal DNA tethers with a defined orientation. A single DNA tether is attached at one end to a 9 μm diameter Protein A/G:anti-digoxigenin IgG functionalized (PAG-AD) microsphere and at the other end to a streptavidin-functionalized superparamagnetic microsphere (SP-MS). The tether is extended horizontally using the force exerted on the superparamagnetic microsphere by a pair of permanent magnets. Fluorescently labeled DNA-bound protein could be observed from below using a long working-distance objective lens and wide-field epifluorescence microscopy

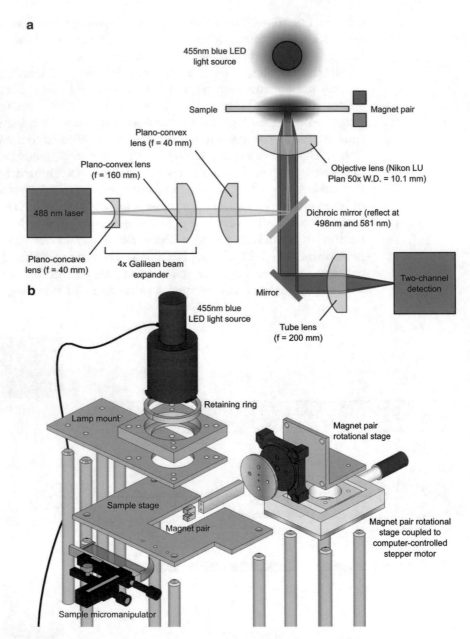

Fig. 2 (**a**) Optical configuration of the transverse magnetic tweezers epifluorescence microscope. Bright-field illumination from a blue LED passes through the laser-coupling dichroic and is focused onto the CMOS camera by the tube lens. The excitation laser beam is expanded 4× using a Galilean beam expander and focussed to the back of the objective lens, whereby it excites fluorophores in the sample. Fluorescence emission follows the same path as transmitted bright-field light, but it is chromatically separated and focussed onto an intensified CCD camera. (**b**) Exploded diagram of sample stage and components for sample and magnet-pair spatial control. Samples are held above the objective lens on a custom-fabricated stage with a commercially purchased micromanipulator for accurate sample translational control. A section cut from the stage allows the magnet pair to be brought into close proximity of the sample. The magnet pair is held in a clamp on the end of a rod connected to a stepper-motor-controlled rotational stage and the entire magnet-control assembly is placed on a one-dimensional micrometer-controlled translational stage, permitting precise movement of the magnets towards the sample. Since magnets are held with friction, magnet-pair separation can be easily adjusted if required

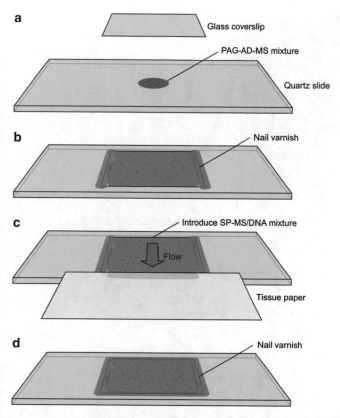

Fig. 3 Sample chamber preparation protocol for transverse magnetic tweezers microscope. (**a**) 10 μl of PAG-AD-MS mixture is deposited on a chemically cleaned quartz slide and trapped beneath a glass coverslip. (**b**) Opposite edges of the channel are sealed with nail varnish to create a flow-cell. (**c**) ~50 μl DNA-[M280]SP-MS mixture is introduced along one open side of the channel and drawn through using a piece of tissue paper applied to the opposite side. (**d**) Following introduction of all reagents, the chamber is sealed along the remaining edges with nail varnish

an easily constructed, thin (~9 μm) sample chamber (Fig. 3). This will allow fluorescently labeled targets to be visualized and tracked on the DNA tether as a function of DNA extension, i.e., applied force. By tracking the bright-field image of the SP-MS at a high sampling frequency (≥60 Hz), the variance of the SP-MS excursions in the lateral direction could be measured and, with the equipartition theorem, used to estimate the applied force on the DNA molecule (Fig. 4a) [2, 12].

The extension of the horizontal DNA was determined directly by measuring the distance between the pedestal microsphere (9 μm diameter, functionalized with Protein A/G:anti-digoxigenin IgG) and the superparamagnetic microsphere ([M280]SP-MS functionalized with streptavidin) (Fig. 1), then subtracting the microsphere radii. The entropic elastic response of long DNA tethers (6000–36,000 base pairs, B-form contour length ≈ 2–12 μm) was

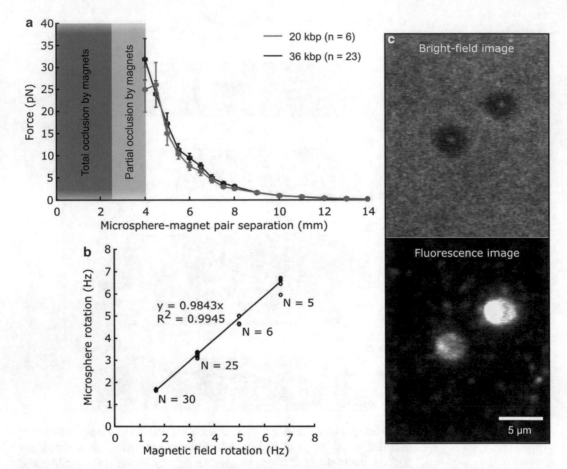

Fig. 4 (**a**) Force applied to DNA tethered (20,000 and 36,000 bp) superparamagnetic microspheres by an external magnetic field as measured through application of the equipartition theorem (*symbols*). This analysis treats DNA tethers as pendulums displaced from their equilibrium positions by thermal motion and relates the magnitude of the magnetic force acting on the tethers to the observed superparamagnetic microsphere lateral displacement sampled at a high video frame rate (60 fps, 1/200 s shutter time). (**b**) Rotation of DNA-tethered superparamagnetic microspheres. The permanent magnets were rotated using a computer-controlled stepper motor. Microsphere rotation was tracked in non-consecutive bright-field images (from video collected at 30 fps). Correlation between frequency of magnetic field rotation and the observed microsphere rotation was observed up to 6.7 Hz. Higher rotational frequencies were not possible with the M280SP-MS. (**c**) Simultaneous bright-field (*top*) and fluorescence (*bottom*) images from the T-MT epifluorescence microscope. Sample containing ~0.1 nM TransFluoSpheres (diameter = 40 nm, λ_{ex} = 488 nm, λ_{em} = 655 nm) and M280SP-MS (diameter = 2.8 μm) was viewed using an intensified CCD camera. The M280SP-MS are intrinsically fluorescent, thus a narrow (655/20) band-pass filter must be used to select the TransFluoSphere fluorescence emission

measured (i.e., applied force versus extension of DNA tether, Fig. 5), and it compared favorably to the predictions of the worm-like chain model for a persistence length of 53 nm [13, 14]. In addition, we show that SP-MS can be spun at up to 6.7 Hz (Fig. 4b) by rotating the magnetic field on an axis coincident with the helical axis of the extended DNA tether. If a torsionally constrained DNA tether were utilized [2, 15], then positive or negative twist

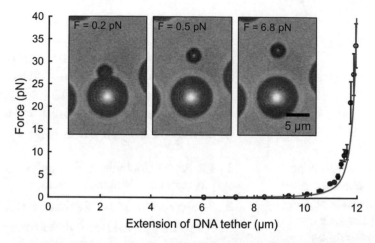

Fig. 5 Plot of measured force as a function of DNA tether extension. A small initial force (<1 pN) is required to achieve a relative extension of 0.8; however, the force necessary to continue extension increases rapidly beyond this point. This entropic elastic response is in good agreement with the theoretical, worm-like chain model (36,000 bp DNA contour length = 12.2 µm, persistence length = 53 nm). Inset bright-field images: Video frames taken from a transverse magnetic tweezers experiment, where increasing force applied by the magnet pair (relatively positioned at the *top* of the image) pulls the smaller superparamagnetic microsphere away from the larger, stationary microsphere (*bottom* of image). Agreement here further demonstrates the successful and reliable manipulation of a single DNA molecule

could be introduced at a constant elongational force to generate DNA supercoils. Simultaneous observation of the DNA tether by epifluorescence microscopy is possible and individual 40 nm diameter TransFluoSpheres can be detected (Fig. 4c). This enables fluorescently labeled proteins to be tracked and their stoichiometry to be quantified while the degree of DNA supercoiling is monitored or actively manipulated in real-time.

2   Materials

2.1   Buffers and Special Reagents

1. 25 mM MES buffer: Dissolve 1.22 g anhydrous 2-[N-morpholino]ethanesulfonic acid (MES, Sigma) in water (heating to 50 °C will aid dissolution) and add 31 ml of 0.1 M NaOH. Allow solution to cool and then increase the volume to 250 ml with water and check pH = 6.

2. Phosphate-buffered saline (PBS): Add 8 g NaCl, 1.44 g Na_2NPO_4, 0.24 g KH_2PO_4, and 0.2 g KCl to 800 ml of ultrapure water (resistivity of 18.2 MΩ cm). Adjust pH to 7.4 and increase volume to 1 L, then sterilize by autoclaving or filtering.

3. Tris–EDTA (TE): 10 mM Tris–HCl and 1 mM EDTA. Adjust pH to 8.0.

4. BSA coat buffer (BCB): 10 mM Tris–HCl, 172 mM NaCl, 1 mM EDTA, and 1 mg/ml acetylated BSA. Adjust pH to 8.0.

5. Tethering buffer (TetB): 10 mM Tris–HCl, 172 mM NaCl, 1 mM EDTA, and 0.1 mg/ml acetylated BSA. Adjust pH to 8.0.

6. 20 mg/ml acetylated BSA (Sigma)

2.2 Preparation of Microspheres Labeled with Anti-digoxigenin (PAG-AD-MS)

1. 4% (w/v) aldehyde-sulfate polystyrene-latex microspheres (~9 μm diameter, Molecular Probes).

2. BSA-passivated 1.5 ml microcentrifuge tubes (*see* **Note 1**).

3. 5 mg/ml Purified Recomb® Protein A/G from *E. coli* (Pierce).

4. 1 M glycine: Dissolved in PBS.

5. 5 mg/ml sheep anti-digoxigenin polyclonal IgG (AbD Serotec).

2.3 Preparation of Oxygen Scavenger System

1. Degassed buffer: Relevant buffer degassed under vacuum with stirring for at least 15 min. Degassed buffer is stored in a plastic syringe fitted with a 25-G needle and used immediately.

2. 1 M dithiothreitol (DTT, Melford).

3. 300 mg/ml glucose (Fisher Scientific).

4. 10 mg/ml glucose oxidase (Sigma) stored as single-use aliquots at –20 °C.

5. 2 mg/ml catalase (Sigma) stored as single-use aliquots at –20 °C.

6. 1 ml plastic syringe fitted with a 25-G needle to minimize air-exposure of buffer

2.4 Preparation of Microscopy Substrates

1. Borosilicate glass coverslips (No. 1, 22 mm×64 mm; Menzel-Gläser).

2. Quartz slides (1 mm thick, 75 mm×25 mm; UQG Optics Ltd.).

3. 2% (v/v) Neutracon (Decon Laboratories Ltd.).

2.5 Preparation of Horizontal DNA Tethers

1. ~2% (w/v) anti-digoxigenin-functionalized ~9 μm diameter polystyrene-latex microspheres (PAG-AD-MS).

2. Dynabeads® M280 streptavidin-labeled superparamagnetic microspheres (M280SP-MS, 2.8 μm diameter; Invitrogen) (alternative SP-MS are also compatible, *see* **Note 2**).

3. Double-stranded DNA template differentially end-labeled with biotin and digoxigenin was prepared according to a published method [16].

4. TransFluoSphere (488/645) streptavidin-labeled microspheres (40 nm diameter; Invitrogen).

5. Cubic gold-plated NdFeB magnet (5 mm×5 mm×5 mm; Supermagnete).

6. Clear nail varnish.

7. Lint-free optical tissue (SPI Supplies, Structure Probe Inc.).

2.6 Combined Magnetic Tweezers and Epifluorescence Microscope

1. DNA is extended and torsionally constrained using a transverse magnetic tweezers (T-MT) setup. The microscope is entirely constructed using a 30 mm cage system (ThorLabs) as detailed elsewhere [17]. This configuration combines wide-field epi-illumination and bright-field illumination to permit simultaneous observation of fluorescently labeled DNA-bound enzymes and measurement of applied force (via equipartition analysis of SP-MS motion [12]).

2. Fluorescence excitation is provided by a diode laser ($\lambda_{ex} = 488$ nm, 75 mW; Coherent Sapphire) with the beam diameter expanded $4\times$ using a lens pair (focal lengths = 40 and 160 mm, diameters = 16 and 25 mm, respectively; Comar) in Galilean beam expander configuration. The laser is focussed to the back aperture of the objective lens and is coupled into the optical path using a dichroic filter (reflection at $\lambda = 498$ and 581 nm, FF498/581; Semrock) (*see* **Note 3**).

3. Bright-field illumination is provided by a blue LED ($\lambda_{max} = 455$ nm; ThorLabs) and is isolated from the fluorescence signal using a second dichroic filter (590 DCXR; Optical Insights) held in a Dual-Cam™ image splitter (Optical Insights). This simultaneously projects two chromatically separated images onto separate cameras for fluorescence (HQ655/20 band pass, Chroma; IC-300B intensified CCD, Photon Technology International) and bright-field (DMK 22BUC03 CMOS; The Imaging Source GmBH) imaging.

4. A long working-distance objective lens (W.D. = 10.1 mm; N.A. = 0.55; CFI LU Plan EPI ELWD, Nikon) is used for sample imaging due to spatial compatibility with the cubic NdFeB magnets, which are placed between the sample and lens.

5. The NdFeB magnets are friction-clamped at the end of an aluminum arm, which is mounted on a rotational stage (*see* **Note 4**). This is mounted on a translational stage, allowing the magnet pair to be rotated next to the sample at a user-defined distance. The magnets are aligned in a parallel, but opposed biaxial configuration with a gap of 0.4 mm, corresponding to the minimum separation possible with the sample chamber able to move freely between them.

6. A modified microscope stage is used, which permits the magnet arm to travel laterally towards the sample, in the plane of the sample.

7. Forces are measured through application of the equipartition function, relating variance of lateral SP-MS excursions to the applied force [12].

3 Methods

3.1 Preparation of Microspheres Labeled with Anti-digoxigenin

1. The 9 μm diameter sulfate-aldehyde functionalized polystyrene-latex microspheres (MS) are washed prior to functionalization in the following manner: 0.6 ml of 4% (w/v) MS is added to 0.6 ml of 25 mM MES buffer (pH 6.0) in a BSA-coated microcentrifuge tube (*see* **Note 1**) and agitated by vortexing at 1200 rpm for 30 s. The suspension in then centrifuged (*see* **Note 5**) at 750 × *g* for 2 min to pellet the MS. The supernatant is removed and is immediately replaced by an equal volume of fresh 25 mM MES buffer (pH 6.0). This process is repeated twice more with the final resuspension in 1.2 ml 25 mM MES buffer (pH 6.0).

2. Add 100 μl 5 mg/ml Protein A/G (final concentration is ~0.385 mg/ml) and incubate overnight at room temperature (~20 °C) on a vertically inclined rotating turntable (or mix in an equivalent gentle manner) to prevent PAG-MS sedimentation.

3. Following incubation, pellet the MS by centrifugation at 750 × *g* for 2 min, then remove the supernatant and resuspend in a 1.2 ml 1 M glycine. Incubate this solution at room temperature for 40 min on a vertically inclined rotating turntable (or mix in an equivalent gentle manner).

4. After incubation with glycine, vortex and centrifuge the MS as described in **step 1**, then remove the supernatant and resuspend in 1080 μl PBS (pH 7.4) and 120 μl 20 mg/ml acetylated BSA (add the PBS first). Repeat this wash step two further times with the final resuspension in 1074 μl PBS (pH 7.4), 120 μl 20 mg/ml acetylated BSA, and 6 μl 2% (w/v) sodium azide.

5. Protein A/G MS (PAG-MS) can be stored for extended durations (up to 6 months) in a fresh BSA-passivated microcentrifuge tube at 4 °C until required.

6. Prior to conjugation of anti-digoxigenin IgG, 100 μl PAG-MS is added to 100 μl TetB in a fresh BSA-passivated 0.5 ml microcentrifuge tube. The PAG-MS are washed three times with 0.2 ml TetB using the vortex, centrifugation and resuspension protocol from **step 1**. Resuspend in 100 μl TetB after the final wash step.

7. Add 3.2 μl 5 mg/ml anti-digoxigenin IgG (final concentration is 0.16 mg/ml) to 100 μl PAG-MS solution and incubate at room temperature for 1 h on a vertically inclined rotating turntable (or mix in an equivalent gentle manner).

8. Following the incubation, the anti-digoxigenin functionalized PAG-MS (PAG-AD-MS) are washed three times with 0.2 ml TetB using the vortex, centrifugation, and resuspension protocol

from **step 1**. Resuspend in 100 μl TetB after the final wash step.

9. Store the ~2 % (w/v) anti-digoxigenin functionalized PAG-MS (PAG-AD-MS) in a fresh BSA-passivated 0.5 ml microcentrifuge tube at 4 °C and use within 24 h (*see* **Note 6**).

3.2 Preparation of Oxygen Scavenger System

1. Mix 960 μl degassed experimental buffer (normally TetB), 20 μl 1 M DTT, 10 μl 300 mg/ml glucose, 5 μl 10 mg/ml glucose oxidase, and 5 μl 2 mg/ml catalase in a 1.5 ml microcentrifuge tube.

2. To minimize solution exposure to air, transfer to a 1 ml plastic syringe fitted with a 25-G needle.

3. Store oxygen scavenger solution on ice (or at 4 °C) and use within 24 h.

3.3 Preparation of Microscopy Substrates

1. Place glass coverslips in a rack inside a water bath-compatible container (*see* **Note 7**).

2. Add 2 % (v/v) Neutracon solution so that coverslips are completely submerged, then sonicate (*see* **Note 8**) coverslips at 50 °C for 10 min.

3. Following sonication remove rack from cleaning solution and rinse thoroughly with deionized water (18.2 MΩ cm), then blow dry with filtered compressed air. Store coverslips in a sealed dust-free container until required.

4. Repeat the process for quartz slides (*see* **Note 9**).

3.4 Preparation of Horizontal DNA Tethers

1. Prior to coupling to DNA, streptavidin-functionalized superparamagnetic M280 microspheres ([M280]SP-MS) are washed using the following process: Add 50 μl of 1 % (w/v) [M280]SP-MS to a 0.5 ml microcentrifuge tube, then increase total volume to 80 μl by adding TetB and mix gently. Hold an NdFeB magnet directly next to the tube and allow [M280]SP-MS to collect on tube wall for 60 s. Gently remove supernatant while the magnet is still in contact with the tube, then remove the magnet and resuspend in 80 μl TetB. Vortex microspheres at 1200 rpm for 30 s to ensure complete resuspension of the [M280]SP-MS pellet. Repeat the process twice more, with the final resuspension in 79 μl TetB to yield a ~0.6 % (w/v) solution.

2. To tether DNA to [M280]SP-MS, add 1 μl 2.8 nM differentially end-labeled DNA (*see* **Note 10**) to the microcentrifuge tube and incubate at room temperature for 1 h on a vertically inclined rotating turntable (or mix in an equivalent gentle manner).

3. Following incubation, any uncoupled DNA is removed from solution using the washing process described in **step 1**, with

each resuspension in 160 μl of TetB. Store the sample on ice (or at 4 °C) and use within 24 h.

4. Take a clean quartz slide and place a 10 μl drop of 2% (w/v) PAG-AD-MS in the center (Fig. 3a). Carefully place a Neutracon-cleaned coverslip over the droplet (Fig. 3a). Through capillary action, the solution should distribute evenly beneath the coverslip.

5. Seal opposite edges of the coverslip to the slide surface using nail varnish (Fig. 3b) (*see* **Note 11**). Allow 10 min for the nail varnish to harden, ensuring the chamber does not dry out during this period via evaporation at the open edges. TetB can be pipetted (~10 μl) along the open edges to prevent this occurring.

6. Once the varnish is dry, 10 μl of the DNA-^{M280}SP-MS sample is pipetted along one of the open edges. A sheet of lint-free optical tissue is placed along the opposite open edge to pull the sample through the chamber (Fig. 3c). Continually replenish the DNA-^{M280}SP-MS until 50 μl of DNA-^{M280}SP-MS sample has passed through the chamber. This process can take up to 10 min (*see* **Note 12**).

7. Add 10 μl TransFluoSphere-labeled DNA-binding protein (incorporating a biotin-tag) containing solution with a pipette along the open edge and use a fresh lint-free optical tissue to pull the sample through the chamber (*see* **Note 13**). The final concentration of TransFluoSpheres should be <1 nM (in experimental buffer with oxygen scavenging system added) to reduce the background fluorescence. A higher concentration of fluorescently labeled DNA-binding protein can be loaded in the chamber to facilitate DNA association; however, the fluorophore-containing buffer in the chamber must be exchanged with fresh experimental buffer until the background fluorescence is reduced enough to resolve single TransFluoSpheres (wash with 50–100 μl buffer, *see* **Note 14**).

8. Use another lint-free optical tissue to remove any excess liquid from the open edges, then seal with nail varnish (Fig. 3d). Wait for 10 min for nail varnish to dry before using sample.

3.5 Manipulation of DNA-Tethered Superparamagnetic Microspheres

1. To prevent premature DNA-shearing, retract the magnet pair to a minimum separation of 10 mm from the nearest sample edge. Rotate the magnets to the vertical position, such that the air gap between them is aligned with the sample (Fig. 2b); this will allow the magnets to pass around the sample when the sample-magnet separation is reduced.

2. Take the assembled sample (from Subheading 3.4) and place coverslip side down on the microscope stage. Clamp in place using the micromanipulator and focus the objective lens on the AD-MS and ^{M280}SP-MS in the chamber.

3. Slowly move the magnet pair towards the sample until the [M280]SP-MS begin to move freely in response to the magnetic field. Leave sample to stand until no further [M280]SP-MS motion is observed. At this point, all remaining [M280]SP-MS in the sample volume should be tethered or nonspecifically immobilized on the chamber surface. Nonspecifically adsorbed [M280]SP-MS can be easily distinguished from DNA tethered [M280]SP-MS by their lack of thermally induced motion at low applied forces ($F < 2$ pN) (see **Note 15**).

4. Measurement of force acting on [M280]SP-MS requires acquisition of high-speed video (≥ 60 fps) of tethered [M280]SP-MS for at least 15 s (see **Note 16**). The [M280]SP-MS centroid is tracked using a particle-tracking algorithm (see **Note 17**) to obtain [M280]SP-MS xy-coordinates. The variance of the lateral [M280]SP-MS displacement (i.e., relative to helical axis of tethered DNA) is translated into applied force using the equipartition theorem [12].

5. The elastic properties of the DNA tether are characterized by obtaining force (F, measured as described above) versus extension (x) data. From this data, it is possible to determine the apparent contour length (L_o) and persistence length (L_p) of the tether, thus confirming whether a single or multiple DNA molecules are forming the tether. In order to obtain the F versus x data, the distance between the microspheres is increased or decreased incrementally by translating the magnet pair. The PAG-AD-MS to [M280]SP-MS distance is determined at discrete molecular extensions and used to obtain x for the DNA molecule after subtracting the microsphere radii. The inextensible worm-like chain model of DNA elasticity [13] is then used to relate F, x, L_o, L_p and thermal energy (kT) at the experimental temperature (T).

4 Notes

1. Add 100 μl 20 mg/ml acetylated BSA to 900 μl of PBS (pH 7.4) in the 1.5 ml microcentrifuge tube to be passivated. Attach tubes to a vertically inclined rotating turntable (or mix in an equivalent gentle manner) while incubating at room temperature (~20 °C) for 1 h. The BSA mixture is discarded and tubes are subsequently washed three times with 1 ml of ultra-pure water (18.2 MΩ cm). Tubes are stored at 4 °C until required.

2. In addition to [M280]SP-MS (Invitrogen), successful tether formation and manipulation was demonstrated using Dynabeads® MyOne streptavidin-labeled T1 superparamagnetic microspheres (1.05 μm diameter; Invitrogen).

3. Specified optical components are also compatible with replacement of 488 nm laser with one centered on 561 nm.

4. The stepper motor (Reliance Cool Muscle, Reliance Precision Limited) coupled to the rotational stage is remotely operated by custom software (5000 positions per revolution) created in Microsoft Visual Studio (Microsoft Corporation). Closed-loop vector drive control ensures motor positioning is ultra smooth.

5. A bench-top microcentrifuge can be used for this centrifugation step.

6. Once functionalized with anti-digoxigenin, microspheres should be used within 24 h. Degradation of functionalization will be evident as a decrease in the frequency of DNA tether formation.

7. Racks for sonication should allow coverslips/slides to be spaced at least 1 mm apart to ensure good access for the cleaning solution. Racks must fit into water bath-compatible containers, such that coverslips/slides can be completely submerged in cleaning solution.

8. A sonicating water bath (Ultrawave Ltd.) is used for cleaning coverslips/slides.

9. Quartz slides can be reused after cleaning. Soak slides overnight in acetone to remove nail varnish and coverslips. The slides are then cleaned as follows: 10 min sonication (*see* **Note 8**) in isopropanol, rinse with deionized water, 10 min sonication in 1 M KOH (no heating), rinse very well with deionized water, immerse in fresh absolute ethanol, transfer to clean slide holder and incubate at 70 °C until dry. Store clean slides in a sealed dust-free container until required.

10. The DNA concentration can be decreased to change the ratio of DNA to ^{M280}SP-MS and reduce the likelihood of multiple DNA tethers forming. For example, DNA concentrations of 3.4 and 10 pM correspond to a 5- and 15-fold excess relative to the ^{M280}SP-MS, respectively.

11. During coverslip placement and edge sealing, motion of the coverslip should be minimized. At 10 μl, the deposited sample droplet should be sufficiently small that the coverslip binds tightly to the slide. If this is not the case, reduce the deposited volume.

12. Progress of the DNA-^{M280}SP-MS sample through the chamber can be observed due to the dark brown color of the ^{M280}SP-MS. If the flow rate is too low, the chamber can be tilted slightly using a pipette tip under one edge. Continued failure to obtain buffer flow is likely an indication that a larger initial droplet of AD-MS is required.

13. Samples containing TransFluoSpheres should be handled in a darkened room in order to minimize fluorophore photobleaching.

14. This step can be omitted if TransFluoSphere labeling is not required. If the step is omitted, the chamber must be flushed with fresh experimental buffer (50–100 μl) to remove untethered SP-MS before proceeding to **step 8** of Subheading 3.4.

15. The rate of nonspecific adsorption is minimized by inclusion of BSA in TetB, which passivates the surface during **step 6** of Subheading 3.4. If excessive adsorption is observed, the chamber can be washed with BCB (50–100 μl) prior to addition of the DNA-^{M280}SP-MS sample.

16. Image acquisition rate must be shorter than the characteristic relaxation time of the system (τ_0) [18]. Acquisition times longer than this will result in blurring of the microsphere image and a perceived reduction in amplitude of oscillation.

17. In each video frame, a small region of interest (ROI) is isolated round the SP-MS to be tracked. This ROI is rotated 180° and spatially shifted relative to the non-rotated ROI using image registration-based cross-correlation (*imregister.m* function; MATLAB, MathWorks) [19]. Localized SP-MS positions in adjacent frames are linked using a nearest-neighbor approach (up to user-defined spatial and temporal thresholds).

Acknowledgements

The authors would like to thank the University of York Biology Electronic and Mechanical Workshops, especially M. Bentley for custom fabrications and S.P. Howarth for stepper motor control software. CGB would like to thank H.K.H. Fung, D. Jones, D.J. Richardson, and J.F. Watson for comments on the manuscript and assistance with method development. SJC and CEB were supported by a BBSRC PhD studentship and Genetics Society Summer Studentship, respectively. T-MT construction and development was supported by the BBSRC and the Department of Biology, University of York.

References

1. De Vlaminck I, Dekker C (2012) Recent advances in magnetic tweezers. Annu Rev Biophys 41:453–472

2. Strick TR, Allemand J-F, Bensimon D, Bensimon A, Croquette V (1996) The elasticity of a single supercoiled DNA molecule. Science 271:1835–1837

3. Bryant Z, Oberstrass FC, Basu A (2012) Recent developments in single-molecule DNA mechanics. Curr Opin Struct Biol 22:304–312

4. Danilowicz C, Coljee VW, Bouzigues C, Lubensky DK, Nelson DR, Prentiss M (2003) DNA unzipping under a constant force exhibits multiple metastable intermediates. Proc Natl Acad Sci U S A 100:1694–1699

5. Graham JS, Johnson RC, Marko JF (2011) Concentration-dependent exchange accelerates turnover of proteins bound to double-stranded DNA. Nucleic Acids Res 39:2249–2259

6. Schwarz FW, Toth J, van Aelst K, Cui G, Clausing S, Szczelkun MD et al (2013) The helicase-like domains of type III restriction enzymes trigger long-range diffusion along DNA. Science 340:353–356

7. van Loenhout MTJ, de Grunt MV, Dekker C (2012) Dynamics of DNA supercoils. Science 338:94–97

8. Haber C, Wirtz D (2000) Magnetic tweezers for DNA micromanipulation. Rev Sci Instrum 71:4561–4570

9. Neuman KC, Nagy A (2008) Single-molecule force spectroscopy: optical tweezers, magnetic tweezers and atomic force microscopy. Nat Methods 5:491–505

10. Chiou C-H, Huang Y-Y, Chiang M-H, Lee H-H, Lee G-B (2006) New magnetic tweezers for investigation of the mechanical properties of single DNA molecules. Nanotechnology 17:1217–1224

11. Baumann CG, Bloomfield VA, Smith SB, Bustamante C, Wang MD, Block SM (2000) Stretching of single collapsed DNA molecules. Biophys J 78:1965–1978

12. Strick TR, Allemand J-F, Bensimon D, Croquette V (1998) Behavior of supercoiled DNA. Biophys J 74:2016–2028

13. Bustamante C, Marko JF, Siggia ED, Smith SB (1994) Entropic elasticity of lambda-phage DNA. Science 265:1599–1600

14. Baumann CG, Smith SB, Bloomfield VA, Bustamante C (1997) Ionic effects on the elasticity of single DNA molecules. Proc Natl Acad Sci U S A 94:6185–6190

15. Seol Y, Neuman KC (2011) Single-molecule measurements of topoisomerase activity with magnetic tweezers. Methods Mol Biol 778:229–241

16. Baumann CG, Cross SJ (2011) Probing the mechanics of the complete DNA transcription cycle in real-time using optical tweezers. Methods Mol Biol 778:175–191

17. Cross SJ (2013) Combining magnetic tweezers and single-molecule fluorescence microscopy to probe transcription-coupled DNA supercoiling. PhD thesis, University of York, York

18. Oliver PM, Park JS, Vezenov D (2011) Quantitative high-resolution sensing of DNA hybridization using magnetic tweezers with evanescent illumination. Nanoscale 3:581–591

19. Cheezum MK, Walker WF, Guilford WH (2001) Quantitative comparison of algorithms for tracking single fluorescent particles. Biophys J 81:2378–2388

Chapter 8

Probing Chromosome Dynamics in *Bacillus subtilis*

Alan Koh and Heath Murray

Abstract

Research over the last two decades has revealed that bacterial genomes are, in fact, highly organized. The goal of future research is to understand the molecular mechanisms underlying bacterial chromosome architecture and dynamics during the cell cycle. Here we discuss techniques that can be used with live cells to analyze chromosome structure and segregation in the gram-positive model organism *Bacillus subtilis*.

Key words Microscopy, Fluorescent protein, Chromosome, DNA replication, DNA segregation, Prokaryote

1 Introduction

Research into genome organization and dynamics was first established in eukaryotic cells where the condensation and segregation of chromosomes could be readily observed using microscopy techniques. Initial approaches with bacterial cells engendered the belief that chromosomes were compacted but largely unstructured, as they did not display the obvious hallmarks of cell cycle condensation and segregation detected in more complex organisms. However, advances in live cell fluorescence microscopy have revealed that, in fact, bacterial chromosomes are highly organized. Furthermore, recent evidence strongly suggests that bacterial genomes are actively segregated and positioned within cells to facilitate accurate genetic inheritance. Bacterial cells, with their relatively small genomes and rapid generation times, provide excellent model systems with which to understand fundamental principles of DNA organization and dynamics.

In most bacteria the critical processes of DNA replication and segregation are coupled during the cell cycle so that following initiation of DNA synthesis the two daughter origin regions are rapidly segregated away from each other [1, 2]. Newly synthesized DNA molecules are thought to be compacted and organized into

Mark C. Leake (ed.), *Chromosome Architecture: Methods and Protocols*, Methods in Molecular Biology, vol. 1431,
DOI 10.1007/978-1-4939-3631-1_8, © Springer Science+Business Media New York 2016

various domain structures to facilitate segregation [3, 4]. Although several factors have been identified that are important for bacterial chromosome organization and segregation (e.g., condensin, ParABS), deletion of such systems often result in either mild or conditional phenotypes, presumably because the overlapping nature of these processes allow the remaining systems to compensate for each other [1, 5–8]. Thus, the aims of future studies will be to identify unknown bacterial chromosome organization and segregation factors and to determine how these systems synergize to ensure accurate genome inheritance. In order to achieve these goals researchers will need tools for the characterization of DNA localization and movement within single cells. Below we describe methods to analyze DNA dynamics in the bacterium *Bacillus subtilis*, a model organism that is particularly advantageous because its chromosome can be easily manipulated using genetic engineering methods and because it has the ability to differentiate into a dormant spore which requires specific developmental regulation of its chromosome copy number and localization (Fig. 1).

The tool used most frequently to study DNA localization in living cells is the green fluorescent protein (GFP), along with its derivatives that have distinct excitation and emission properties to allow multicolor imaging (cyan = CFP, yellow = YFP, red = RFP). These reporters can be genetically fused to a protein of interest in order to assess its position within the cell. No fixation or permeabilization is required for this approach; thus, the signal detected can be observed during live cell growth and development. Although it is possible to use fluorescent intercalating dyes to stain DNA in live cells (Fig. 2a), we have found that there are several drawbacks: (a) the most commonly used stain DAPI is excited using short wavelengths of light which can damage DNA upon prolonged exposure; (b) alternative stains excited with longer wavelengths are available but more expensive; (c) most significantly we have observed that staining is often heterogeneous within a population of cells, impeding quantitative analysis.

To easily visualize the entire bacterial nucleoid, FPs can be fused to the highly abundant nucleoid associated histone-like protein (HBsu) (Fig. 2a) [9]. Coupling this with lipophilic membrane dyes (e.g., FM5-95, Nile red) allow bulk chromosome localization and dynamics to be studied in individual cells.

For more specific labeling of the *B. subtilis* chromosome at the DNA replication origin and terminus regions, the endogenous Spo0J/ParB and replication terminator protein (RTP) proteins can be tagged with FPs, respectively. These DNA binding proteins localize to multiple recognition motifs within these regions and generate a punctate fluorescent signal within cells (Fig. 3a, b) [10–12]. Furthermore, by measuring the position of the FP tagged origins/terminus or counting the number of origins within each cell; one could quickly determine the location of

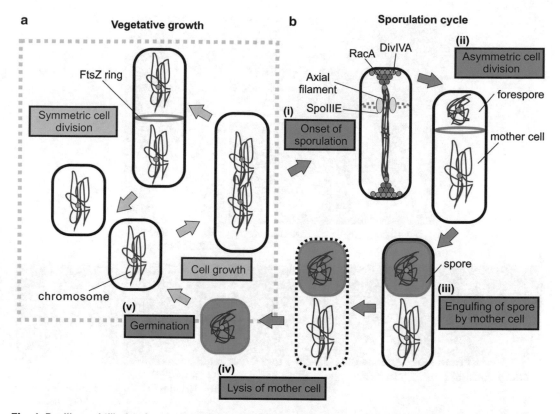

Fig. 1 *Bacillus subtilis* developmental pathways. Cartoon representation showing the different growth patterns of *Bacillus subtilis*. (**a**) Under favorable conditions, *B. subtilis* undergoes vegetative growth and divides by binary fission (*Green dotted box*). (**b**) During conditions of nutrient deprivation and high cell density, *B. subtilis* undergoes a differentiation process that involves the formation of a stress resistant spore. (*i* and *ii*) Sporulation requires a diploid state where the chromosomes form an axial filament and the replication origin regions (*green circle*) are anchored to the cell poles by RacA and DivIVA. Formation of the asymmetric septum (*orange dotted ring*) near one pole leads to the capture of ~25 % of the chromosome surrounding *oriC* in the forespore. The remaining ~75 % of the chromosome in the mother cell is then pumped into the forespore by the translocase, SpoIIIE. (*iii*) As sporulation proceeds, the forespore is engulfed by the mother cell. (*iv*) Following spore maturation the mother cell will lyse, releasing the spore into the environment. (*v*) Spores remain dormant until conditions favorable for growth are encountered, whereupon they will germinate and resume vegetative growth

these tagged regions and the rate of DNA replication initiation respectively (Fig. 3c–e).

In addition to visualizing the replication origin and terminus regions using endogenous proteins, any genetic locus of interest can be investigated by integrating arrays of operator sites that are recognized by fluorescently labeled DNA binding proteins. The two commonly used systems in *B. subtilis* are based on the repressor proteins TetR (binding *tetO*) and LacI (binding *lacO*) (Fig. 4) [13, 14]. We wish to highlight the systems constructed by the Sherratt Lab in which the repeated operator sites within the arrays are separated by randomized 10 base pair sequences to reduce

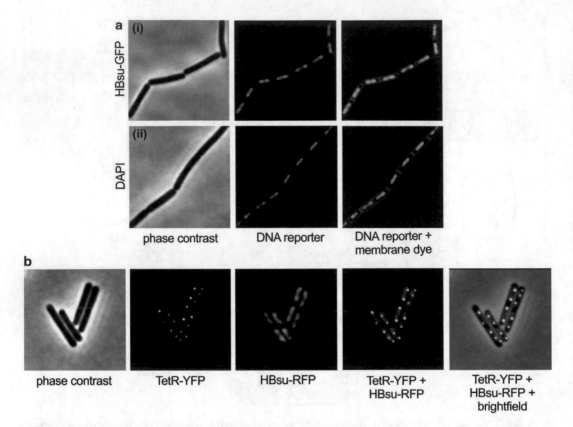

Fig. 2 Bulk chromosome localization within the cell. Strains were grown at either 30 or 37 °C until mid-exponential phase. Cell membranes were stained with FM5-95 dye to distinguish individual cells. (**a**) Bulk chromosome morphology was visualized with (*i*) the nucleoid associated DNA binding protein HBsu-GFP or (*ii*) the DNA stain DAPI. (**b**) The origin region and the nucleoid were visualized simultaneously using TetR-YFP binding to a *tetO* array (~150 operator sites) inserted near the replication origin (359°) and the nucleoid visualized with HBsu-RFP

recombination and the tetramerization domains of the repressors have been removed to prevent DNA looping [15]. Moreover, by fusing DNA binding proteins to different FPs with distinct spectral properties (e.g., GFP/RFP or CFP/YFP) allowed multiple chromosomal features to be visualized simultaneously (Fig. 5) [6, 15].

At this point it is important to note that each of the DNA labeling strategies outlined above have potential shortcomings. First, FP-tags on endogenous proteins will always alter activity to a degree, so although cell growth and chromosome organization/segregation may appear normal in an otherwise wild-type strain background, combining multiple FP-tagged proteins in one strain or combining FP-tagged proteins with other mutants may result in synthetic phenotypes [16]. Second, the repressor/operator arrays have the capacity to block replisome progression [17]. This problem can be mitigated by using arrays containing a small

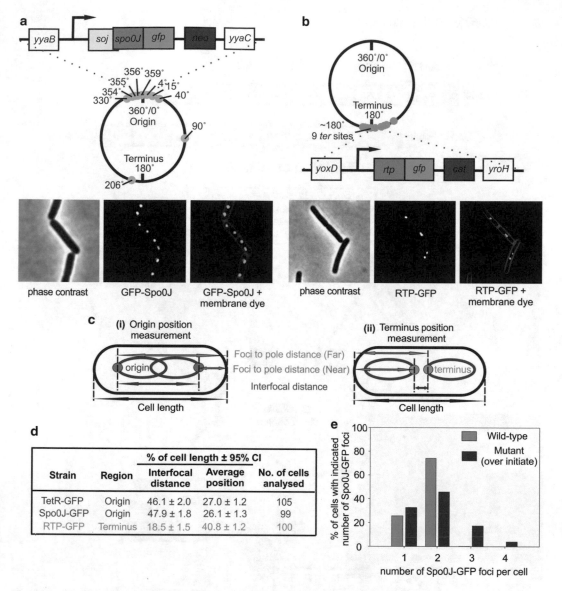

Fig. 3 Visualization of the replication origin and terminus with fluorescently labeled proteins. Strains were grown at 37 °C until exponential phase. Cell membranes were stained with FM5-95 dye to distinguish individual cells. (**a**) The origin can be visualized using SpoOJ-GFP binding to origin proximal *parS* sites (*grey dots*). The *spoOJ-gfp* fusion was expressed from its native locus at 359°. (**b**) The terminus can be visualized using RTP-GFP binding to nine *ter* sites located at the terminus region (*green dots*). The *rtp-gfp* fusion was expressed from its native locus located at 178°. (**c**) The origin/terminus localization assay was used to determine the position of each chromosome region within the long axis of the cell. The origin position was determined by visualizing the *oriC* region using either SpoOJ-GFP binding to origin proximal *parS* sites or TetR-GFP binding to a *tetO* array near the replication origin. Schematic diagrams illustrate the measurements for either the (*i*) origin or (*ii*) terminus position in cells with two foci. For a detailed explanation of the measurement, please *see* Subheading 3.6. (**d**) Quantification of origin and terminus localization within the cell. Approximately 100 cells were measured for each reporter strain. The 95 % confidence intervals for the mean were calculated. (**e**) The origin counting assay was used to determine the average rate of DNA replication initiation. Reporter strains using SpoOJ-GFP binding to origin proximal *parS* sites were grown at 37°. Cell membranes were stained with FM5-95 dye to distinguish individual cells. Qualification of SpoOJ-GFP foci per cell in the wild-type strain (*green bar*) and a mutant that overinitiates DNA replication (*red bar*) reveals the mutant phenotype (for each strain approximately 500 cells were analyzed). For a detailed explanation of the measurement, please *see* Subheading 3.7

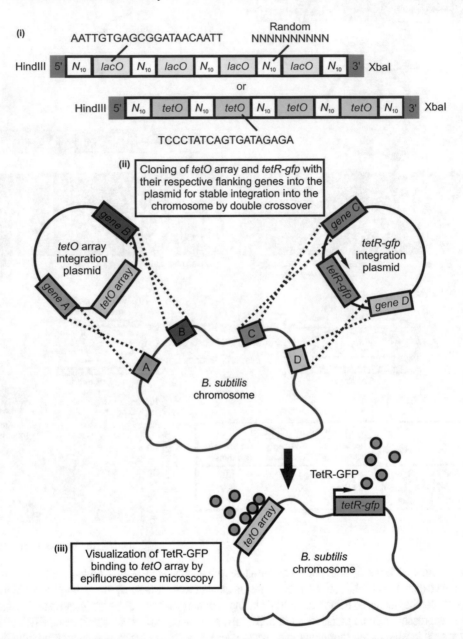

Fig. 4 Construction of the TetR/*tetO* and LacI/*lacO* reporter system in *B. subtilis*. Cartoon representation showing the construction of the reporter systems. (*i*) Organization of the *lacO/tetO* operator sequence (up to 240 operator repeats) arranged into arrays that contains 10 base pairs of randomized nucleotide sequence between each operator sequence. (*ii*) Plasmids containing either the *tetO* array or *tetR-gfp* are stably integrated into the chromosome by double-crossover. (*iii*) Successful construction allows visualization of the *tetO*-proximal locus bound by TetR-GFP using epifluorescence microscopy

number of binding sites or lowering the expression level of the FP-tagged repressor, although the trade-off is that the fluorescent signal will also be diminished. Since no single labeling technique is without caveats, it is advisable to utilize multiple approaches where possible.

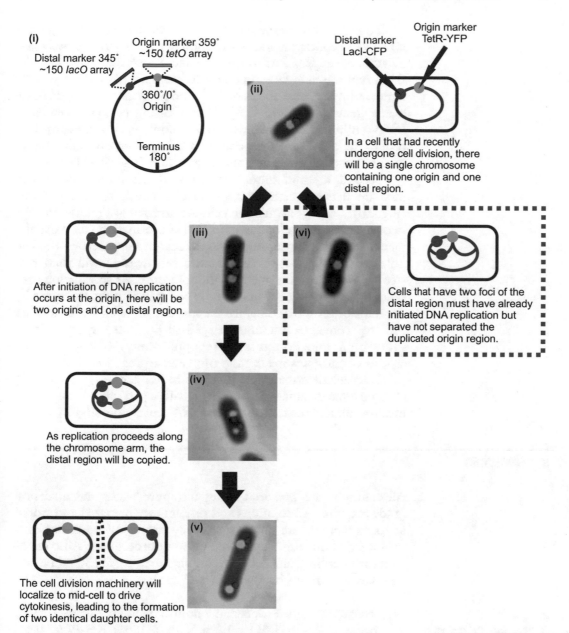

Fig. 5 The origin separation assay. Strains were grown at 30 °C in minimal growth media to avoid overlapping rounds of DNA replication. (*i*) Schematic diagram showing the location of the *tetO* array (~150) inserted near the replication origin (359°) (visualized using TetR-YFP; *green dot*) and the location of the *lacO* array (~150) inserted ~150 kb down the left chromosome arm at 345° (visualized using LacI-CFP; *red dot*). (*ii*) A newborn cell that recently underwent cell division. (*iii*) A cell has initiated DNA replication and segregated the duplicated origin regions. (*iv*) DNA replication and segregation proceeds normally. (*v*) Successful formation of two identical daughter cells. (*vi*) A cell displaying a defect in separation of sister origins

To study chromosome dynamics it can be useful to synchronize DNA replication and segregation events. There are two readily available approaches to synchronize *B. subtilis* cells. First, the DNA replication cycle can be arrested at the initiation stage using temperature sensitive alleles of initiation proteins (e.g., the helicase loader gene *dnaB134ts*) [18]. After allowing ongoing rounds of DNA synthesis and segregation to be completed, dropping the culture to the permissive temperature produces a synchronous round of chromosome replication and segregation (Fig. 6b) [19].

Second, a liquid culture of *B. subtilis* can be resuspended in medium that stimulates the sporulation developmental pathway (Fig. 1b). During sporulation cells are arrested as diploids and the two chromosomes adopt an extended conformation (the axial filament) with the chromosome origin region anchored to the cell pole by RacA [20–23]. Asymmetric cell division will then trap ~25% of the chromosome into the forespore. As sporulation proceeds the remaining chromosome is pumped into the forespore by the translocase SpoIIIE before the spore is engulfed by the mother cell to complete maturation [23–25]. Thus, synchronizing sporulation initiation offers the opportunity to study unique aspects of chromosome organization and segregation (Fig. 7b).

Here we describe methodologies in live cell imaging to study chromosome dynamics in *B. subtilis*, with a particular focus on the localization and separation of the DNA replication origin.

2 Materials

All solutions are prepared using ultrapure water and analytical grade reagents. All solutions and reagents are prepared and stored at room temperature unless specifically stated. All waste disposals were carried out using approved disposal procedures. All components are sterilized either by autoclaving at 15 psi for 30 min or for heat-labile solutions by filtering (0.45 μm).

2.1 Origin Separation, Counting, and Positioning Assay

1. Overnight culture Spizizen minimal medium (SMM) based media: 0.2% NH_4SO_4, 1.4% K_2PO_4, 0.6% KH_2PO_4, 0.1% sodium citrate dehydrate, 0.02% $MgSO_4$, 0.01 mg/ml Fe-NH_4-citrate, 6 mM $MgSO_4$, 0.1 mM $CaCl_2$, 0.13 mM $MnSO_4$, 1 μM $ZnCl_2$, 2 μM thiamine, 0.1% glutamate, 0.02 mg/ml tryptophan, 200 μg/ml casein hydrolysate, 2.0% succinate, and inducers as needed (1 μg/ml tetracycline, 500 ng/ml anhydrotetracycline, or 1 mM IPTG).

2. SMM based media supplemented with the following carbon source: 2% succinate for slow growth, 2% glucose for medium growth or 2% glucose + 200 μg/ml casein hydrolysate for fast growth. Note that no inducer should be added into the fresh media.

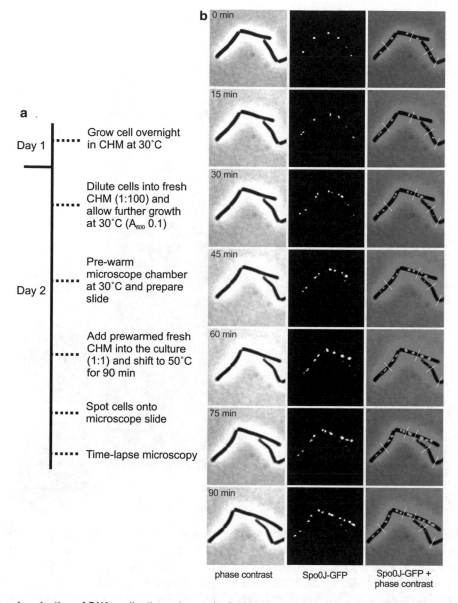

a

Day 1 ..... Grow cell overnight in CHM at 30°C

..... Dilute cells into fresh CHM (1:100) and allow further growth at 30°C (A$_{600}$ 0.1)

Day 2 ..... Pre-warm microscope chamber at 30°C and prepare slide

..... Add prewarmed fresh CHM into the culture (1:1) and shift to 50°C for 90 min

..... Spot cells onto microscope slide

..... Time-lapse microscopy

b 0 min / 15 min / 30 min / 45 min / 60 min / 75 min / 90 min

phase contrast   Spo0J-GFP   Spo0J-GFP + phase contrast

Fig. 6 Synchronization of DNA replication using a *dnaB134ts* mutant and localization of the replication origin using Spo0J-GFP. (**a**) Experimental overview showing the major steps involved in synchronizing DNA replication in a *dnaB134ts* mutant. For a detailed explanation of the procedure, *see* Subheading 3.2. (**b**) The origin region was visualized using Spo0J-GFP binding to origin proximal *parS* sites in a *dnaB134ts* mutant after synchronizing DNA replication. Cells were imaged every 15 min after shifting to the permissible temperature (30 °C), displaying a synchronous increase in Spo0J-GFP foci per cell as replication proceeds. A *white line* (−) denotes boundary between cells

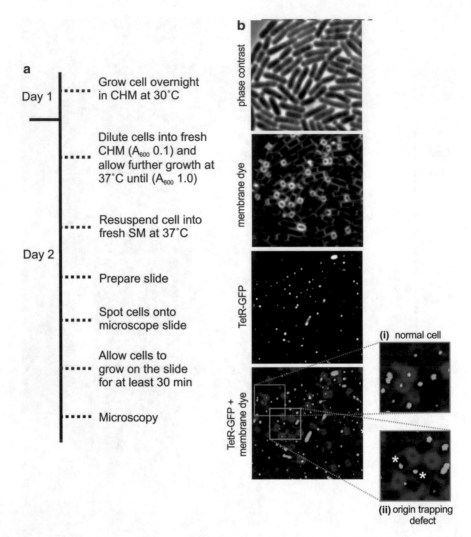

Fig. 7 The replication origin trapping assay during sporulation using the TetR/*tetO* reporter system. (**a**) Experimental overview showing the major steps involved in the sporulation assay. For a detailed explanation of the procedure, *see* Subheading 3.3. (**b**) The origin region was localized by visualizing TetR-GFP binding to a *tetO* array (~25) inserted near the replication origin (353°). TetR-GFP localization was determined during sporulation of *B. subtilis* cells 120 min post resuspension in sporulation medium. Cell membranes were stained with FM5-95 dye to identify individual cells undergoing spore development. Enlarged images highlight cells displaying either (*i*) normal origin localization or (*ii*) origin trapping defects (denoted with an *asterisk*)

3. Test-tubes or 125 ml conical flasks.

4. Shaking incubator with temperature setting.

2.2 Sporulation Assay

1. Casein hydrolysate media (CHM): 1% casein hydrolysate, 0.46% L-glutamic acid sodium salt, 0.13% L-alanine, 0.14% L-asparagine, 0.14% KH_2PO_4, 0.05% NH_4Cl, 0.01% Na_2SO_4, 0.01% NH_4NO_3, 0.98 mg $FeCl_3 \cdot 6H_2O$ and adjusted

to pH 7.0 with NaOH or HCl. After that add 0.1 mM $CaCl_2$, 0.4 mM $MgSO_4$, 0.13 mM $MnSO_4$, 0.02 mg/ml tryptophan and inducers as needed (1 µg/ml tetracycline, 500 ng/ml anhydrotetracycline, or 1 mM IPTG).

2. Sporulation salts solution (Solution A): 4 mM $FeCl_3$, 40 mM $MgSO_4$, and 100 mM $MgCl_2$.

3. Sporulation salts solution (Solution B): 1 M NH_4Cl, 75 mM Na_2SO_4, 50 mM KH_2PO_4, and 120 mM NH_4NO_3 adjusted to pH 7.0 with HCl or NaOH. Sterile filter both solutions and store at 4 °C.

4. Sporulation salts solution (Solution A + B): Mix 1 ml of solution A with 10 ml of solution B and top up with water to make 1 L. Autoclave the sporulation salts solution.

5. Sporulation media (SM): Sporulation salts (solution A + B) supplemented with 0.2% glutamate, 1 mM $CaCl_2$, 40 mM $MgSO_4$, and 0.02 mg/ml tryptophan.

6. Test tubes or 125 ml conical flasks.

7. Shaking incubator with temperature setting.

2.3 General Microscopy

1. Prepare ~1.5% agarose gel in the media that is used for the cell culture (*see* **Notes 1** and **2**).

2. Prepare 200 µg/ml of stock FM5-95 membrane dye and mix it with the molten agarose to a final concentration of 0.5 µg/ml (*see* **Note 3**).

3. If desired prepare 10 µg/ml of stock DAPI stain and mix it with cells to stain the DNA to a final concentration of 0.6 µg/ml.

4. Multi-spot microscope slide (Fig. 8a) or a Gene Frame (Life Technologies, cat no: AB-0578; 17 mm × 28 mm) mounted on a clear microscope slide (Fig. 8b).

5. Glass coverslip.

6. Surgical scalpel blades.

7. Prepare 70% ethanol.

8. Epifluorescence microscope with appropriate filter sets.

9. METAMORPH software (version V.6.2r6) for image capture.

10. ImageJ software (1.49n) can be downloaded at the following URL: http://imagej.nih.gov/ij/.

11. ImageJ plugin for cell counter can be downloaded at the following URL: http://imagej.nih.gov/ij/plugins/cell-counter.html.

12. ImageJ plugin for ObjectJ can be downloaded at the following URL: https://sils.fnwi.uva.nl/bcb/objectj/.

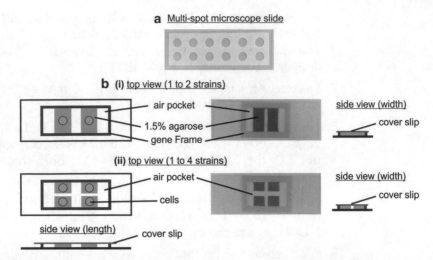

Fig. 8 Layout of a multi-spot microscope slide and a gene frame on a microscope slide. (**a**) Image showing a multi-spot microscope slide. (**b**) Schematic diagrams showing the layout of a gene frame microscope slide for either (*i*) two or (*ii*) four different strains. Note that the agarose pads have been stained with brilliant blue dye to allow their visualization in the images shown

3 Methods

3.1 Growth Conditions for Origin Separation, Counting, and Positioning Assay

1. To visualize cells during exponential growth, 2 ml of starter culture is grown overnight at either 30 or 37 °C in SMM based media (*see* **Notes 4–8**).

2. The next day, 1 ml cultures are washed twice with fresh SMM based media to remove any remaining inducer molecules (this step can be skipped if no inducer is used for the overnight culture).

3. Dilute culture 1:100 into fresh SMM based media supplemented with 2.0% succinate, 2.0% glucose, or 2.0% glucose + 200 µg/ml casein hydrolysate (*see* **Notes 9–11**).

4. Allow cultures to achieve at least three mass doublings (A_{600} 0.3–0.5) before observation by microscopy (*see* Subheadings 3.4 and 3.5).

3.2 Synchronization of DNA Replication

1. To visualize a synchronized DNA replication and segregation cycle, 5 ml of starter culture is grown overnight at the permissible temperature of 30 °C in CHM with inducer as needed (*see* **Notes 4–8**) (Fig. 6a; flowchart).

2. The next day, 1 ml cultures are washed twice with fresh CHM to remove any remaining inducer molecule (this step can be skipped if no inducer is used for the overnight) before being diluted 1:100 into fresh CHM.

3. At an A_{600} of 0.1, 5 ml of fresh CHM that has been prewarmed to 70 °C is added into the culture. This will rapidly equilibrate

the culture temperature to the nonpermissive temperature (~50 °C) and allow further growth at this temperature for 90 min to allow ongoing rounds of replication to complete.

4. To initiate DNA replication, the culture is shifted back to the permissible temperature (30 °C).

5. Observe DNA replication by microscopy (*see* Subheadings 3.4 and 3.5).

3.3 Sporulation Assay

1. To visualize cells during sporulation, 2 ml of starter culture is grown overnight at 30 °C in CHM media (*see* **Notes 4** and **8**) (Fig. 7a; flowchart).

2. The next day the overnight cultures are diluted into 2 ml of fresh CHM media to achieve a starting A_{600} of 0.1, and then incubated at 37 °C until they reach an A_{600} of 1.0.

3. The cultures are then centrifuged at $16,000 \times g$ for 10 min and the cell pellet is resuspended in 2 ml of fresh SM.

4. Transfer 2 ml of the resuspended culture back into the same test tube to induce sporulation according to the resuspension method of Sterlini and Mandelstam [26] and modified by Partridge and Errington [27] for at least 120 min before observation by microscopy (*see* Subheadings 3.4 and 3.5).

3.4 Preparation of Multi-spot Microscope Slide

1. Clean the multi-spot microscope slide with 70 % ethanol and ensure that it is dry and free of dust.

2. Pipette 750 μl of molten agarose onto the middle of the slide. Ensure that there is no air bubble in the agarose as this might interfere with how the agarose pad will harden (*see* **Note 12**).

3. Quickly place a standard microscope slide on top of the molten agarose and squeeze any excess agarose out by gently pressing down on the slide (*see* **Note 13**).

4. Allow the agarose pad to harden. This normally takes about 5 min (*see* **Note 14**).

5. Carefully remove the standard microscope slide on top of the multi-spot microscope slide to reveal the agarose.

6. Pipette ~1 μl of cell culture onto the agarose pad (*see* **Note 15**).

7. Air-dry to allow the media to absorb into the pad. This normally takes about 5 min (*see* **Note 14**).

8. Place a clean coverslip on top of the cells (*see* **Note 16**).

9. The microscope sample is now ready for imaging (Table 1).

3.5 Preparation of Microscope Slide (Gene Frame)

1. Clean the microscope slide with 70 % ethanol and ensure that it is dry and free of dust.

2. Carefully remove the plastic cover from the gene frame (i.e., the side with the solid plastic covering the whole gene frame) which will reveal the sticky pad.

Table 1
Suggested growth conditions and exposure times for fluorescent reporters

Fluorophore	Array size	Average exposure time	Optimum growth temperature (°C)	Repressor/Reagent concentration
TetR-GFP TetR-YFP	~25 tetO ~150 tetO	3–5 s 5 s	30–37 30	Tetracycline (1 μg/ml) or Anhydrotetracycline (500 ng/ml)
LacI-CFP	~150 lacO	5 s	30–37	IPTG (1 mM)
Spo0J-GFP	parS sites	3–5 s	30–37	Nil
RTP-GFP	ter sites	5 s	30–37	Nil
DAPI	Chromosome	3–5 s	30–37	DAPI (0.6 μg/ml)
HBsu-GFP	Chromosome	3–5 s	30–37	Nil
HBsu-RFP	Chromosome	3–5 s	30–37	Nil
FM5-95	Cell membrane	3 s	Nil	Add FM5-95 (0.5 μg/ml to agarose)
Brightfield	Whole cell	10 ms	Nil	Nil

Table showing the suggested growth conditions and exposure times for each fluorescent reporter used in this paper

3. Attach the gene frame with the sticky pad onto the middle of a standard microscope slide. Use the edge of a pen and move along the frame ensuring that there are no air bubbles between the frame and the slide (note that the upper side of the sticky gene frame will remain covered with a plastic mask).

4. Pipette 500 μl of molten agarose onto the middle of the gene frame. Ensure that the agarose exceeds the volume of the gene frame and that there are no air bubbles in the agarose (*see* **Note 12**).

5. Quickly place a standard microscope slide on top of the molten agarose. Squeeze excess agarose out by gently pressing down on the slide (*see* **Note 13**).

6. To harden the agarose, place the gene frame horizontally into a petri dish that contains a small ball of wet tissue (to prevent desiccation). Cover the petri dish and store it in the refrigerator at 4 °C for at least 30 min (*see* **Note 14**).

7. To prepare the slides for microscopy, warm the microscope slides by shifting the petri dishes into the desired temperature (depending on experimental requirements) for at least 30 min (*see* **Note 12**).

8. Carefully remove the clear microscope slide on top of the gene frame to reveal the agarose (*see* **Note 14**).

9. To provide a source of oxygen create air pockets using a scalpel to cut out agar strips (Fig. 8b).

10. Pipette ~1 μl of cell culture onto the agarose pad (*see* **Note 15**).

11. Air-dry to allow the media to absorb into the pad. This normally takes about 5 min (*see* **Note 14**).

12. Remove the mask from the gene frame and firmly attach a clean coverslip, ensuring no gaps are present (*see* **Note 16**).

13. The microscope sample is now ready for imaging (Table 1).

14. For time lapse microscopy incubate the prepared microscope slide at the desired temperature for at least **30 min**.

15. The microscopy chambers should also be prewarmed to the desired temperature for at least 1 h before commencing the time lapse experiment.

3.6 Measurement of Focus Position Within Cells with Two Foci (Replication Origin and Terminus Positioning)

1. Cells are grown as described in (Subheading 3.1).

2. ImageJ software with ObjectJ plugin was utilized for determining the focus position within the cell (Fig. 3c).

3. For each cell, the focus closest to an arbitrarily selected pole was designated "near", and the other focus was designated "far". Three measurements were made: (a) the distance from the pole to the center of the proximal focus (near); (b) the distance from the same pole to the center of the distal focus (far); and (c) the distance between the two poles (cell length).

4. To determine the position of the near focus within the cell, the measured distance was divided by the cell length and multiplied by 100 to give the focus position as a percentage of cell length. To determine the position of the far focus within the cell, the measured distance was subtracted from the cell length before being divided by the cell length, then multiplied by 100 to give the focus position as a percentage of cell length. These numbers were averaged for all cells in a sample. The 95 % confidence intervals for the mean were calculated.

5. Interfocal distance was calculated by subtracting the position of the near focus from the far focus, then dividing by cell length and multiplying by 100 to give the interfocal distance as a percentage of cell length. These numbers were averaged for all cells in a sample. The 95 % confidence intervals for the mean were calculated.

3.7 Counting the Number of Different Class of Cells (Origin Separation) and the Number of Origin per Cell (Origin Counting)

1. Cells are growth as described in (Subheading 3.1).

2. ImageJ software with cell counter plugin was utilized to determine the number of different type of cells or the number of origins per cell.

4   Notes

1. Minimize the use of complex media such as PAB, LB, and CH, which produce high autofluorescence. While minimal media has a lower autofluorescence level.

2. Always prepare fresh agarose solution on the day of the experiment and ensure that the agarose is completely dissolved to prevent agarose crystallization and store the solution at ~60 °C to prevent it from solidifying.

3. Mix the membrane dye with the agarose solution ~1 h before the anticipated microscopy session; in our hands this produces the most uniform straining. Note that exposing the dye to light and high temperature will reduce its efficacy over time.

4. *B. subtilis* requires thorough aeration for optimum growth and development; therefore ensure vigorous shaking of the culture. Normally a >1:20 ratio (culture volume–container volume) is desired.

5. Maintain and grow overnight culture of strains that harbor the large ~150 *tetO* array with 1 μg/ml tetracycline (only if the strain is resistance to tetracycline) or 500 ng/ml anhydrotetracycline and large ~150 *lacO* array with 1 mM IPTG to inhibit TetR and LacI binding to its operator sites, respectively.

6. Use fresh colonies streaked onto nutrient agar plates for each experiment.

7. Allow strains that exhibit slower growth rates a longer overnight incubation period to allow the overnight culture to achieve a high density.

8. Prewarm media before use to prevent temperature shock to the bacteria.

9. Care should be taken to prevent *B. subtilis* from entering the sporulation developmental pathway as this could interfere with the positioning of the chromosome and thus the origin.

10. There is a positive correlation between DNA replication initiation and nutrient-mediated growth rates. Therefore in complex media such as PAB, LB, and CH, cells undergo faster growth rate as compared to minimal media supplemented with the various type of carbon sources.

11. Media such as minimal media which support slower growth rate will result in cells having fewer origins/chromosomes per cell, therefore making analysis less complicated.

12. Reduce exposing the sample and the microscope slide to rapid temperature changes. Try to do all steps in the desired experimental temperature.

13. Ensure that the agarose pad is evenly spread onto the microscope slide to achieve best imagining for the field of cells. To achieve this, it is recommended that the gene frame be used.

14. Avoid exposing the agarose pad to the external environment for too long as this will cause excessive drying.

15. Agitate the culture before removing samples for imaging to reduce cells from clumping together.

16. To prevent air bubbles from accumulating under the coverslip, use the edge of the pen and moves it firmly from one end of the coverslip to the other. This will force any air pockets between the coverslip and agarose pad out.

Acknowledgement

This work was supported by a grant from the BBSRC (BB/K017527/1) and a Royal Society University Research Fellowship to H.M.

References

1. Wang XD, Llopis PM, Rudner DZ (2014) *Bacillus subtilis* chromosome organization oscillates between two distinct patterns. Proc Natl Acad Sci U S A 111:12877–12882

2. Viollier PH, Thanbichler M, Mcgrath PT et al (2004) Rapid and sequential movement of individual chromosomal loci to specific subcellular locations during bacterial DNA replication. Proc Natl Acad Sci U S A 101:9257–9262

3. Mercier R, Petit MA, Schbath S et al (2008) The MatP/*matS* site-specific system organizes the terminus region of the *E. coli* chromosome into a macrodomain. Cell 135:475–485

4. Valens M, Penaud S, Rossignol M et al (2004) Macrodomain organization of the *Escherichia coli* chromosome. EMBO J 23:4330–4341

5. Ireton K, Gunther NW, Grossman AD (1994) Spo0j is required for normal chromosome segregation as well as the initiation of sporulation in *Bacillus subtilis*. J Bacteriol 176:5320–5329

6. Lee PS, Grossman AD (2006) The chromosome partitioning proteins Soj (ParA) and Spo0J (ParB) contribute to accurate chromosome partitioning, separation of replicated sister origins, and regulation of replication initiation in *Bacillus subtilis*. Mol Microbiol 60:853–869

7. Gruber S, Veening JW, Bach J et al (2014) Interlinked sister chromosomes arise in the absence of condensin during fast replication in *B. subtilis*. Curr Biol 24:293–298

8. Britton RA, Lin DC, Grossman AD (1998) Characterization of a prokaryotic SMC protein involved in chromosome partitioning. Gene Dev 12:1254–1259

9. Kohler P, Marahiel MA (1997) Association of the histone-like protein HBsu with the nucleoid of *Bacillus subtilis*. J Bacteriol 179:2060–2064

10. Lee PS, Lin DCH, Moriya S et al (2003) Effects of the chromosome partitioning protein Spo0J (ParB) on *oriC* of positioning and replication initiation *Bacillus subtilis*. J Bacteriol 185:1326–1337

11. Teleman AA, Graumann PL, Lin DCH et al (1998) Chromosome arrangement within a bacterium. Curr Biol 8:1102–1109

12. Lin DC, Levin PA, Grossman AD (1997) Bipolar localization of a chromosome partition protein in *Bacillus subtilis*. Proc Natl Acad Sci U S A 94:4721–4726

13. Dworkin J, Losick R (2002) Does RNA polymerase help drive chromosome segregation in bacteria? Proc Natl Acad Sci U S A 99:14089–14094

14. Gordon GS, Sitnikov D, Webb CD et al (1997) Chromosome and low copy plasmid segregation in *E. coli*: visual evidence for distinct mechanisms. Cell 90:1113–1121

15. Lau IF, Filipe SR, Soballe B et al (2003) Spatial and temporal organization of replicating *Escherichia coli* chromosomes. Mol Microbiol 49:731–743

16. Gruber S, Errington J (2009) Recruitment of condensin to replication origin regions by ParB/Spo0J promotes chromosome segregation in *B. subtilis*. Cell 137:685–696

17. Possoz C, Filipe SR, Grainge I et al (2006) Tracking of controlled *Escherichia coli* replication fork stalling and restart at repressor-bound DNA *in vivo*. EMBO J 25:2596–2604

18. Mendelson NH, Gross JD (1967) Characterization of a temperature-sensitive mutant of *Bacillus subtilis* defective in deoxyribonucleic acid replication. J Bacteriol 94:1603–1608

19. Su'etsugu M, Errington J (2011) The replicase sliding clamp dynamically accumulates behind progressing replication forks in *Bacillus subtilis* cells. Mol Cell 41:720–732

20. Ben-Yehuda S, Fujita M, Liu XS et al (2005) Defining a centromere-like element in *Bacillus subtilis* by identifying the binding sites for the chromosome-anchoring protein RacA. Mol Cell 17:773–782

21. Ben-Yehuda S, Rudner DZ, Losick R (2003) RacA, a bacterial protein that anchors chromosomes to the cell poles. Science 299:532–536

22. Wu LJ, Errington J (2003) RacA and the Soj-Spo0J system combine to effect polar chromosome segregation in sporulating *Bacillus subtilis*. Mol Microbiol 49:1463–1475

23. Wu LJ, Errington J (1994) *Bacillus subtilis* SpoIIIE protein required for DNA segregation during asymmetric cell-division. Science 264:572–575

24. Bath J, Wu LJ, Errington J et al (2000) Role of Bacillus subtilis SpoIIIE in DNA transport across the mother cell-prespore division septum. Science 290:995–997

25. Wu LJ, Errington J (1997) Septal localization of the SpoIIIE chromosome partitioning protein in *Bacillus subtilis*. EMBO J 16:2161–2169

26. Sterlini JM, Mandelstam J (1969) Commitment to sporulation in *Bacillus subtilis* and its relationship to development of actinomycin resistance. Biochem J 113:29–37

27. Partridge SR, Errington J (1993) The importance of morphological events and intercellular interactions in the regulation of prespore-specific gene expression during sporulation in *Bacillus subtilis*. Mol Microbiol 8:945–955

Chapter 9

Systems Biology Approaches for Understanding Genome Architecture

Sven Sewitz and Karen Lipkow

Abstract

The linear and three-dimensional arrangement and composition of chromatin in eukaryotic genomes underlies the mechanisms directing gene regulation. Understanding this organization requires the integration of many data types and experimental results. Here we describe the approach of integrating genome-wide protein–DNA binding data to determine chromatin states. To investigate spatial aspects of genome organization, we present a detailed description of how to run stochastic simulations of protein movements within a simulated nucleus in 3D. This systems level approach enables the development of novel questions aimed at understanding the basic mechanisms that regulate genome dynamics.

Key words Genome organization, Systems biology, Stochastic spatial simulations, Hidden Markov models, Chromatin states

1 Introduction

Eukaryotic gene regulation is a process dependent on a large number of proteins and epigenetic marks [1] occurring on the complex three-dimensional structure of the stochastic yet organized genome [2]. This regulatory complexity is evident from the fact that many gene regulatory events are hard to attribute to the specific functions of individual proteins or histone modifications. For this reason, the concept of chromatin states is gaining increasing adoption in understanding the mechanisms responsible for gene regulation during normal growth, development, or cancer [3, 4]. Additionally, 3D genome organization is known to be important in regulating gene expression [5, 6] and alterations therein lead to severe disease [7]. Both methods described here focus on protein–DNA interactions.

Mark C. Leake (ed.), *Chromosome Architecture: Methods and Protocols*, Methods in Molecular Biology, vol. 1431,
DOI 10.1007/978-1-4939-3631-1_9, © Springer Science+Business Media New York 2016

1.1 Chromatin States Chromatin describes the nuclear fiber composed of DNA, histones, and a large variety of other proteins that bind DNA, either sequence specifically or sequence nonspecifically. Their function can broadly be described as being important for gene regulation. Their molecular functions are diverse, ranging from sequence specific transcription factors (TFs), to ATP-dependent chromatin remodelers, protein components of the transcription machinery, initiation factors, and chromatin modifiers, that together regulate chromatin structure and accessibility of genetic features such as promoters and enhancers [6]. Together, these factors are called "chromatin associated proteins". The structure and detailed composition of the chromatin fiber has been investigated for decades, with different models for the structure being proposed [8, 9]. The reason for the fact that no unequivocal structure has been determined lies in the diverse nature of the fiber, which, depending on regulatory state, can adopt different conformations and be bound by different proteins. Some consensus has emerged, with for example constitutive promoters adopting "open" promoter structures, and regulated genes being described as having "covered" promoters [10]. Due to the regulatory complexity inherent in eukaryotic transcription, it is not surprising that these functions are mediated by different sets of proteins. The analysis of this complexity is challenging, and has resulted in the concept of chromatin states. Here, the distinct pattern of histone marks or binding of chromatin-associated proteins is classified computationally [11–13]. A lot of research has focused on the distribution of histone modifications to identify regulatory elements [14], or to determine co-regulated or active genes [15], and these methods have been applied to data from numerous organisms [11–13]. Chromatin states derived from data of eight histone modifications, DNAse hypersensitivity sites and locations of CTCF binding can now be accessed through the Ensembl Regulatory Build [16]. This is indication that there is growing understanding that chromatin states represent a valid and important approach to understanding the above-mentioned biological processes. In addition, chromatin states have been speculatively linked to 3D genome organization [17].

The methods described here are an alternative approach to arriving at chromatin states. They do not rely on histone modification data, but start with genome-wide binding patterns for chromatin associated proteins. Both approaches have been shown to result in a classification of the genome that lends itself to further fruitful analysis [18, 19]: Chromatin states are characterized by covering genes that are co-regulated or belong to similar gene ontologies, and share similar expression patterns. For a meaningful characterization, the number of histone modifications that need to be queried is much lower than the number of proteins. But only by using protein–DNA binding data does one retain the relative levels of protein occupancy at a given locus. This has unique advantages that result in the ability to perform significantly different downstream analyses (*see* Subheading 3.1.5).

1.2 Spatial Organization

A rapidly expanding field is the study of three dimensional aspects of nuclear genome architecture [20–22]. In particular, the movement of transcription factors (TFs) within the genome has been intensely studied, experimentally [23–25], theoretically [26], and, more recently, computationally [27–29]. The movement of transcription factors occurs by four basic modes of motion: (a) 1D diffusion along DNA, (b) 3D Brownian diffusion, (c) intersegmental transfer, and (d) hopping [26]. From an observer's point of view, these modes of motion can be differentiated by their distance dependence. In 1D diffusion, the time a TF takes to find its target gene (TG) is a function of the linear distance, and scales with the square of this distance [30]. As a result, sequences located in close proximity to the DNA-bound TF are found relatively quickly, while sequences at greater distances are reached at progressively longer times. It is thus an inefficient way to locate DNA sequences on a genome scale. Diffusion in 3D, on the other hand, is effectively distance independent. This means that the time to locate a given target site is not a function of the distance between binding site and target site. It is the slowest form of motion, but allows equal access to all binding sites within the genome [31–33]. It is most effective to combine all four modes of motion [29].

Spatial, particle-based simulations provide a good means to quantitatively analyze which aspects of nuclear architecture, and which properties of nuclear proteins, have a significant effect on the efficiency of proteins to move among the chromosomes and find their target sequences [29]. We here describe the use of Smoldyn, which is the most advanced and accurate particle-based simulator. Each molecule of the system is modeled as a point, which diffuses and reacts with other molecules and surfaces much as real molecules do. Space is continuous, rather than a lattice, and can be structured with the aid of surfaces. Using Smoldyn, we recently determined the length of the antenna effect on finding of target genes, which coincided with the length of the nucleosome free region (NFR) at eukaryotic promoters [29].

2 Materials

2.1 R packages Required for the Determination of Chromatin States

The implementation of the Baum–Welch algorithm and the method to derive the Viterbi-path are contained in an R package available on GitHub (https://www.github.com/guillaume/HMMt/) [18]. This implementation runs on UNIX based systems (Mac OS X, Linux). Methods for data normalization are contained within the Limma package [34], and are available via Bioconductor [35]. In addition, the HMMt implementation requires scripts to preprocess the data, such as averaging duplicate samples and running of the binary HMM. These scripts, developed for ChIP-chip data from yeast, will be available upon request (Sewitz et al., in preparation).

2.2 Software for Spatial Simulations

Smoldyn is open-source, publicly available, and multi-platform (Mac OS X, Linux, or Windows). Smoldyn simulations benefit from fast processors, but require only moderate amounts of RAM. The Smoldyn software and documentation can be downloaded free of charge from Steve Andrews' website: www.smoldyn.org.

In addition, general tools for programming and visualization are necessary, namely

- A Terminal application.
- A text editor for programming with line numbers and paths, such as TextWrangler or Sublime Text.
- A scripting language for creating arrays of molecule or surface positions, such as perl, Python, C (optional).
- Data analysis software such as MATLAB, Octave, R, or Mathematica; simple spreadsheets are not recommended.
- Media software such as QuickTime Pro for creating movies (optional).

---

3 Methods

3.1 Determination of Chromatin States

The starting point for the analyses described here are genome-wide protein occupancy data of chromatin-associated proteins. The source can be ChIP-chip data, ChIP-seq data, or DamID data. Depending on the nature of the experiment, the raw data will either be $\log_2$-enrichment values or read counts per binding site. The methods described below are applicable to raw data from ChIP-chip experiments. For the analysis of ChIP-seq or DamID data, the same general principles apply [16, 18], but the details of the methodology have to be adapted and are not described here.

3.1.1 Raw Data Normalization

The raw data is used as a matrix of $\log_2$-ratios (with antibody: without); protein names are column headers and genomic locations are row headers. The first step is to average replicate probes. Limma [36] is then used to perform background correction and loess normalization.

3.1.2 Principal Component Analysis

The data from a typical experiment consists of signals from several thousand hybridization probes and dozens to hundreds of proteins (Fig. 1a). To reduce the dimensionality of this data, while preserving the maximum of information, principal component analysis

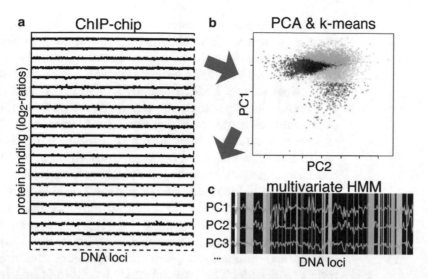

Fig. 1 Overview of the computational steps to determine chromatin states. (**a**) The log$_2$-enrichment values of the DNA bound proteins are taken for PCA analysis. (**b**) A selection of principal components (PC) is k-means clustered. (**c**) The clustered PCs (*grey lines*) are the emission values analyzed by a multivariate Hidden Markov Model (HMM). The chromatin states are then mapped back onto the genome (shown as colors along the *x*-axis of genomic loci)

(PCA) of the data has to be applied. Different implementations exist. We used R, and the function prcomp, which is part of the base {stats} package. The eigenvectors are contained in the $rotation matrix of the prcomp object, and are needed for clustering and the Hidden Markov Model (*see* below, Subheadings 3.1.3 and 3.1.4).

It is essential to optimize both the number of principal components (c) and the number of states (K) for the HMM. To achieve this, we performed the entire analysis with a varying number of PCs and states and optimized for maximum difference in the fraction bound values, described below (Subheading 3.1.5).

3.1.3 K-Means Clustering and Initialization

The matrix of the first c principal components has to be k-means clustered. This is done using the R function kmeans, with K, the number of states, being a user-defined variable. This results in all datapoints belonging to one cluster appearing as an individual lobe or cloud in a scatterplot of the PCs. In Fig. 1b, the positions of the points are determined by the PCA, while the colors of the lobes are determined by k-means clustering.

From the k-means results, two types of matrices are required for initialization of the segmentation: (1) The [$K \times c$] mean matrix is accessed by calling $centers on the kmeans result. (2) The [$c \times c$] correlation matrices are calculated for each of the K clouds using the cor function, which is supplied with the R {stats} package.

3.1.4 Segmentation of the Genome Using a Hidden Markov Model

The values of the principal component analysis are specific to each position of a chip-probe: At each genomic location where a chip-probe is located, we now have a vector of the values of the c first principal components, calculated from the $\log_2$-values of the protein occupancy. The chromatin state at each position is the hidden variable that we wish to determine, and the c principal component values are the observed values. These are the assumptions when using a Hidden Markov Model (HMM) and allow us to computationally recognize patterns that arise from the binding of a group of proteins. A discrete-time Markov chain models a process as a series of states with a transition matrix defining the probability of moving from one state to another. An HMM extends this basic concept by allowing each state to output, with a defined probability, a hidden value (single variable) or hidden values (multivariate). In our application, the equivalent notion of a time step are discrete positions on the genome (Fig. 1c). In this case, the c principal component values PC1, PC2, ... PCc are the (multivariate, continuous) output signals, also called emissions, that the HMM is trying to decode. The Baum–Welch algorithm is one method to derive the hidden state from multivariate values [37, 38].

An implementation of the Baum–Welch algorithm exists as the function BaumWelchT in the R package HMMt [18]. It estimates the model parameters that are most likely to have generated the observed outputs, and determines the most probable sequence of states. This sequence is known as the Viterbi path [39] and is accessible through the $ViterbiPath variable, contained in the result of the BaumWelchT function. This completes the segmentation of the genome into chromatin states.

3.1.5 Distribution of Proteins Between Chromatin States

The successful definition of chromatin states and the assignment of each gene locus to one of the states enable a large number of subsequent analyses. For example, gene expression levels of the genes in each state can be queried, and patterns of histone modifications, or the gene ontology of the genes of a given state can be determined. This type of analysis helps to understand what differentiates the states. Additionally, when the states have been determined from protein binding data as here, the same raw dataset can be queried to calculate the distribution of proteins between chromatin states. It is insightful to determine the fraction of loci of each state that are bound by a particular protein. This fraction is characteristic for each protein, and shows the composition of a chromatin state.

The first step is to convert the $\log_2$-ratios into binary information, determining whether a locus is bound or not bound by a particular protein. To achieve this, a 2-state (binary) HMM is used to classify a protein's binding profile into regions of bound and unbound. This provides a probabilistic model, where the state at a given genomic position is dependent on the state at the previous position. This results in the noisy ChIP-chip-data being discretized, and produces more robust results with respect to protein localization (Fig. 2). The HMM is parameterized by a 2×2 transition matrix containing the probabilities of changing binding state, or

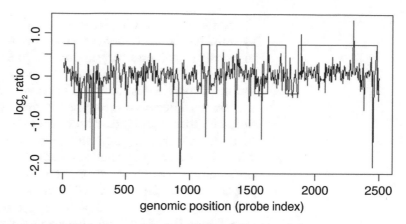

Fig. 2 Determination of the bound or unbound state of chromosomal loci. The experimental log$_2$-ratios of binding for one factor are shown across a segment of chromatin (*black lines*). Superimposed in *red* are the binary values from the two-state HMM, indicating whether the protein was calculated to be either bound (high value) or unbound (low value)

staying in the same binding state. Setting a probability of 0.9 down the diagonal of the transition matrix ensures that once in a bound (unbound) state, there is a greater probability of staying in that state. This binary HMM is run independently for each protein's binding profile. This results in a matrix, with proteins as column headers and chip-probe locations as row headers, containing values 0 and 1 corresponding to being either unbound or bound.

To calculate the fraction bound, the results from the binary HMM (above) and the state HMM (Subheading 3.1.4) are combined: First, the number of gene loci of a given state that a given protein binds to is counted. This is then divided by the total number of gene loci in that state. Each protein factor will be bound to a particular percentage of all loci of one state, and this percentage varies for each protein. Comparisons can now be made between factors, and also between states.

3.2 Spatial Simulations

In the previous sections we described bioinformatic methods to analyze existing datasets. With computational simulations, we can generate new data that serve to test hypotheses or propose new mechanisms. For example, it is possible to test arrangements of gene segments and the effects of using only certain modes of motion of transcription factors, such as allowing or disallowing intersegmental transfer [29].

3.2.1 Smoldyn

A method of choice is Smoldyn, a particle-based simulator which excels at modeling spatial, stochastic processes at the molecular scale, up to organelles, in a small number of cells [40, 41]. As a general guide, the steps to successful models are firstly to clearly identify the questions at hand. As an example, even though flexible filaments are not yet implemented, and it is not currently possible to simulate the movements and self-organization of DNA strands or cytoskeletal fibers, many important questions relating to genome organization can be addressed [29]. Once the questions have been set, our concrete tips for using Smoldyn can be used to implement the model. They do not replace the user manual. We strongly recommend that you first read Steve Andrews' excellent overview and methods paper [42] and the user manual Smoldyn_doc1.pdf, which is constantly updated and included in the download package on smoldyn.org. Other inspiration can be gained from the ~30 publications to date that use Smoldyn to model various aspects of cell biology (e.g., [43–48]). For large systems, we recommend considering the use of Smoldyn's new multiscale features [49].

Briefly, Smoldyn is called from a Terminal application, with a configuration file written by the user. The outputs are live graphics of the current cell architecture and/or text files. At the very least, the configuration file needs to define the dimensionality of the system (dim), the system's boundaries, a list of molecule species, the time_start, time_stop, and time_step, and end with end_file. Units are not entered in the configuration file; instead, the user decides on a space unit and a time unit, and then adheres to them. For intracellular and intranuclear simulations, the combinations μm–ms, 10 nm–ms (as in the examples given below), and nm–μs have proven to be useful unit combinations. *See* ref. 42 for a discussion of the choice of the time_step length. A good first estimate is 0.1 ms.

3.2.2 *Graphics*

Setting up the System

Choose graphics opengl (fastest and simplest; small square molecules) or graphics opengl_good (resonably fast; larger, flat, circular molecules). This will quickly allow you to check whether everything is as you intended it to be or whether you have made any mistakes during the setup. Start the simulation, increase the size of window and object if required, and observe the simulation. Check that all molecules and surfaces are at the correct position, no molecules escape the system, etc.

Running Long Quantitative Simulations

Remove or comment out (#) the graphics statement. This will shorten the simulation time significantly. Remote computer grids usually cannot display graphics; here, the graphics statement should also be removed in order to avoid errors. Important: Some statements about graphics, such as frame_thickness, trigger graphics even in the absence of any graphics statement. These must be removed or commented out. Other statements, such as color and display_size are ignored in the absence of graphics, and it does not matter whether they are still present. For grids, remove any statement that requires user interaction, such as pause.

Creating Figures or Movies of Publication Quality

- Choose opengl_better (slow; lit spheres of the same size as in opengl_good). Here, all molecules appear black unless they are lit by a light source.

- Good light settings for a white background are these:

  background_color 1 1 1

  light 0 position -50 50 0

  light 0 diffuse 1 1 1

  light 0 ambient 0.05 0.05 0.05

  light 0 specular 1 1 1

- Insert the command cmd b pause. This will allow you to expand the graphics window, expand the size of the object (shift +) and rotate the object (arrow keys, or x, y, z) to the desired position. Then press the space bar to start the simulation.

- For movies, avoid unnecessary white space and frame size. If the image files are too large, the movie will not run smoothly on laptops with limited RAM.

- For movies, think ahead which time resolution you require. We find that 12 frames per second (fps) is sufficient for smooth movies. Taking into account by which factor you wish to slow down or speed up the movie with respect to simulated time, choose the frequency of graphic display and image acquisition accordingly (graphic_iter and tiff_iter).

- When tiff_iter is not zero, Smoldyn saves a series of numbered TIFF files. These are large, and good for figures. For movies, we batch convert them to PNG using GraphicConverter. We then create a movie using QuickTime Pro (Open Image Sequence, 12 fps).

  Note that Smoldyn graphics only displays and records snapshots of the simulation. For dynamic figures, such as diffusion traces (Fig. 3), you need to overlay a Smoldyn snapshot of the cell with a plot of the trace created from the Smoldyn text output with the aid of an analysis program, as described in Subheading 3.2.4.

3.2.3 Nuclear Structure and Reactions

Nuclear Envelope

Define a sphere of experimentally determined radius, usually with reflective inner and transmissive outer surface to keep all molecules enclosed (Fig. 3).

```
start_surface
    name nuclear_envelope
    action front all transmit
    action back all reflect
    color both 0.2 0.2 0.2
    polygon both edge
    panel s 100 100 100 75 20 20
end_surface
```

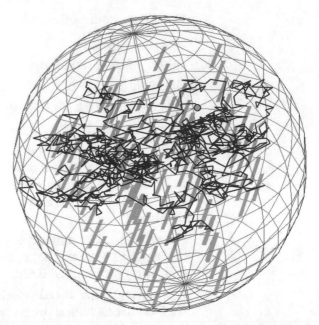

Fig. 3 Diffusion trace of a protein moving through the eukaryotic nucleus (*blue line*), shown for the duration of 100 ms. The start point of the trace is highlighted by a *cyan circle*, the end point, a binding site on a chromosome, by an *orange hexagon*. Chromosome sections are represented as *gray panels*, arranged throughout the nucleus (modified from [29])

Nucleoplasm

Define the inside of the sphere as a compartment. The definition needs to include the bounding surface and one or more interior defining points (point), such that a straight line can be drawn between any position in the compartment and at least one of these points without crossing a bounding surface.

```
start_compartment
    name nucleus
    surface nuclear_envelope
    point 100 100 100
end_compartment
```

Chromosomes

Thin, long rectangles can be used to model chromosomes, with the front and back surface representing the major and minor groove of the double helix. Nonintuitively but conveniently, a surface can be composed of a number of panels, which do not have to be in contact with each other. Defining all chromosomes as one surface is extremely useful, as it allows to define (and change) their properties and reactions all at once.

Nonspecific binding can be implemented by defining binding reactions between the diffusing protein species (here: P) and the entire surface of the rectangle.

```
start_surface
  name chromosome
  rate P fsoln front 0.17
  rate P front fsoln 0.0116
  rate P bsoln front 0.17
  rate P front bsoln 0.0116
  color front 0.35 0.35 0.35
  color back 0.2 0.2 0.2
  thickness 0.5
  panel rect +2 100 90 502 25.6 a1
  panel rect +2 100 90 602 25.6 a2
  panel rect +2 80 90 90 2 25.6 d5
  ...
end_surface
```

Specific binding sites are best defined as surface-bound molecules:

```
surface_mol 1 B(front) chromosome rect d5
80.13 102.5 90
```

Different panels can be joined by neighbors statements to allow continuous diffusion on the surface. This will work whether or not the panels are touching each other.

```
neighbors a1 b1
```

Proteins

Monomeres and reasonably small complexes of proteins are modeled as dimensionless points. They can be given specific or random starting positions and can be placed on surfaces using surface_mol, in free space using mol, or randomly inside the compartment using compartment_mol:

```
mol 1 P 81 82 83
```

```
compartment_mol 100 P nucleus
```

We recommend that long lists of surfaces and molecules are created using an external scripting programme, and that they are placed in one or more files separate to the main configuration file. These are loaded by including a readfile statement in the configuration file, e.g.:

```
readfile positions.txt
```

Protein Movements

- 3D isotropic diffusion in solution is defined using difc.
- 1D diffusion can be defined using difm and a one-dimensional diffusion matrix. For diffusion along chromosomes, we found it more useful to allow isotropic diffusion on the surface of the

chromosome-representing rectangles. Strictly speaking, this is 2D diffusion, but as the rectangles are very thin, there is very little difference.

```
difc P(solution) 27
difc P(front) 0.27
difc B(all) 0
```

- Intersegmental transfer is the movement of proteins from one part of a chromosome to another, or to a different chromosome, by transiently binding both sites simultaneously. In biological cells, this requires the protein or protein complex to have two or more distinct DNA binding sites, and the chromosomal sites to come close together in 3D space. As mentioned above (Subheading 3.2.1), movement of chromosomes is not implemented in Smoldyn 2.x. A workaround is to estimate the rate by which such intersegmental transfer is successful between two chromosomal regions (or panels), and to then define the transfer using movesurfacemol.

```
cmd E movesurfacemol P(all) 0.1 chromosome:b1
    chromosome:b2
cmd E movesurfacemol P(all) 0.1 chromosome:b2
    chromosome:b3
...
```

Reactions

- If required, protein expression can be simulated using zeroth order reactions. A rate, listed at the end of the `reaction` statement, is the number of new molecules per spatial unit^3 per time unit. In this context, it can be more useful to define `reaction_production` directly, which is given per system per time step. Note that the overall reaction rate will then change with a change of the `time_step`.

```
reaction Pexpr 0 ->P 10
reaction Qexpr 0 ->Q
    reaction_production Qexpr 2
```

- First order reactions in the context of the nucleus are protein degradation, autocatalytic protein modification, dissociation of protein complexes, and dissociation of a protein from a surface. If the rate is listed at the end of the reaction statement, Smoldyn calculates from this and the time step length the probability of the reaction at each time step. This reaction_probability can also be entered directly; the overall reaction rate will then change with a change of the time_step.

```
reaction Pdegr P ->0 5
reaction Qphos Q ->Qp 0.002
reaction PQdissoc PQ ->P+Q 5e-6
```

```
reaction unbindP PB(front) ->B(front)+P(solution)
    2.89e-18
```

```
reaction unbindQ QB(front) ->B(front)+Q(front)
    reaction_probability unbindQ 0.2
```

- Second order reactions are binding events of proteins to each other or to surfaces, and enzymatic reactions that are approximated to occur immediately after two molecules encounter each other. To use an experimentally determined bimolecular rate, make sure to convert it from M^{-1} s^{-1} to your chosen spatial and time units (*see* Table "Unit conversion" in Smoldyn_doc1.pdf) and include it at the end of the reaction statement. Smoldyn will then calculate the appropriate binding radius from this rate and the time step length, and reactants that diffuse within this radius will always react. Alternatively, the binding_radius can be defined directly. For some applications, this can be very useful: For example, when a chromosome-bound binding site has a binding radius that exceeds the width of the chromosome, *all* surface-bound proteins that diffuse into it will bind, without the possibility of passing it by.

```
reaction PQassoc P+Q ->PQ 2
reaction QEphos Q+E ->Qp+E
    binding_radius QEphos 0.1
reaction bindP B(front)+P(all) ->BP(front) 0.17
reaction bindQ B(front)+Q(front) ->BQ(front)
    binding_radius bindQ 3
```

3.2.4 Results and Analysis

Smoldyn has a long list of "virtual experimenter" commands that allow the user to manipulate or observe the simulation. All observation commands write into an output file each, which first has to be initialized. The list of commands is well worth a careful read and consideration of how they can help to get more out of the simulation. For our purposes, the most useful commands have been the following:

- `molcount` counts the current number of all molecule species at user-defined time points or intervals. Often, this is the only output needed, as a lot can be learnt from the time profile of the formation and resolution of complexes and other binding events, especially when comparing and further analyzing the results of a multitude of simulations (Fig. 4). Even when the ultimate aim of a simulation is to plot something different than molecule numbers, it is useful to record them in order to check that reactions have been set up correctly.

```
output_files out_mols.txt
cmd n 100 molcount out_mols.txt
```

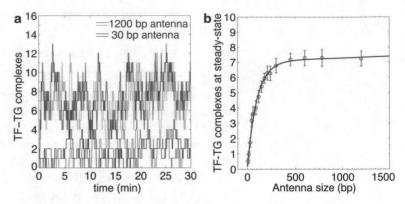

Fig. 4 (**a**) Timecourse of four individual Smoldyn simulations, in which 50 transcription factors (TF) are released in a nucleus that contains 20 chromosomes with a target gene (TG) placed in each center. The chromosomes have the equivalent of either 1200 bp (*blue/cyan* traces) or 30 bp (*red/orange* traces) nonspecific sequence adjacent to the specific binding site (TG). The surface of the chromosome provides nonspecific binding space for transcription factors, acting as an antenna. The number of all molecule species was recorded with the mol-count command at one-second intervals. Shown is the time profile of complex numbers of transcription factors with their target genes, for two individual stochastic simulations of each chromosome length. (**b**) Plot summarizing the results of 16 chromosome lengths with the length of the antenna given on the *x*-axis. Twenty individual simulations were run for each chromosome length. For each of the individual simulations, the steady-state complex number was calculated from the mean of the last 20 minutes. For each set of 20 simulations of a particular chromosome length, the mean and standard error were calculated and plotted, and a curve fitted through the values. All analyses were done with MATLAB. (Simulation results and panel (**b**) from [29])

- `listmols3` lists the position of each individual molecule of one specified species at user-defined intervals.

    For Fig. 3, we ran a simulation with a single diffusing protein molecule for tens of millions of time steps, and recorded its position at every time step. To select a trace suitable for publication, we used a MATLAB script to find binding events to the target gene, and to then plot the positions of the preceding 1000 time steps using plot3D. The most appealing of these traces was then placed on top of a Smoldyn snapshot of the same nucleus using Adobe Illustrator.

```
cmd n 1 listmols3 P out_trace.txt
```

- `replacecmptmol` replaces molecules of a given species within a compartment by another species with a defined probability. This can be used to simulate Fluorescence Recovery After Photobleaching (FRAP) [43, 44]. If the bleaching compartment is bounded by transmissive surfaces, it will not act as a diffusion barrier.

```
cmd @ 199.9 replacecmptmol P D 0.8 FRAPregion
```

- molcountincmpt counts the numbers of molecules in a specified compartment.

```
output_files out_mols.txt out_FRAP.txt
cmd N 20 molcount out_mols.txt
cmd N 20 molcountincmpt FRAPregion out_FRAP.txt
```

- molcountspace counts the numbers of molecules of a defined species in a defined spatial volume. This can for example be used to plot an intracellular gradient.

```
cmd i 2000 3000 10 molcountspace P 0 -50 230
    28 -50 50 -50 50 0 out_slice_P.txt
```

4   Notes

1. In Smoldyn, the default random seed for the random number generator is the time of the simulation start. This is fine when starting simulations individually, but when submitting a set of simulations to a computer grid with the aid of a submit script, the entire set will have the same random seed, leading to identical outcomes. A solution is to define random_seed SIMNUM or random_seed SEED in the configuration file, and to set a different seed for each simulation using a scripting language. An example of a short Python script is given in Smoldyn_doc1. pdf.

2. When running many simulations of the same kind, we recommend numbering each simulation and its output with the same number, defined once at the top of the file or with the aid of a script.

```
output_files    out_mols_SIMNUM.txt    out_trace_
    SIMNUM.txt
```

3. For very long simulations, we recommend the command savesim, which writes down the entire state of the simulation, including all molecules and their positions. With minor editing, it can be used to restart a crashed simulation. As the saved files are very large, however, it makes most sense to call the command only every couple of hours in real time.

```
cmd n 1000000 savesim out_save_nSIMNUM.txt
```

4. Common Errors:
   - file not found: Are all files (configuration file, read-files) in the current directory?
   - file not found: Check the exact name of the file, incl. extensions (.txt)—the extensions are not always displayed but might still be present.

- `file cannot be read`: Check whether the line endings of the configuration file match the computer's operating system—Unix, Windows, or Mac.

5. Common Warnings:

   `boxsize too small`: This will lead to errors, as some bimolecular reactions will be missed. OK for setting up the system, but should be avoided for quantitative simulations. Change either the `boxsize` or the `time_step`.

   `boxsize too large`: Inefficient simulation, but quantitatively fine.

Acknowledgements

We would like to thank Guillaume Filion for providing the HMMt package and for advice on using it, Jeremy Bancroft for work on the implementation of HMMt to work with ChIP-chip data, and Hugo Schmidt and Zsuzsanna Sükösd Etches for their Smoldyn models of the nucleus. We thank Steve Andrews for development and continued support of Smoldyn, some of the cited code snippets, and many fruitful discussions over the years.

SS was supported by the Biotechnology and Biological Sciences Research Council UK grant BBS/E/B/000C0405; KL was supported by a Royal Society University Research Fellowship and a Microsoft Research Faculty Fellowship.

References

1. Ernst J, Kellis M (2015) Large-scale imputation of epigenomic datasets for systematic annotation of diverse human tissues. Nat Biotechnol 33(4):364–376

2. Cavalli G, Misteli T (2013) Functional implications of genome topology. Nat Struct Mol Biol 20(3):290–299

3. Polak P, Karlić R, Koren A, Thurman R, Sandstrom R, Lawrence MS et al (2015) Cell-of-origin chromatin organization shapes the mutational landscape of cancer. Nature 518(7539):360–364

4. Farh KK-H, Marson A, Zhu J, Kleinewietfeld M, Housley WJ, Beik S et al (2015) Genetic and epigenetic fine mapping of causal autoimmune disease variants. Nature 518(7539): 337–343

5. Sanyal A, Lajoie BR, Jain G, Dekker J (2013) The long-range interaction landscape of gene promoters. Nature 489(7414):109–113

6. Phillips-Cremins JE, Sauria MEG, Sanyal A, Gerasimova TI, Lajoie BR, Bell JSK et al (2013) Architectural protein subclasses shape 3D organization of genomes during lineage commitment. Cell 153(6):1281–1295

7. McCord RP, Nazario-Toole A, Zhang H, Chines PS, Zhan Y, Erdos MR et al (2013) Correlated alterations in genome organization, histone methylation, and DNA-lamin A/C interactions in Hutchinson-Gilford progeria syndrome. Genome Res 23(2):260–269

8. Robinson PJJ, Fairall L, Huynh VAT, Rhodes D (2006) EM measurements define the dimensions of the "30-nm" chromatin fiber: evidence for a compact, interdigitated structure. Proc Natl Acad Sci U S A 103(17):6506–6511

9. Nishino Y, Eltsov M, Joti Y, Ito K, Takata H, Takahashi Y et al (2012) Human mitotic chromosomes consist predominantly of irregularly folded nucleosome fibres without a 30-nm chromatin structure. EMBO J 31(7):1644–1653

10. Cairns BR (2009) The logic of chromatin architecture and remodelling at promoters. Nature 461(7261):193–198

11. modENCODE Consortium, Roy S, Ernst J, Kharchenko PV, Kheradpour P, Nègre N et al (2010) Identification of functional elements and regulatory circuits by Drosophila modEN-CODE. Science 330(6012):1787–1797

12. Kharchenko PV, Alekseyenko AA, Schwartz YB, Minoda A, Riddle NC, Ernst J et al (2011) Comprehensive analysis of the chromatin landscape in Drosophila melanogaster. Nature 471(7339):480–485

13. Ernst J, Kheradpour P, Mikkelsen TS, Shoresh N, Ward LD, Epstein CB et al (2011) Mapping and analysis of chromatin state dynamics in nine human cell types. Nature 473(7345): 43–49

14. Ram O, Goren A, Amit I, Shoresh N, Yosef N, Ernst J et al (2011) Combinatorial patterning of chromatin regulators uncovered by genome-wide location analysis in human cells. Cell 147(7):1628–1639

15. Larson JL, Yuan G-C (2012) Chromatin states accurately classify cell differentiation stages. PLoS One 7(2), e31414

16. Zerbino DR, Wilder SP, Johnson N, Juettemann T, Flicek PR (2015) The Ensembl regulatory build. Genome Biol 16:56

17. de Graaf CA, van Steensel B (2013) Chromatin organization: form to function. Curr Opin Genet Dev 23(2):185–190

18. Filion GJ, van Bemmel JG, Braunschweig U, Talhout W, Kind J, Ward LD et al (2010) Systematic protein location mapping reveals five principal chromatin types in drosophila cells. Cell 143(2):212–224

19. Ernst J, Kellis M (2010) Discovery and characterization of chromatin states for systematic annotation of the human genome. Nat Biotechnol 28(8):817–825

20. Schoenfelder S, Clay I, Fraser P (2010) The transcriptional interactome: gene expression in 3D. Curr Opin Genet Dev 20(2):127–133

21. Schoenfelder S, Sexton T, Chakalova L, Cope NF, Horton A, Andrews S et al (2010) Preferential associations between co-regulated genes reveal a transcriptional interactome in erythroid cells. Nat Genet 42(1):53–61

22. Dekker J, Marti-Renom MA, Mirny LA (2013) Exploring the three-dimensional organization of genomes: interpreting chromatin interaction data. Nat Rev Genet 14(6):390–403

23. Gowers DM, Wilson GG, Halford SE (2005) Measurement of the contributions of 1D and 3D pathways to the translocation of a protein along DNA. Proc Natl Acad Sci U S A 102(44):15883–15888

24. Gowers DM, Halford SE (2003) Protein motion from non-specific to specific DNA by three-dimensional routes aided by supercoiling. EMBO J 22(6):1410–1418

25. Elf J, Li G-W, Xie XS (2007) Probing transcription factor dynamics at the single-molecule level in a living cell. Science 316(5828): 1191–1194

26. Berg OG, von Hippel PH (1985) Diffusion-controlled macromolecular interactions. Annu Rev Biophys Biophys Chem 14:131–160

27. Isaacson SA, Larabell CA, Le Gros MA, McQueen DM, Peskin CS (2013) The influence of spatial variation in chromatin density determined by X-ray tomograms on the time to find DNA binding sites. Bull Math Biol 75(11):2093–2117

28. Ando T, Skolnick J (2014) Sliding of proteins non-specifically bound to DNA: Brownian dynamics studies with coarse-grained protein and DNA models. PLoS Comp Biol 10(12), e1003990

29. Schmidt HG, Sewitz S, Andrews SS, Lipkow K (2014) An integrated model of transcription factor diffusion shows the importance of inter-segmental transfer and quaternary protein structure for target site finding. PLoS One 9(10), e108575

30. Veksler A, Kolomeisky AB (2013) Speed-selectivity paradox in the protein search for targets on DNA: is it real or not? J Phys Chem B 117(42):12695–12701

31. Berg OG, Winter RB, von Hippel PH (1981) Diffusion-driven mechanisms of protein translocation on nucleic acids. 1. Models and theory. Biochemistry 20(24):6929–6948

32. Seksek O, Biwersi J, Verkman AS (1997) Translational diffusion of macromolecule-sized solutes in cytoplasm and nucleus. J Cell Biol 138(1):131–142

33. Dross N, Spriet C, Zwerger M, Müller G, Waldeck W, Langowski J (2009) Mapping eGFP oligomer mobility in living cell nuclei. PLoS One 4(4), e5041

34. Ritchie ME, Phipson B, Wu D, Hu Y, Law CW, Shi W et al (2015) Limma powers differential expression analyses for RNA sequencing and microarray studies. Nucleic Acids Res 43(7):47

35. Gentleman RC, Carey VJ, Bates DM, Bolstad B, Dettling M, Dudoit S et al (2004) Bioconductor: open software development for computational biology and bioinformatics. Genome Biol 5(10):R80

36. Smyth GK (2004) Linear models and empirical Bayes methods for assessing differential

expression in microarray experiments. Stat Appl Genet Mol Biol 3:Art. 3, 29 pages

37. Baum LE (1972) An equality and associated maximization technique in statistical estimation for probabilistic functions of Markov processes. Inequalities 3:1–8

38. Miklós I, Meyer IM (2005) A linear memory algorithm for Baum-Welch training. BMC Bioinformatics 6:231

39. Viterbi A (1967) Error bounds for convolutional codes and an asymptotically optimum decoding algorithm. IEEE Trans Inform Theory 13(2):260–269

40. Andrews SS, Bray D (2004) Stochastic simulation of chemical reactions with spatial resolution and single molecule detail. Phys Biol 1(3-4):137–151

41. Andrews SS, Addy NJ, Brent R, Arkin AP (2010) Detailed simulations of cell biology with Smoldyn 2.1. PLoS Comp Biol 6(3): e1000705

42. Andrews SS (2012) Spatial and stochastic cellular modeling with the Smoldyn simulator. In: van Helden et al (eds) Bacterial molecular networks: methods and protocols. Methods Mol Biol 804:519–542

43. DePristo MA, Chang L, Vale RD, Khan SM, Lipkow K (2009) Introducing simulated cellular architecture to the quantitative analysis of fluorescent microscopy. Prog Biophys Mol Biol 100(1-3):25–32

44. Sewitz S, Lipkow K (2013) Simulating bacterial chemotaxis at high spatio-temporal detail. Curr Chem Biol 7(3):214–223

45. Lipkow K, Andrews SS, Bray D (2005) Simulated diffusion of phosphorylated CheY through the cytoplasm of Escherichia coli. J Bacteriol 187:45–53

46. Hoffmann M, Schwarz US (2014) Oscillations of Min-proteins in micropatterned environments: a three-dimensional particle-based stochastic simulation approach. Soft Matter 10:2388

47. Zavala E, Marquez-Lago TT (2014) The long and viscous road: uncovering nuclear diffusion barriers in closed mitosis. PLoS Comp Biol 10, e1003725

48. Singh P, Hockenberry AJ, Tiruvadi V, Meaney DF (2011) Computational investigation of the changing patterns of subtype specific NMDA receptor activation during physiological glutamatergic neurotransmission. PLoS Comp Biol 7:1002106

49. Robinson M, Andrews SS, Erban R (2015) Multiscale reaction-diffusion simulations with Smoldyn. Bioinformatics 31:2406–2408

Chapter 10

In Vivo and In Situ Replication Labeling Methods for Super-resolution Structured Illumination Microscopy of Chromosome Territories and Chromatin Domains

Ezequiel Miron, Cassandravictoria Innocent, Sophia Heyde, and Lothar Schermelleh

Abstract

Recent advances in super-resolution microscopy enable the study of subchromosomal chromatin organization in single cells with unprecedented detail. Here we describe refined methods for pulse-chase replication labeling of individual chromosome territories (CTs) and replication domain units in mammalian cell nuclei, with specific focus on their application to three-dimensional structured illumination microscopy (3D-SIM). We provide detailed protocols for highly efficient electroporation-based delivery or scratch loading of cell impermeable fluorescent nucleotides for live cell studies. Furthermore we describe the application of (2′S)-2′-deoxy-2′-fluoro-5-ethynyluridine (F-ara-EdU) for the in situ detection of segregated chromosome territories with minimized cytotoxic side effects.

Key words Chromosome territories, Chromatin, Replication domains, Super-resolution imaging, Structured illumination microscopy, Replication labeling, F-ara-EdU

1 Introduction

The three-dimensional (3D) organization of chromatin in mammalian interphase cell nuclei is important to the epigenetic regulation of genome function [1–4]. Microscopic observations have long identified spatially separated chromosome territories [5], and more recent studies of chromatin architecture in mammalian genomes by chromatin conformation capturing (3C) based techniques (4C, 5C, Hi-C, reviewed in ref. 6) have supported these observations with increasing genomic and spatial resolution. These techniques have identified topologically associated domains (TADs) in the size range of ~0.5–1 Mb, defined on the linear genome by increased chromatin interaction frequencies within single domains [7]. Studies on replication timing have described the near synchronous firing of replication origins clustered on the linear scale to domains of similar size [8]. Strong correlation has been found

Mark C. Leake (ed.), *Chromosome Architecture: Methods and Protocols*, Methods in Molecular Biology, vol. 1431, DOI 10.1007/978-1-4939-3631-1_10, © Springer Science+Business Media New York 2016

between TAD boundaries and the boundaries separating early and late replication timing chromatin [9], suggesting that these refer to the same unit of genome organization.

Analysis of fluorescence microscopy can add information on the absolute three-dimensional positioning of chromatin architecture to complement genomic techniques [10]. Nevertheless, segmentation of chromatin in single territories or in domain topologies on scales below the Abbe diffraction limit of ~200 nm is not possible with conventional microscopy. Technical advancements over recent years have lead to the development of multiple super-resolution microscopy techniques that can bypass Abbe's diffraction limit. Of these, 3D structured illumination microscopy (3D-SIM) has an eightfold increase in volumetric resolution (twofold in the x, y, and z-dimension) over conventional wide-field deconvolved imaging [11]. 3D-SIM is capable of resolving a three-dimensional chromatin landscape that has intricate networks of chromatin-void channels pervading from nuclear pores to the inside of condensed Barr body chromatin, and to resolve and quantify individual replication subunits [12, 13].

Here we describe various replication (pulse) labeling methodologies compatible with 3D-SIM imaging for the subsequent segmentation of individual chromosome territories or replication domains in both live cell experiments and fixed mammalian cell samples. This is achieved through the incorporation of fluorescent or traceable thymidine analogs via nascent replication and fine-tuning of labeling pulse lengths and chase timing before imaging. Combination of different labels at separate times allows us to explore the sequential nature of chromatin replication in 3D space and which mechanisms establish linear sequences as stable 3D domains. Moreover, simultaneous immunofluorescence protocols targeting transcription factors, chromatin binding proteins and histone posttranslational modifications can help elucidate how active and repressive chromatin is organized and maintained in whole chromosomes down to TADs. Whilst this protocol is concerned with optimization for super-resolution imaging, many steps also have general applicability to wide-field, confocal, and other fluorescent imaging methods.

2 Materials

2.1 Cell Culture and Labeling

1. Cell culture growth media: Dulbecco's modified Eagle medium (DMEM), 10 % fetal bovine serum (FBS), 1 % penicillin–streptomycin.

2. 10 cm cell culture dish with treated surface for adherent cells (Nunclon Delta surface, Thermo Scientific).

3. Coverslips: 18×18 mm or 22×22 mm No 1.5H high precision 170 ± 5 μm (Marienfeld Superior) (see **Note 1**).

4. 6-well cell culture dish with treated surface for adherent cells (Nunclon Delta surface, Thermo Scientific).

5. 0.05–0.25 % Trypsin in PBS or 1× trypsin replacement solution (TrypLE express, Gibco).

6. Thymidine stock solution: 100 mM in PBS.

7. PBS (phosphate buffered saline): 0.01 M sodium hydrogen phosphate (Na_2HPO_4), 0.137 M sodium chloride (NaCl), 1.8 mM potassium hydrogen phosphate (KH_2PO_4), 2.7 mM potassium chloride (KCl) adjusted to pH 7.4 with hydrogen chloride (HCl) in double distilled water (ddH_2O) (*see* **Note 2**).

8. 10 mM EdU: 5-ethynyl-2′-deoxyuridine, dissolved in dimethyl sulfoxide (DMSO, *see* **Note 3**).

9. 10 mM F-ara-EdU: (2′S)-2′-deoxy-2′-fluoro-5-ethynyluridine, dissolved in DMSO.

10. 100 mM fluorescent dUTP dyes (*see* **Note 4**).

11. Tweezers: fine, stainless steel.

12. Hypodermic needles (e.g., 20 g × 1 in.; BD Microlance).

2.2 Sample Staining, Fixation, and Microscopy

1. Fixation solution: 2 % or 4 % formaldehyde/PBS freshly made either from electron microscopy grade 16 % formaldehyde ampules (Thermo Scientific) or from molecular biology grade 37 % solution stabilized with 10 % methanol.

2. Washing solution: 0.02 % Tween-20/PBS (PBST).

3. Permeabilization solution: 0.2 % Triton X-100/PBS.

4. Blocking medium: 2 % bovine serum albumin (BSA), 0.5 % fish skin gelatin (FSG) in PBST; or Maxblock, nonmammalian blocking agent in PBS, pH 7.4, 0.09 % sodium azide (Active Motif) (*see* **Note 5**).

5. Click reaction solution (per 100 μl): 55 μl ddH₂O, 10 μl Tris–HCl buffer (1 M, pH 7), 10 μl sodium ascorbate (500 mM), 5 μl copper sulfate (100 mM), 20 μl fluorescent azide dye (0.1 mM) (*see* **Note 6**).

6. Counterstaining solution: 4′,6-diamidino-2-phenylindole (DAPI) or SYTOX Green (Thermo Fisher Scientific) counterstains (*see* **Note 7**).

7. Mounting medium (*see* **Note 8**).

8. Small glass beaker.

9. Delicate task wiper tissues (e.g., Kimwipes).

10. Paraffin based film (Parafilm).

11. Dark chamber: light-tight plastic or metal container, capable of holding 6-well dish lid.

12. Microscope slide.

13. Nail varnish for sealing.

14. Cotton swabs (*see* **Note 9**).

15. Ethanol.

16. Chloroform.

17. Immersion oil with appropriate refractive index (*see* **Note 10**).

18. Optional for live cell imaging: μ-Dish 35 mm live cell dishes, high precision No. 1.5 glass bottom (Ibidi), and Opti-MEM reduced serum, indicator free medium (Thermo Fisher Scientific).

3   Methods

Perform all steps at room temperature unless specified. Use standard tissue culture techniques and cell type-specific growth medium and splitting ratios (*see* **Note 11**).

3.1   F-ara-EdU Labeling of Individual Chromosome Territories

1. Grow cells in a 10 cm tissue culture dish in growth media incubating at 37 °C, 5 % CO_2 in humidified incubator at 25–40 % confluence. Synchronize cell cycles in cultured population at G1/S transition with double thymidine block. Add thymidine to a final concentration of 2 mM to the media and incubate for 20 h (*see* **Note 12**). Wash thrice with 10 ml of PBS followed by a final wash in culture media before exchanging with medium (thymidine-free) and incubating for a further 12 h. Transfer to media with 2 mM thymidine for a further 20 h.

2. Release cells from thymidine block by triple wash with 10 ml of PBS exchanging with label-free media and immediately add F-ara-EdU to final concentration of 10 μM. For labeling entire chromosomes incubate for at least 10 h to cover the length of an entire S-phase, before exchange with label-free media (Fig. 1, *see* **Note 13**).

3. Split and culture labeled cells for up to 4 days to allow segregation of labeled and unlabeled chromosomes over several

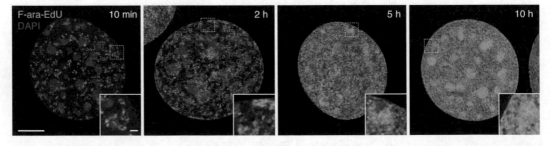

Fig. 1 Replication label incorporation. 3D-SIM super-resolution imaging of C127 cells incubated with 10 μM F-ara-EdU showing progressive extension of label incorporation as labeling pulse length is increased from 10 min to 10 h. Note that after 5 h the majority of chromatin has been labeled via F-ara-EdU with the exception of heterochromatin-dense chromocenters, compare inset at 5 and 10 h. Maximum intensity projections are shown. Scale bar, 5 μm (*inset* 0.5 μm)

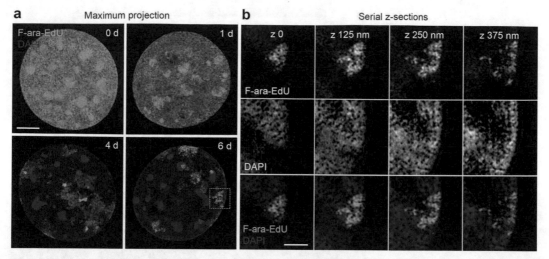

Fig. 2 Chromosome territory segregation imaged with 3D-SIM. (**a**) Segregation of F-ara-EdU labeled chromosome territories in mouse C127 cells over the course of up 6 days after 10 h pulse labeling. At day 4 individual territories can be distinguished. Scale bar, 5 μm. (**b**) Magnified view of consecutive z-sections through the structure of a single chromosome territory (*boxed* region in **a**). Scale bar 2 μm

post-labeling replication cycles to reach a desired average number of labeled chromosome territories per nucleus (Fig. 2, *see* **Note 14**).

4. At least 1 day prior to fixation seed cells on 18×18 mm or 22×22 mm high precision coverslip in 6-well plate dishes (alternatively in 35 mm dishes). Use appropriate dilution ratio to let cells reach 60–80 % confluency at time of fixation.

5. Fill small glass beaker with 50–100 ml of PBS. Fold tissue lengthwise and place it on the bench next to the beaker. For each coverslip fill 2 ml fixation solution in any dish of a new 6-well plate (alternatively 35 mm dish may be used).

6. Carefully pick up coverslip by its edge with fine tweezers; gently dab the side of coverslip on the tissue to remove excess medium and wash shortly by dipping 2–3 times in PBS. Dab again and immediately transfer to the well with fixation solution (*see* **Note 15**).

7. Agitate gently by hand; then incubate for 10 min with closed lid under a hood.

8. Aspirate solution with bench-top pump and simultaneously refill well with 2–5 ml of PBST avoiding drying of sample from formaldehyde evaporation (*see* **Note 16**). Repeat 2–3 times until fixation solution is fully exchanged with washing buffer (*see* **Note 17**).

9. Exchange PBST with 2 ml 0.2 % Triton X-100 in PBS. Agitate shortly, and then incubate for 10 min. Exchange with PBST (*see* **Note 18**).

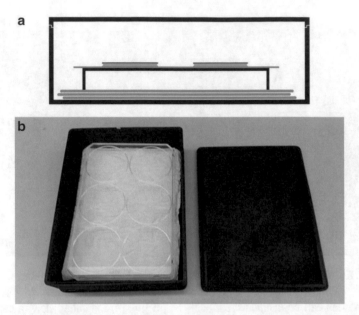

Fig. 3 (**a**) Schematic of humidified dark chamber incubation assembly. From *center*: Two coverslips incubating (cells down) over media (*green*). Incubation rests over a layer of Parafilm (*grey*) flattened over the top of a 6-well dish lid (or other flat surface). Lid sits over multiple layers of humidified tissue inside a solid black plastic container. (**b**) 3D-printed black ABS plastic humidified chamber, designed to hold one 6-well lid over tissue, as shown. Small printing tolerances generate airtight seal between inner lid rim and case

10. Cut Parafilm to 6-well format and press it, to create a flat coating, on the top of the 6-well lid to be placed in a humidified dark chamber (Fig. 3).

    (*Optional for additional immunostaining after click reaction: for each coverslip pipette 100 μl of blocking solution, according to the well position onto the film. Pick up coverslip, dab on tissue and place on the drop with cell side down. Incubate in a humidified dark chamber for 30 min*)

11. Pipette a 100 μl drop of the click reaction mix for each coverslip onto Parafilm applied on a 6-well lid as described above. Pick up coverslip with the tweezers, dab on tissue and place on the drop with cell side down. Incubate in a humidified dark chamber for 30 min (*see* **Note 19**).

12. For washing fill two small glass beakers with 50–100 ml of PBST, fill dishes of 6-well plate (cleaned with H_2O demin. for reuse) with 2 ml PBST for each coverslip, and place tissue on the bench. Carefully pick up coverslip by its edge with tweezers; gently dab the side of coverslip on tissue to remove excess; wash by dipping in the beaker 1, dab again, dip in beaker 2, dab again before placing the coverslip back into the 6-well dish (*see* **Note 15**).

(At this point an additional immunostaining can be performed. We recommend thorough washing as described above after each incubation step and post-fixation with 4 % formaldehyde/PBS after secondary antibody incubation and washing)

13. For optional counterstaining, add 100 μl of DAPI solution (2 μg/ml) or SYTOX Green solution (1 μM) on Parafilm on lid and incubate in a humidified dark chamber for 10 min (*see* **Note 7**). Wash and dab coverslip as described in **step 4**.

14. Wash 1× in PBST as described above followed by a final wash in ddH$_2$O to remove salts, dab again and immediately place on a 30 μl drop of mounting medium on Parafilm for 2 min (*see* **Note 20**). Add 10 μl of mounting medium in the center of a pre-cleaned microscope slide (if frosted, use non-frosted side; *see* **Note 21**). Pick up coverslip, dab excess dilute mounting medium on tissue and mount carefully onto the drop of mounting medium on the slide. Let the mounting medium settle for 2 min, then dry excess by covering with a fine tissue and applying mild pressure. If necessary repeat with new tissue. Only when all excess has been removed, seal edges with appropriate amount of nail varnish (*see* **Note 22**).

15. For storage and clean maintenance of slides *see* **Note 23**.

3.2 Replication Domains and Origins for Fixed/Live Samples

1. For cell synchronization follow **step 1** from Subheading 3.1.

2. Release cells from thymidine block by triple wash with 10 ml of PBS exchanging with culture media.

3. Wait until desired S phase stage can be labeled and incubate for 5 min with addition of 10 μM EdU or of F-ara-EdU, then exchange with label-free media (Fig. 4a, *see* **Note 24**). Alternatively, for live cell imaging, transfer coverslip to a 6 cm dish, and immediately cover cells (to avoid drying) with 20 μl of fluorescent conjugated dUTPs (10–20 μM) (Fig. 4b). Scratch surface of coverslip thoroughly with light pressure using a Microlance needle, wait 2 min and return coverslip to media-filled well (*see* **Note 25**). Another method to deliver cell-impermeable dyes at higher efficiency is based on electroporation and requires the commercially available 4D Nucleofector (Lonza, *see* **Note 26**). Over 85 % of cells in S phase within an unsynchronized population can be efficiently labeled using this approach compared to EdU control (data not shown). Furthermore the compatibility of labeling with cell permeable and impermeable dyes introduces temporal resolution for determining replication directionality in super-resolution imaging (Fig. 4c).

4. For fixed samples, follow **steps 4–12** from Subheading 3.1, including or omitting **step 9** dependent on dUTP analog incorporated (*see* **Note 27**).

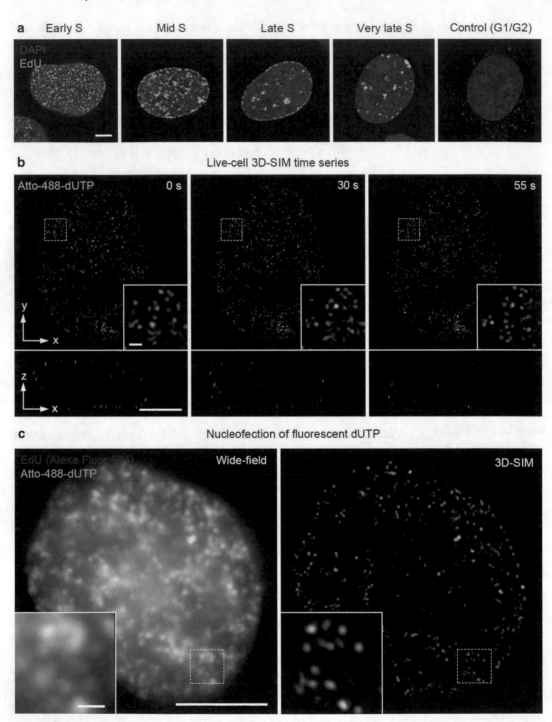

Fig. 4 S-phase pattern, live-cell imaging and nucleofection labeling compatibility with 3D-SIM. (**a**) From *left* to *right*, wide-field deconvolved images of 10 μM EdU with 30 min labeling pulse after 30 min, or 1, 6, 8, and 16 h after release from thymidine block. Note the changing three-dimensional pattern of chromatin replicated at each time point (*green*) and that no labeling occurs after exit from S phase, 16 h (control). Scale bar, 5 μm. (**b**) Single z-section live-cell 3D-SIM data of Atto-488-dUTP scratch-replication labeled HeLa cell. Note the increase in high frequency background signal from 55 s after start of time series. (**c**) Single z-section wide-field

5. For live-cell imaging, trypsinize cells and seed in live cell imaging dish. After cells become adherent and before imaging, exchange media with indicator-free Opti-MEM.

4 Notes

1. Super-resolution imaging requires coverslips of uniform thickness and high precision to ensure consistency of the optical path. We recommend pre-cleaning in H_2O (demineralized), to remove residual dust particles and storage in 100 % ethanol until use. Air-dry coverslips prior to use, as flaming may cause bending of the glass.

2. For convenience, we recommend dissolving one phosphate buffered saline tablet (Dulbecco A) in 100 ml of ddH_2O and autoclave.

3. Reagent can be stored at 4 °C but DMSO will crystallize at this temperature. Reagent should be pre-warmed and agitated by vortex before use.

4. For this protocol we have tested Alexa Fluor 594-azide, Alexa Fluor 488-azide, and CF405M-azide, as well as Atto-488-dUTP, Cy3-dUTP, and Alexa Fluor 647-dUTP. Note that nucleotides conjugated to other fluorophores (e.g., Alexa Fluor 488-dUTP) may be incorporated with lower efficiency. Hence thorough testing is required when using other nucleotide-dye combinations.

5. Blocking is only required for combined immuno-labeling, not for click-reaction and/or counterstaining alone. To our experience, dependent on the selected antibody, a mixture of blocking reagents is often more effective than using BSA alone.

6. We recommend making fresh every time. Stock solutions for Tris–HCl buffer, copper sulfate and fluorescent azide dyes can be kept for prolonged periods at 4 °C, However sodium ascorbate is a strong reducing agent and should optimally be made fresh every time. If stocks of sodium ascorbate are to be made we recommend only storing for up to one month at 4 °C. Visual inspection should confirm deterioration from a light translucent yellow to a deep red amber solution.

Fig. 4 (continued) versus 3D-SIM image of C127 cells labeled with Atto-488-dUTP (*green*) using nucleofector approach, followed by 30 min chase and subsequent 15 min EdU incorporation before wash, fixation and Click chemistry with Alexa Fluor 594-azide dye (*red*). It can be clearly observed from the wide-field image that both labels overlap significantly given their incorporation at the same early stage in S-phase. However, 3D-SIM reveals that only some foci remain overlaid whilst many *red labels* have migrated further from the original dUTP nucleofection incorporation, opening possibilities to study replication directionality in 3D space. Scale bar, 5 μm

7. Unlike DAPI, SYTOX Green does not have a bias towards binding AT-rich sequences. However, it has a weak affinity to bind RNA at high concentrations. To avoid residual RNA binding, we recommend incubation with 1–10 U RNAse I/PBS at 37 °C for at least 30 min prior to counterstaining (1 U RNAse I will degrade 100 ng of RNA per second in optimal condition).

8. We recommend non-hardening Vectashield (Vector Laboratories) as a mounting and anti-fade medium. An exception is use with Alexa Fluor 647 or Cy5, as Vectashield promotes reversible dark-state formation of this class of dyes [14]. In this case we recommend the use of alternative glycerol-based mounting media (e.g., DABCO-glycerol: 1 % 1,4-diaz-abicyclo-octane in 90 % glycerol/PBS). Hardening media such as Prolong Gold may be used depending on the sample, but its polymerization can artificially flatten the specimen. In all cases, avoid mounting media containing DAPI or propidium iodide counterstains, unless this is desired for a particular application.

9. Cotton swabs mounted on plastic or with adhesive that dissolves in chloroform are to be avoided.

10. The 3D-SIM reconstruction algorithm is particularly susceptible to artifacts caused by mismatch between the optical transfer function (OTF = Fourier transform of the point spread function, PSF) that encodes the assumed optical properties of the system for a given wavelength and the effective optical conditions within the sample's volume of interest. For multicolor experiments on DeltaVision OMX system (GE Healthcare), we strongly recommend the use of channel-specific measured OTFs. Note that OTF sets for different colors should be recorded with the same refractive index (RI) immersion oil. The RI should be selected to provide a symmetric PSF for the middle wavelength of interest (e.g., 1.512 RI for green emitting beads). Using immersion oil with higher refractive index for the sample acquisition will shift the region of best match from near the coverslip deeper into the sample (a +0.002 higher RI will shift the optimum a few μm deeper, e.g., to achieve optimal reconstruction inside mammalian nuclei).

11. This protocol is implemented primarily on immortalized mammalian adherent tissue culture cell lines. It may also be used for primary lines and embryonic stem cells but consideration should be given to their respective cell morphology, and the imaging depth away from the coverslip. Imaging depth is a limiting factor in achieving optimal resolution and avoiding super-resolution image reconstruction artifacts by light scattering and spherical aberrations.

12. This protocol can also be applied in an asynchronous cell population. However we recommend synchronization in order to maximize labeling efficiency.

13. The incubation duration depends on the S-phase length of the respective cell line. Some cells may experience some lag from block release. Given the reduced toxicity of the F-ara-EdU compared to EdU, it is possible to incubate cells for 12 h or overnight to ensure maximum coverage [15]. For full S-phase labeling, the F-ara-EdU concentration may be reduced to 1 μM to further minimize adverse effects. This method is suitable for bulk chromatin labeling as an alternative for counterstaining with standard dyes.

14. As with labeling pulse length, chase length is dependent on the cell cycle of the respective cell line. Given the high label coverage throughout the genome, cytotoxic long-term effects cannot be ruled out. A chase time of four post-labeling cell division can be sufficient for segregation of individual territories in a per-cell basis.

15. Washes can be performed by aspiration and immediate replacement of solution in the same well repeatedly; nevertheless we recommend the use of a dipping beaker as we find the excess volume of PBS (>50 ml) is more effective than that of a single well (~2–5 ml).

16. Avoid aspiration of all formaldehyde solution from over the coverslip, as its rapid evaporation will cause fixation artifacts apparent as shriveled and creased nuclear outlines.

17. Samples can be stored in PBST overnight at 4 °C after fixation if required.

18. For a combined Click/immunofluorescence labeling it is possible to incorporate a primary and secondary antibody incubation protocol, to label desired targets and their relative position to chromatin. Note that the Click reaction can be detrimental to imaging GFP protein fusions. Kits with optimized buffer condition to avoid this are commercially available; alternatively one can use anti-GFP antibodies or nanobodies (GFP-booster) in a combined Click/immunofluorescence labeling protocol.

19. We recommend the use of a secondary pair of tweezers as backstop supports for careful lifting of coverslips from Parafilm. Controlled lifting of the coverslip avoids shearing cells from coverslips due to capillary surface tension created between the sample and the Parafilm.

20. The addition of this step between the last wash and mounting coverslips on microscopy slides ensures an excess of mounting medium over water in the final sealed volume of the sample. This equilibration step essentially reduces the dilution of

mounting media and ensures the desired refractive index is maintained in the final sample for imaging.

21. If using microscope slides with frosted coating for labeling it is recommended to mount on unfrosted side as frosting can create a small but noticeable tilt of the sample when mounted on the stage, leading to large focus point variations at opposing ends of the coverslip.

22. Excess mounting medium should be carefully removed without moving the coverslips. We recommend the use of fine tissue (or a single layer of double layered Kimwipes) placed evenly over the coverslip and removed vertically after absorption. This may need to be repeated once or twice with the application of soft pressure with the fingertip along the edges of the coverslip to ensure that all excess mounting medium has been absorbed before proceeding to sealing samples. Thorough removal of excess mounting medium will prevent the coverslip from moving during the sealing procedure and helps the nail varnish attach cleanly to the slide surface. A small amount of nail polish applied with a single stroke along each side of the coverslip is usually sufficient for sealing, and can be repeated after the first coat has dried if necessary.

23. Sealed slides can be stored in slide-boxes at 4 °C. Coverslips should be cleaned from residual medium and, after imaging, from immersion oil using 80 % ethanol/H_2O demin. and fine tissue. Directly before imaging, chloroform dipped cotton swabs may be used to remove residual dirt off the coverslip. Note that repeated cleaning with ethanol or chloroform may dissolve nail polish. In this case old nail varnish may be peeled off using fine tweezers and new nail varnished reapplied.

24. Progression of DNA synthesis through S phase occurs in distinct stages. Early S phase short labeling pulse produces a punctate pattern throughout the nucleus, mid S phase labeling shows a dotted ring at the nuclear and nucleoli periphery, and late S phase pulses label regions of constitutive heterochromatin (such as mouse chromocenters). Incubation times for labeling can extend to 20–30 min and punctate pattern will still be conserved nevertheless individual spots may contain multiple replication domains. Incubation should not last for less than 5 min, as this is the approximate lag time for entry of the dye molecule into cells. Incubations shorter than 5 min may label smaller genomic regions, but can compromise efficiency of label incorporation and density. EdU or F-ara-EdU can be used, as the absolute incorporation is far lower than for whole chromosome territories, reducing the chance of observing cytotoxic effects.

25. The scratching procedure leads to transient permeabilization of the membranes of cells along the scratch wound site due to

mechanical shearing, allowing the uptake of cell impermeable dyes for a few seconds [16, 17].

26. A method for incorporation of cell impermeable dyes via electroporation is currently available commercially using a Lonza Nucleofector and nucleofection kit buffers optimized for multiple cell lines. This requires harvesting cells in suspension or in a 24-well plate format, mixing with nucleofection buffer and 1 μl of fluorescently labeled dUTP (for 20 μl reaction mix), and selecting a shock program suitable for the chosen cell line. This procedure has the advantage of delivering nucleotides to the majority of the cell population, although incorporated only by cells currently in S phase. The procedure is typically more efficient (providing a more reproducible and higher fraction of labeled cells) than scratch labeling, which only affects cells along the scratch wound site.

27. Sites of active replication show local and transient chromatin de-compaction [18]. Hence an appropriate chase time after pulse labeling before fixation should be considered to avoid local remodeling effects.

Acknowledgements

This work was supported by the Wellcome Trust Strategic Award 091911, funding advanced microscopy at Micron Oxford and the John Fell Oxford University Press (OUP) Research Fund 143/064. We thank Justin Demmerle for valuable comments on the manuscript.

References

1. Cremer T, Cremer M, Hübner B et al (2015) The 4D nucleome: evidence for a dynamic nuclear landscape based on co-aligned active and inactive nuclear compartments. FEBS Lett 589: 2931–2943. doi:10.1016/j.febslet.2015.05.037

2. Lemaître C, Bickmore WA (2015) Chromatin at the nuclear periphery and the regulation of genome functions. Histochem Cell Biol 144:111–122. doi:10.1007/s00418-015-1346-y

3. Bickmore WA, van Steensel B (2013) Genome architecture: domain organization of interphase chromosomes. Cell 152:1270–1284. doi:10.1016/j.cell.2013.02.001

4. Cavalli G, Misteli T (2013) Functional implications of genome topology. Nat Struct Mol Biol 20:290–299. doi:10.1038/nsmb.2474

5. Cremer M, von Hase J, Volm T et al (2001) Non-random radial higher-order chromatin arrangements in nuclei of diploid human cells. Chromosome Res 9:541–567. doi:10.1023/A:1012495201697

6. de Laat W, Dekker J (2012) 3C-based technologies to study the shape of the genome. Methods 58:189–191. doi:10.1016/j.ymeth.2012.11.005

7. Lieberman-Aiden E, van Berkum NL, Williams L et al (2009) Comprehensive mapping of long-range interactions reveals folding principles of the human genome. Science 326:289–293. doi:10.1126/science.1181369

8. Jackson DA, Pombo A (1998) Replicon clusters are stable units of chromosome structure: evidence that nuclear organization contributes to the efficient activation and propagation of S phase in human cells. J Cell Biol 140:1285–1295. doi: 10.1083/jcb.140.6.1285

9. Pope BD, Ryba T, Dileep V et al (2014) Topologically associating domains are stable

units of replication-timing regulation. Nature 515:402–405. doi:10.1038/nature13986

10. Williamson I, Berlivet S, Eskeland R et al (2014) Spatial genome organization: contrasting views from chromosome conformation capture and fluorescence in situ hybridization. Genes Dev 28:2778–2791. doi:10.1101/gad.251694.114

11. Schermelleh L, Heintzmann R, Leonhardt H (2010) A guide to super-resolution fluorescence microscopy. J Cell Biol 190:165–175. doi:10.1083/jcb.201002018

12. Markaki Y, Gunkel M, Schermelleh L et al (2010) Functional nuclear organization of transcription and DNA replication: a topographical marriage between chromatin domains and the interchromatin compartment. Cold Spring Harb Symp Quant Biol 75:475–492. doi:10.1101/sqb.2010.75.042

13. Baddeley D, Chagin VO, Schermelleh L et al (2010) Measurement of replication structures at the nanometer scale using super-resolution light microscopy. Nucleic Acids Res 38, e8. doi:10.1093/nar/gkp901

14. Olivier N, Keller D, Rajan VS, Gönczy P, Maneley S (2013) Simple buffers for 3D STORM microscopy. Biomed Opt Express 4:885–899. doi:10.1364/BOE.4.000885

15. Neef AB, Luedtke NW (2011) Dynamic metabolic labeling of DNA in vivo with arabinosyl nucleosides. Proc Natl Acad Sci U S A 108:20404–20409. doi:10.1073/pnas.1101126108

16. Schermelleh L, Solovei I, Zink D, Cremer T (2001) Two-color fluorescence labeling of early and mid-to-late replicating chromatin in living cells. Chromosome Res 9:77–80. doi:10.1023/A:1026799818566

17. Schermelleh L (2006) In vivo replication labeling. In: Celis JE (eds), Cell Biology: A Laboratory Handbook, 3rd edition, Elsevier Science, vol. 1, pp 301–303

18. Schneider K, Fuchs C, Dobay A et al (2013) Dissection of cell cycle-dependent dynamics of Dnmt1 by FRAP and diffusion-coupled modeling. Nucleic Acids Res 41:4860–4876. doi:10.1093/nar/gkt191

Chapter 11

DNA–Protein Interactions Studied Directly Using Single Molecule Fluorescence Imaging of Quantum Dot Tagged Proteins Moving on DNA Tightropes

Luke Springall, Alessio V. Inchingolo, and Neil M. Kad

Abstract

Many protein interactions with DNA require specific sequences; however, how these sequences are located remains uncertain. DNA normally appears bundled in solution but, to study DNA–protein interactions, the DNA needs to be elongated. Using fluidics single DNA strands can be efficiently and rapidly elongated between beads immobilized on a microscope slide surface. Such "DNA tightropes" offer a valuable method to study protein search mechanisms. Real-time fluorescence imaging of these interactions provides quantitative descriptions of search mechanism at the single molecule level. In our lab, we use this method to study the complex process of nucleotide excision DNA repair to determine mechanisms of damage detection, lesion removal, and DNA excision.

Key words Single molecule imaging, DNA tightropes, Quantum dots, Diffusion, DNA repair, Search mechanisms, Nucleotide excision repair

1 Introduction

In this chapter we will describe the method that we use to prepare DNA tightropes, which are single molecules of DNA suspended between surface immobilized beads. DNA tightropes offer a unique, powerful single molecule method for studying DNA–protein interactions. Silica beads are fixed to a flow cell surface, when DNA is flowed through the chamber single DNA molecules efficiently bind to these beads and achieve ~90% elongation as they suspend between beads [1]. Tightropes are formed using 5 μm beads, offering the following main advantages: (a) Tightropes are not in contact with a surface, reducing artifacts, (b) fluorescence observed in the focal plane can only derive from proteins bound to DNA tightropes; this reduces background [1, 2].

Proteins can be labeled with any fluorescent moiety, we prefer quantum dot (Qdot) conjugation through antibodies or directly to

Mark C. Leake (ed.), *Chromosome Architecture: Methods and Protocols*, Methods in Molecular Biology, vol. 1431,
DOI 10.1007/978-1-4939-3631-1_11, © Springer Science+Business Media New York 2016

a biotinylated protein at a Qdot–protein ratio of >3:1 [3]. Previous investigations have shown that Qdots are unable to bind to the DNA tightropes without protein conjugation [2]. This approach yields bright fluorescent proteins that strongly resist photobleaching. As a result only low concentrations (nanomolar) of protein and Qdots are required for DNA binding experiments.

Specific flow cells can be customized to the experimental requirement, altering parameters such as volume and number of ports. Along with the range of available Qdot colors this represents a versatile yet simple system to study DNA–protein interactions.

Videos of individual protein motion can be simply converted into kymographs, displaying position against time. Gaussian fits to single fluorescent particle kymographs can then be analyzed to calculate diffusion constants and diffusive exponents (which provide the mode of motion) of the protein. These algorithms are freely available for download. Thus, direct visualization of protein motion on DNA tightropes offers an unmatched insight into numerous protein DNA transactions.

2   Materials

All procedures are performed at room temperature unless otherwise stated, and high quality reagents are required including water which must be of resistivity >10 MΩ cm.

2.1   5× ABC Buffer

1. 250 mM Tris–HCl, pH 7.5, 250 mM KCl, 50 mM $MgCl_2$, 0.1% NaN_3.

2.2   ABT Buffer

2. 1× ABC buffer, 10 mg/ml BSA, 0.1% Tween 20 (see **Note 1**).

2.3   Concatermerized λ DNA

1. 2 μL of 10× ligase buffer, 7 μL of water, 10 μL of DNA, 1 μL of T4 DNA Ligase.

2. Leave at room temperature overnight, then store at 4 °C.

2.4   DNA Mix

1. 5 ng/μL of λ DNA in 1× ABC buffer.

2.5   mPEG Solution

1. 25 mg/ml $mPEG_{5000}$ in 250 mM $NaHCO_3$, pH 8.15–8.3 (see **Notes 1** and **2**).

2.6   5 μm Diameter Poly-L-Lysine Coated Silica Beads

1. Add 100 μL of beads to 500 μL of water and vortex.

2. Spin at 14 k rpm for 2 min using a microfuge.

3. Remove water and resuspend in 400 μL of 350 μg/mL poly-L-lysine (P5899, Sigma-Aldrich).

2.7   YOYO Solution

1. 10 mM DTT, 1× ABC buffer, 5 nM of YOYO-1 (Invitrogen) dye (see **Notes 3** and **4**).

3 Methods

3.1 PEGylation and Flow Cell Preparation

1. Figure 1 depicts a schematic of a flow cell. It consists of a few basic elements, a standard glass slide with two 1 mm diameter holes drilled 12 mm apart, an adhesive gasket, a glass coverslip, and two small tubes (inlet and outlet) for connecting to the flow chamber (*see* **Note 5**).

2. The cell is assembled starting with the glass slide into which the inlet and outlet tubes are glued, ensuring no access for air.

3. Once the glue has set, any excess tubing protruding from the bottom of the glass slide should be removed with a scalpel blade.

4. Apply the adhesive gasket (*see* **Note 6**).

5. Attach the glass coverslip completing the flow cell (*see* **Note 7**).

6. Incubate flow cell overnight in mPEG solution.

7. Wash the chamber with 400 μL of water.

8. Incubate overnight in ABT buffer (*see* **Note 8**).

3.2 Preparation of a Bead Covered Surface

1. Add 10 μL of poly-L-lysine coated silica beads to 500 μL water and vortex.

2. Spin at 14 k rpm for 2 min using a microfuge.

3. Remove water and add another 500 μL water of and vortex (*see* **Note 9**).

4. Spin at 14 k rpm for 2 min using a microfuge.

5. Remove water and add another 100 μL water of and vortex.

6. Sonicate the solution at 80 % amplitude for 1 s bursts, four times (*see* **Note 10**).

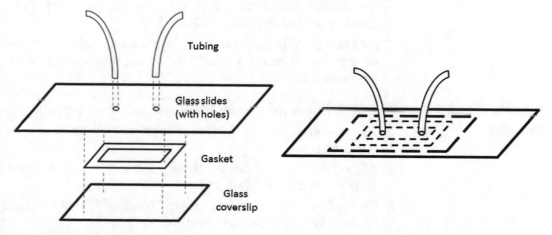

Fig. 1 Schematic of a flow cell

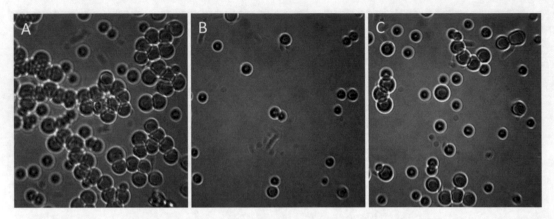

Fig. 2 Bead density images. (**a**) Beads too dense for suitable tightropes to form. (**b**) Beads too sparsely distributed for DNA tightropes to form. (**c**) Good density of beads for DNA tightropes to form

7. Immediately inject beads into the flow cell.

8. Check the bead density on a microscope (*see* **Note 11**).

9. Add 100 µL of water to flow cell and re-check density (Fig. 2) (*see* **Note 12**).

10. Store at 4 °C or continue with next stage.

11. Withdraw 2 mL of 1× ABC buffer into a syringe, attach a length of perfusion tubing and completely fill the tubing with buffer.

12. Attach the perfusion tubing to the outlet tube on the flow cell being careful not to introduce any air bubbles.

13. Attach a second perfusion tube of known length (and therefore volume) to the inlet tube on flow cell.

14. Perfuse 500 µL of 1× ABC buffer through the flow cell from the syringe into a microfuge tube via the perfusion tube attached to the inlet tube (*see* **Note 13**).

15. Add 500 µL of 1× ABC buffer to the microfuge tube and withdraw all liquid except a small amount to prevent entry of air (*see* **Note 13**).

3.3 DNA Tightrope Formation

1. Add DNA mix to microfuge tube and withdraw to empty.

2. Add a volume of 1× ABC buffer to microfuge tube (*see* **Note 14**).

3. Allow DNA to flow back and forth for any period between 20 min and 2 h (*see* **Note 15**).

4. To check the presence of tightropes 100 µL of YOYO solution can be added (Fig. 3a) (*see* **Note 16**).

5. Withdraw liquid from perfusion tube leaving a small amount (*see* **Note 17**).

6. The air-tight system is now set up and the flow cell is ready for experimental work.

7. 100 mM DTT should be added to 1× ABC buffer before imaging (*see* **Note 18**).

8. Quantum dot labeled protein sample can now be added for imaging.

9. Figure 3b shows the situation when too much labeled protein is added to the flow cell. The optimal saturation is shown in Fig. 3c.

10. Figure 4 depicts the optical setup we use to view DNA tightropes (*see* **Note 19**).

3.4 Data Analysis

1. From the videos collected on tightropes a kymograph can be constructed using the ImageJ stacks > reslice command (*see* **Note 20**).

2. The kymograph can be analyzed using a sliding window Gaussian fit macro for ImageJ. This is summarized in Fig. 5 (*see* **Note 21**).

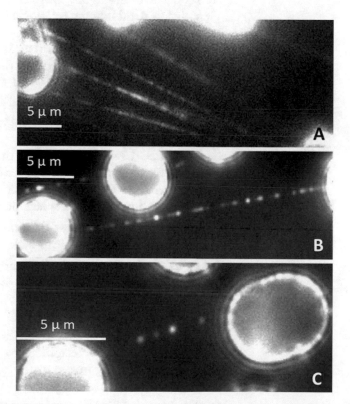

Fig. 3 DNA tightrope images. (**a**) DNA tightropes visualized with YOYO solution (*see* **Notes 3**, **4** and **16**). (**b**) DNA tightropes over saturated with Qdot–protein complexes. (**c**) Optimal Qdot–protein concentration on DNA tightropes

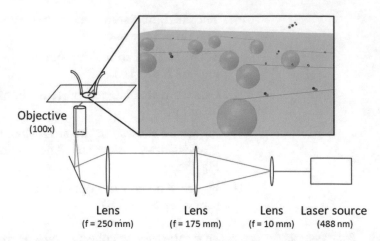

Fig. 4 Schematic of a microscope set up to view DNA tightropes

3. From the Gaussian fit, the mean position is used for analysis.

4. To convert from pixels to position we use this equation: Position (Pixel) × Pixel size (nm) = Position (nm).

5. To calculate the mean squared displacement (MSD) for each molecule the following relationship is used for the first 10–20 % of the data [4].

   where N is the total number of frames in the kymograph, n the frame, xi is the position of the protein in one dimension (along the DNA tightrope), and t is the time window [4].

$$\text{MSD}(n\Delta t)\frac{1}{N-n}\sum_{i-1}^{N-n}\left[\left(x_{i+n}-x_i\right)^2\right]$$

6. From $<x> = 2Dt\alpha$ [5], we know that displacement is related to the diffusion constant. Where $<x>$ is the scalar displacement in nm over time t, D is the diffusion constant in $\mu m^2/s$, and α relates to the mode of displacement (Fig. 6a).

7. By plotting MSD against time one can extract D and the diffusive exponent α (*see* **Note 22**).

8. To ascertain how much data should be used to calculate D and α within the window of 10–20 % of the data, a threshold of linear fit quality is applied; the R^2 value must remain above 0.7.

9. Once the amount of data for analysis is ascertained D and α can more simply be determined by plotting log(MSD) versus log(t): the y-axis intercept is log($2D$) and the slope is α (Fig. 6b).

10. Plotting the diffusion constant against the corresponding alpha value provides an independent view of the data and is used to calculate means in both dimensions (Fig. 7) (*see* **Note 23**).

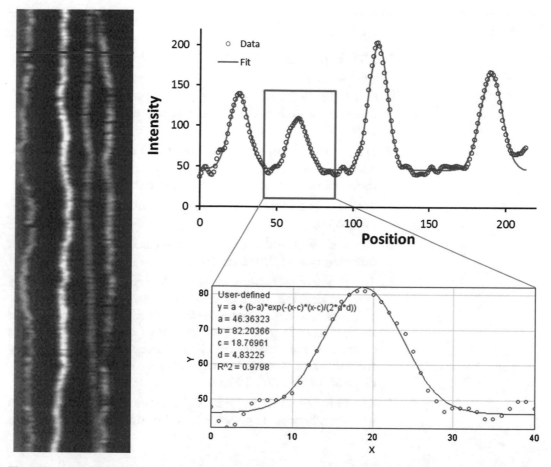

Fig. 5 Raw data analysis. (**a**) Kymograph constructed from movie obtained of Qdot–protein movement on DNA tightrope. The *red line* indicates section of the kymograph used in (**b**). (**b**) Intensity profile along *red line* in (**a**), overlaid with a multiple Gaussian fit. (**c**) Enlarged section for Gaussian fitting (*see* **Note 21**)

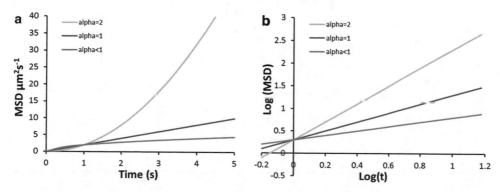

Fig. 6 Assessing the mode of motion for single molecules on tightropes. (**a**) is a linear plot of MSD versus time showing three dependencies on the diffusive exponent α (*see* **Note 21**). (**b**) Log(MSD) versus Log(time) allows for D and α to be determined: the y-axis intercept is log($2D$) and the slope is α. For these example graphs $D = 1$ $\mu m^2/s$ and alpha is indicated

4   Notes

1. ABT buffer and mPEG solution should be remade every 2 weeks.

2. 350 μg/mL: 28 μL of 5 mg/mL stock added to 372 μL of water and stored at –20 °C. Add 21 mg of $NaHCO_3$ per 25 mg of mPEG.

3. DTT is a reducing agent that prevents formation of disulphide bonds. It also mops up free radicals produced by exposure to the excitation beam preventing photodamage to the sample.

4. YOYO-1 is a DNA intercalating dye used to stain the DNA tightropes.

5. Holes are best drilled using a Dremel electric hand drill with a diamond coated dental drill tip.

6. The gasket is cut using a scalpel blade from double-sided sticky tape. In our case we use an adhesive layer of width 180 μm. The gasket controls the final volume of the flow cell and can be shaped according to the experiment (even accommodating changes in the number of inlets if necessary), as long as they are consistent throughout experiments. We cut a rectangle of dimensions 15 mm × 10 mm.

7. The flow cell needs to be air-tight to prevent any liquid losses while incubating the proteins under study or while imaging, as

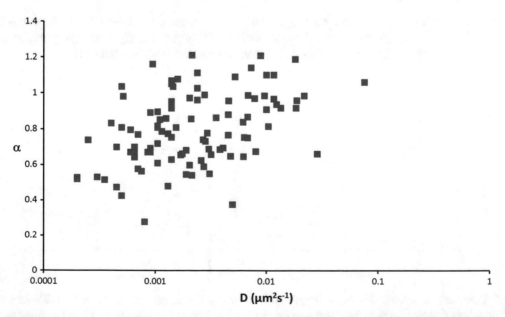

Fig. 7 Alpha distributes normally in linear space whereas *D* distributes normally in logarithmic space. Such plots are used to determine subpopulations of molecules that possess reduced or enhanced mobility (*see* ref. 4)

any sudden change in the volume or pressure within the flow cell will most likely disrupt the tightropes. This also prevents oxygenation of the sample which results in photodamage.

8. ABT and mPEG solutions are used to reduce the number of Qdot–protein conjugates sticking to the surface therefore reducing the background noise.

9. Removing water after vortexing and adding more water removes excess poly-L-lysine.

10. Sonication helps to separate the beads reducing clumping.

11. Checking the bead density is essential for the construction of useable DNA tightropes.

12. Addition of water further washes the beads to remove excess poly-L-lysine which could adhere DNA to the coverslip surface. This is also a good test for the quality of the coated beads; any movement of the beads at this stage likely indicates the lifetime of the poly-L-lysine coating is coming to an end.

13. Removal of air from the system is essential, if air bubbles enter the flow cell chamber they will render the flow cell useless by displacing beads thus destroying tightropes.

14. The volume of 1× ABC buffer is directly related to the length of tubing used, enough volume should be added so that the DNA is comfortably allowed to flow back and forth with no air bubbles entering the system.

15. Less than 20 min is not enough time for a sufficient number of tightropes to form, longer than 2 h has no additional benefit.

16. If YOYO solution is used this must be removed as much as possible by flowing 1× ABC buffer through the system as it can destabilize DNA tightropes. YOYO-1 has not been seen to affect protein binding [2].

17. After the sample is withdrawn a volume of 1× ABC buffer should be added to ensure the system can be flowed back and forth if necessary.

18. Addition of DTT reduces "Qdot blinking" which can interfere with imaging and also reduces fluorophore photobleaching [6]. Be aware that "vivid" labeled Qdots (Invitrogen) are quenched by high concentrations of DTT. If these Qdots are used then reduce [DTT] to below 10 mM.

19. The optical setup uses a 488 nm DPSS laser to illuminate the sample at an oblique angle. This is achieved by focusing the incident laser beam to the edge of the objective's back-focal plane producing a subcritically angled collimated beam on exit. Compared with a standard epi-fluorescent illumination scheme, the signal to noise ratio is improved ~8-fold [7], since a smaller proportion of background fluorophores are not illuminated [4].

20. Kymographs plot position versus time. ImageJ is available as a free download from http://imagej.nih.gov/ij/download.html.

21. Gaussian fits produce five values: baseline, maximum height, mean peak position, standard deviation, and r^2. This macro is available from: http://kadlab.mechanicsanddynamics.com/images/Downloads/Gaussian_Fit.txt.

22. For immobile particles α approaches zero, for unbiased random walkers α approaches 1 and particles showing directed motion α approaches 2 [1, 2].

23. The diffusion constant follows a normal distribution in logarithmic space and should be plotted to represent this. Subpopulations in the distribution can inform about pauses or periods of directed motion [4].

Acknowledgements

This work was supported by the BBSRC [BB/I003460/1] and [BB/M019144/1] to N.M.K., BHF [FS/13/69/30504] to A.V.I., and University of Kent for L.S.

References

1. Dunn AR, Kad NM, Nelson SR, Warshaw DM, Wallace SS (2011) Single Qdot-labeled glycosylase molecules use a wedge amino acid to probe for lesions while scanning along DNA. Nucleic Acids Res 39:7487–7498

2. Kad NM, Wang H, Kennedy GG, Warshaw DM, Van Houten B (2010) Collaborative dynamic DNA scanning by nucleotide excision repair proteins investigated by single- molecule imaging of quantum-dot-labeled proteins. Mol Cell 37:702–713

3. Wang H, Tessmer I, Croteau DL, Erie DA, Van Houten B (2008) Functional characterization and atomic force microscopy of a DNA repair protein conjugated to a quantum dot. Nano Lett 8:1631–1637

4. Hughes CD, Wang H, Ghodke H, Simons M, Towheed A, Peng Y, Van Houten B, Kad NM (2013) Real-time single-molecule imaging reveals a direct interaction between UvrC and UvrB on DNA tightropes. Nucleic Acids Res 41:4901–4912

5. Berg HC (1993) Random walks in biology. Princeton University Press, Princeton, NJ

6. Hohng S, Ha T (2004) Near-complete suppression of quantum dot blinking in ambient conditions. J Am Chem Soc 126:1324–1325

7. Tokunaga M, Imamoto N, Sakata-Sogawa K (2008) Highly inclined thin illumination enables clear single-molecule imaging in cells. Nat Methods 5:159–161

Chapter 12

Escherichia coli Chromosome Copy Number Measurement Using Flow Cytometry Analysis

Michelle Hawkins, John Atkinson, and Peter McGlynn

Abstract

Flow cytometry is a high-throughput technique that analyzes individual particles as they pass through a laser beam. These particles can be individual cells and by detecting cell-scattered light their number and relative size can be measured as they pass through the beam. Labeling of molecules, usually via a fluorescent reporter, allows the amount of these molecules per cell to be quantified. DNA content can be estimated using this approach and here we describe how flow cytometry can be used to assess the DNA content of *Escherichia coli* cells.

Key words Flow cytometry, Genome copy number, Genome content, *Escherichia coli*, Replication, Chromosome, DnaA

1 Introduction

The start sites of DNA replication are called origins and *E. coli* has a single circular chromosome with one origin called *oriC*. Origin activity is predominantly regulated by the DnaA initiator protein. DnaA binds to 9bp repeat elements near *oriC* and mediates unwinding of the origin region so that helicase loading can occur [1]. Once *oriC* fires, two replication forks travel in opposite directions until they reach the terminus region and complete genome replication (Fig. 1a). In optimal conditions the average genome replication time of cells in an exponentially growing population (~40 min) can be longer than the doubling time of *E. coli* (~20 min) [2]. This is possible because *oriC* can reinitiate before previous sets of replication forks have finished replicating the genome [3]. The resulting concurrent rounds of replication mean that multiple sets of replisomes can be active in a single cell (Fig. 1a). The number of active replisomes in a cell is a useful readout for replication and fork progression defects whilst the ability of cells to complete ongoing rounds of replication can also report on the efficiency of fork progression. Here we describe how to quantify active replisome

Mark C. Leake (ed.), *Chromosome Architecture: Methods and Protocols*, Methods in Molecular Biology, vol. 1431,
DOI 10.1007/978-1-4939-3631-1_12, © Springer Science+Business Media New York 2016

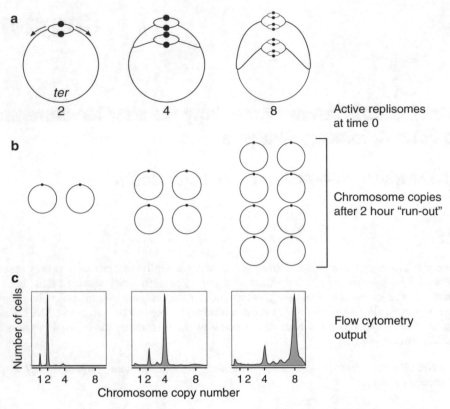

Fig. 1 "Run-out" experiment principle and output. (**a**) *E. coli* chromosome schematics showing concurrent rounds of DNA replication and how this alters active replisome numbers. *Black circles* represent *oriC*. *Arrows* indicate replisome direction. (**b**) After 2 h of "run-out" conditions where origin initiation and cell division are inhibited, all the forks will have finished replicating their template and the final number of chromosome copies will equal the number of active replication forks at the time of antibiotic addition. (**c**) Representative chromosome copy number profiles with fluorescence measurement as a proxy for total DNA content

number by inhibiting replication initiation and cell division before using flow cytometry to assess total genome content.

In this method origin initiation in an exponentially growing population is inhibited using rifampicin. Rifampicin inhibits DNA-dependent RNA synthesis by binding to RNA polymerase and blocking elongation [4]. Inhibition of transcription prevents any further initiation from *oriC* but active replication forks are not disrupted. Since we are interested in measuring genome content, cell division must be prevented in order to avoid a reduction of the number of chromosomes per cell. Cephalexin is a β-lactam antibiotic that disrupts cell division by binding to peptidoglycans in the cell wall. This inhibits cross–linking of membrane peptidoglycans and the downstream septation events that lead to cell division [5]. The DNA replication apparatus is unaffected by both these antibiotics so replication forks can continue and complete chromosome duplication. A similar method was originally employed by Steen and colleagues to study initiation timing [6] and this technique is generally known as a "run-out" experiment. In this protocol cells are grown in the absence of the above antibiotics and then at a given time point these antibiotics are added to enable all active replication forks to complete genome replication but without cell division occurring. Cells are then stained with a dye that fluoresces only when bound to DNA and then analyzed using flow cytometry to measure the DNA content in individual cells. This DNA content can then be used to estimate the total number of chromosomes present within cells. This estimation requires comparison with cells grown under conditions known to favour the presence of only a single pair of replication forks at any one time. The majority of these cells will therefore have a fluorescence signal equivalent to two chromosomes. The final number of genome copies estimated using this benchmark fluorescence signal enables the number of active replication forks in a cell upon addition of rifampicin and cephalexin to be inferred (Fig. 1b).

Here we describe how to perform "run-out" experiments for standard *E. coli* strains (Subheading 3.1) and temperature sensitive DnaA mutants (Subheading 3.2). The method detailed in Subheading 3.2 is for strains where the mutant DnaA is active at 30 °C but non-functional at 42 °C due to instability at higher temperatures [7]. Temperature-based control of origin initiation enables synchronization of cells by extended growth in non-permissive conditions where initiation is prevented. Once all cells have completed ongoing rounds of replication a brief return to permissive conditions is employed to allow DnaA to function and initiate a new round of replication from *oriC*, after which the cells are returned to a higher temperature to inhibit further rounds of initiation. This approach allows the majority of cells to initiate one round of chromosome replication within a short (10 min) time window. Tracking the DNA content as a function of time using flow cytometry then allows progression of the newly initiated replication forks to be followed. Approximate rates of replication fork movement between different strains can thus be compared as the DNA content increases from one to two chromosomes (Fig. 2).

Flow cytometry relies on particles flowing in a narrow stream through a laser. Measurements of scattered light are recorded as "events." These events can be confused by debris in the cell suspension and by neighbouring particles being detected as a single event, termed doublets. To avoid debris being recorded as an event it is important to filter all reagents used in preparation of your sample suspension. Doublets can be avoided by using a homogenous sample preparation and can be excluded during and post-analysis. Most flow cytometry takes advantage of a fluorescent indicator dye that binds to a cell or molecule of interest. When the laser excites these fluorophores they emit light and this fluorescence serves as a proxy for the relative amount of the cell or molecule being interrogated. The wide variety of fluorescent dyes and laser

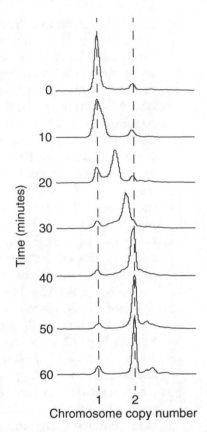

Fig. 2 Monitoring progression of genome duplication using an *E. coli dnaA* temperature-sensitive mutant. Strain HB159 [10] was grown at 42 °C for 2 h and then shifted to 30 °C at time 0. At this time point the majority of cells contained a single chromosome equivalent since cell division could proceed after completion of ongoing rounds of replication but replication could not be reinitiated during the 42 °C incubation period. After 10 min at 30 °C the culture was then shifted back to 42 °C. The DNA content of the majority of cells increased as a function of time, reflecting the speed with which the chromosome was duplicated

wavelengths available make cytometry a versatile method that can be used for a range of prokaryotic and eukaryotic species. Here we are interested in total bacterial DNA content as a measure of genome copy number after "run-out." We stain our fixed cells with SYTOX® Green but other suitable dyes are available. SYTOX® Green only permeates dead cells and binds to all nucleic acid. RNaseA is used to remove RNA in the sample and avoid unwanted nucleic acid binding. When SYTOX® Green is bound to DNA it has absorption and emission maxima of 502 and 523 nm respectively and so can be excited by a 488 nm argon-ion laser or another 450–490 nm source [8]. We use a Beckman Coulter CyAn™ ADP Analyzer for our analysis but most flow cytometers are equipped to excite and detect at these wavelengths.

Here we describe how to prepare *E. coli* cells for flow cytometry with SYTOX® Green as the fluorophore (Subheading 3.3). Protocol alterations are required to stain eukaryotes with SYTOX® Green and may also be required for other bacterial species. A full description of optimizing flow cytometry parameters for analysis is beyond the scope of this method since they vary depending on the cytometer set up and software. The key considerations are to account for any debris and cell autofluorescence by running buffer and unstained cell control samples. Detectable events in these samples are background readings and should be minimal in order to proceed. The sensor voltage parameters should be optimized so that fluorescence levels corresponding to $1n$ and at least $8n$ genome copies can be displayed simultaneously on the x axis. Some mutant strains can contain cells with 16 genome copies. We count at least 10,000 events but routinely collect data for samples of 100,000. For an excellent overview of flow cytometry mechanics and outputs please refer to Givan, 2011 [9].

2   Materials

1. LB medium: 10 g/L tryptone, 5 g/L yeast extract, 5 g/L NaCl. pH to 7.0 with NaOH.

2. Minimal medium (MM): 2.64 g/L KH_2PO_4, 4.34 g/L $Na_2HPO_4 \cdot 12H_2O$, 1 g/L $(NH_4)_2SO_4$, 0.02% $MgSO_4 \cdot 7H_2O$, 0.001% $Ca(NO_3)_2 \cdot 4H_2O$, 0.00005% $FeSO_4 \cdot 7H_2O$. Prepare 150 mL batches of 56 salts (5.28 g/L KH_2PO_4, 8.68 g/L $Na_2HPO_4 \cdot 12H_2O$, 2 g/L $(NH_4)_2SO_4$, 2 mL 10% $MgSO_4 \cdot 7H_2O$, 1 mL 1% $Ca(NO_3)_2 \cdot 4H_2O$, 50 μL 1% $FeSO_4 \cdot 7H_2O$. Make $FeSO_4$ just prior to use. Autoclave and add an equal volume of sterile distilled water. A carbon source and any necessary supplements can then be added. For our MG1655 strain background we add 4.8 mL 20% glucose (0.32% final concentration) and 300 μL of 0.1% thiamine/ Vitamin B1 (0.0001% final concentration) before use.

3. 1× PBS: 137 mM NaCl, 2.7 mM KCl, 4.3 mM Na_2HPO_4, 1.47 mM KH_2PO_4 adjusted to a pH of 7.4. The solution should be filtered twice with 0.22 μm filters to avoid debris that could interfere with flow cytometry.

4. Rifampicin: 10 mg/mL in dimethyl formamide wrapped in foil and stored at −20 °C.

5. Cephalexin: 10 mg/mL in dH_2O wrapped in foil and stored at −20 °C.

6. SYTOX® Green (Invitrogen). Dilute from 5 mM stock to 50 μM working stock in DMF. Store wrapped in foil at −20 °C (*see* **Note 1**).

7. RNase A. Make up 1 mg/mL in dH$_2$O working stock and store at –20 °C (*see* **Note 1**).

8. SYTOX mix: 1 µM SYTOX® Green, 50 µg/mL RNase A, made up in 1× PBS (*see* **Note 1**).

9. Flow cytometer: Analyzer with a 450–490 nm source for use with SYTOX® Green and the appropriate flow cytometry tubes. We use a Beckman Coulter CyAn™ ADP Analyzer.

3   Methods

3.1   Standard Strains

All of our *E. coli* growth is carried out at 37 °C in an air incubator shaking at 170 rpm.

1. Inoculate 10 mL of LB with a single colony of your strain of interest. Pre-warm 10 mL of LB per strain in a 37 °C incubator to prepare for **step 2**.

2. After the culture has grown to an OD$_{650}$ of 0.4, dilute the culture to an OD$_{650}$ of 0.01 in 10 mL of LB pre-warmed to 37 °C (*see* **Note 2**).

3. Grow the culture to mid-exponential phase (OD$_{650}$ of 0.4–0.6) (*see* **Note 3**).

4. Take a 100 µL sample and transfer to a 1.5 mL tube. Spin the sample down for 1 min in a bench-top centrifuge at 17,000×*g*. Remove the supernatant and resuspend the pellet in 100 µL of 1×PBS. Add 400 µL of 100% methanol, touch vortex and store at –20 °C (*see* **Note 4**).

5. Add rifampicin to the cell culture to a final concentration of 100 µg/mL and cephalexin to a final concentration of 15 µg/mL. Touch vortex. For antibiotic concentrations adjust the current volume by subtracting the amount of any culture removed to measure absorbance. Antibiotic addition is time 0.

6. Grow the culture for two hours in the presence of rifampicin and cephalexin and then take a sample as in **step 4** (*see* **Note 5**).

7. For a genome copy number control grow wild-type *E. coli* in 5 mL minimal media containing 0.32% glycerol. Grow to stationary phase (overnight growth) and then carry out **steps 5** and **6**. These cells provide a $1n+2n$ genome copy number control reflecting cells in the population prior to antibiotic addition that contained either no replication forks or two forks (Fig. 1c, left panel).

3.2   dnaA^{ts} Mutants

Steps **3–9** should be carried out as quickly as possible.

1. Inoculate 5 mL of LB with a single colony of your *dnaA^{ts}* strain. We have tested several different *dnaA^{ts}* alleles and have found that *dnaA46* [10] provides the highest fraction of cells

that initiate replication within the permissive temperature time window (*see* **step 6** below). Grow at 30 °C to an OD_{650} of 0.2–0.3.

2. Transfer tubes to a 42 °C shaking (180 rpm) water bath and grow for 2 h. At this point move LB to an 18 and a 55 °C incubator to prepare for **steps 4** and 7 (5 and 10 mL per strain respectively).

3. Take a 100 μL sample and transfer to a 1.5 mL tube.

4. Add 5 mL of LB pre-chilled to 18 °C directly to the culture and move to the 30 °C water bath.

5. Process the sample taken in **step 3**. Spin the sample down for 1 min in a bench-top centrifuge at $17,000 \times g$. Remove the supernatant and resuspend the pellet in 100 μL of 1× PBS. Add 400 μL of 100 % methanol, touch vortex and store at −20 °C.

6. After 10 min incubation at 30 °C, take a 100 μL sample and transfer to a 1.5 mL tube.

7. Add 10 mL of LB pre-warmed to 55 °C directly to the culture and transfer to the 42 °C water bath.

8. Process the sample taken in **step 6** as in **step 5**.

9. Take 400 μL samples (as in **step 5**) at 10 min intervals for 70 min (80 min after the shift to 30 °C in **step 4**). An optional sample can be taken 2 h after **step 4** (*see* **Note 5**).

3.3 Staining Cells for Flow Cytometry

1. Spin the fixed samples for 1 min in a bench-top centrifuge at $17,000 \times g$.

2. Remove the supernatant and resuspend the pellet in 500 μL of 1× PBS.

3. Spin the samples for 1 min in a bench-top centrifuge at $17,000 \times g$.

4. Remove the supernatant and resuspend pellets in 1 mL of SYTOX mix (*see* **Note 6**).

5. Transfer the samples to flow cytometry tubes. All stained cells should be kept out of the light using dark tubes or foil and stored at 4 °C (*see* **Note 7**).

4 Notes

1. Make up the working stocks (50 μM SYTOX® Green in DMF, 1 mg/mL RNase A in dH_2O) the night before they are required for the SYTOX mix. The working stocks can be kept for 1 week at −20 °C.

2. Depending on your strain background, it may not be necessary to grow the culture to exponential phase twice. In such cases proceed to **step 3** after **step 1**.

3. Growth to exponential phase takes 2–3 h for wild–type *E. coli* strains.

4. This sample is from an exponential phase population. Since the population will contain cells at every stage of genome replication it will produce a continuous distribution of genome content. This is not informative in most cases and probably only needs carrying out once per strain to check for gross replication defects such as abnormal overall DNA content.

5. Once cells have been fixed with methanol they can be stored at –20 °C indefinitely before processing and staining.

6. At this stage the pellet is invisible. Depending on the specifications of the flow cytometer used for analysis, you may need to dilute samples to avoid exceeding the flow rate at which data collection is accurate. An appropriate dilution should be optimized empirically but for guidance a recommended suspension density is 5×10^5 to 5×10^6 cells/mL [9]. In our experience diluting cells two-fold in SYTOX mix gives good results with a Beckman Coulter CyAn™ ADP Analyzer. We dilute half the stained cells so that we can also run undiluted samples if necessary later.

7. Stained cells kept in the dark will still eventually bleach. We recommend storing stained *E. coli* for no longer than 2 months. Touch vortex samples before flow cytometry analysis to avoid cell clumps.

Acknowledgements

We thank Karen Hogg and the Imaging and Cytometry Laboratory in the Technology Facility at the University of York for technical assistance and support. This work was supported by BBSRC grant BB/I001859/1 and the University of York.

References

1. Mott ML, Berger JM (2007) DNA replication initiation: mechanisms and regulation in bacteria. Nat Rev Microbiol 5(5):343–354, doi:nrmicro1640 [pii]. 10.1038/nrmicro1640

2. Helmstetter CE, Cooper S (1968) DNA synthesis during the division cycle of rapidly growing *Escherichia coli* B/r. J Mol Biol 31(3):507–518

3. O'Donnell M, Langston L, Stillman B (2013) Principles and concepts of DNA replication in bacteria, archaea, and eukarya. Cold Spring Harb Perspect Biol 5(7):pii: a010108. doi:10.1101/cshperspect.a010108

4. Campbell EA, Korzheva N, Mustaev A, Murakami K, Nair S, Goldfarb A, Darst SA (2001) Structural mechanism for rifampicin inhibition of bacterial RNA polymerase. Cell 104(6):901–912

5. Bush K (2012) Antimicrobial agents targeting bacterial cell walls and cell membranes. Rev Sci Tech 31(1):43–56

6. Skarstad K, Boye E, Steen HB (1986) Timing of initiation of chromosome replication in individual Escherichia coli cells. EMBO J 5(7):1711–1717

7. Hansen FG, Koefoed S, Atlung T (1992) Cloning and nucleotide sequence determination of twelve mutant dnaA genes of Escherichia coli. Mol Gen Genet 234(1):14–21

8. Roth BL, Poot M, Yue ST, Millard PJ (1997) Bacterial viability and antibiotic susceptibility testing with SYTOX green nucleic acid stain. Appl Environ Microbiol 63(6):2421–2431

9. Givan AL (2011) Flow cytometry: an introduction. Methods Mol Biol 699:1–29. doi:10.1007/978-1-61737-950-5_1

10. Atkinson J, Gupta MK, Rudolph CJ, Bell H, Lloyd RG, McGlynn P (2011) Localization of an accessory helicase at the replisome is critical in sustaining efficient genome duplication. Nucleic Acids Res 39(3):949–957, doi:gkq889 [pii]

Chapter 13

Bacterial Chromosome Dynamics by Locus Tracking in Fluorescence Microscopy

Avelino Javer, Marco Cosentino Lagomarsino, and Pietro Cicuta

Abstract

Bacterial chromosomes have been shown in the last two decades to have remarkable spatial organization at various scales, and also well-defined movements during the cell cycle, for example, to reliably segregate daughter chromosomes. More recently, various labs have begun investigating the short-time dynamics (displacements during time intervals of 0.1–100 s), which one hopes to link to structure, in analogy to "microrheology" approaches applied successfully to study mechanical response of complex fluids. These studies of chromosome fluctuation dynamics have revealed differences of fluctuation amplitude across the chromosome, and different characters of motion depending on the time window of interest. The highly nontrivial motion at the shortest experimentally accessible times is still not fully understood in terms of physical models of DNA and cytosol. We describe how to carry out tracking experiments of single locus and how to analyze locus motility. We point out the importance of considering in the analysis the number of GFP molecules per fluorescent locus.

Key words Chromatin, Bacterial nucleoid, Loci and foci, Fluorescence imaging, Mean-squared displacement, Polymer dynamics

1 Introduction to Live-Cell Locus Tracking at High Frame Rate

In recent years, it has started to be recognized that the physical structure of the bacterial nucleoid plays an important role in fundamental biological processes, e.g. segregation and transcription. This chapter focuses on the methods to characterize chromosomal dynamics at short timescales (0.1–100 s), where it is possible to explore the state of the nucleo-protein complex and its environment, without being dominated by large-scale motions related to the genome segregation and cell growth. The movement of fluorescent chromosomal labels in live *Escherichia coli* can be obtained by a custom-designed single-particle tracking program. The collection of a large number of trajectories is crucial, making it possible to characterize not just average chromosomal dynamics, but by

Mark C. Leake (ed.), *Chromosome Architecture: Methods and Protocols*, Methods in Molecular Biology, vol. 1431, DOI 10.1007/978-1-4939-3631-1_13, © Springer Science+Business Media New York 2016

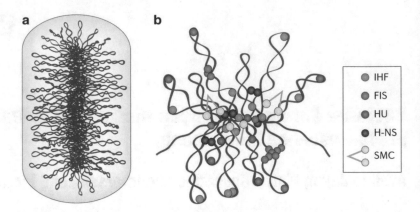

Fig. 1 (a) Schematic illustration of supercoiled chromosome sections, giving a branched spatial structure; (b) illustration of the structure and condensation inducing role of nucleoid-associated proteins (NAP). Adapted from ref. 17

binning for time in the cell cycle, or subcellular localization, to tease apart some of the diverse factors that affect chromosome mobility [1, 2].

The bacterial chromosome spontaneously condenses, together with its associated RNA and proteins, into the cell's central region to form a structure called "nucleoid" [3, 4], which is a highly organized and dynamic structure [5–8], *see* Fig. 1. In recent years, the idea that the physical properties and organization of the nucleoid are intimately related to important cellular functions, particularly chromosomal segregation [6, 9–12] and gene expression [13, 14] has grown in importance. Bacteria are particularly interesting organisms for a variety of reasons, including a "physics" perspective. Indeed, they are in some ways simpler than eukaryotic cells: They do not have organelles or internal membranes, they are three orders of magnitude smaller in volume than a typical eukaryote cell, and have a very compact genome [15], and yet have the extraordinary complexity of life. *E. coli* is by far the best characterized bacterium. Its genetics and molecular biology are well understood, it is easy to maintain and a large collection of strains and tools for manipulation is available. Therefore *E. coli* is very often the first choice in studies of any general aspect in bacterial biology.

The development of systems that allow tagging-specific chromosomal regions, using fluorescent proteins through genetic engineering, has allowed the in vivo exploration of the dynamics of specific chromosomal regions [16, 17]. Most of the studies of chromosomal markers have focussed on the segregation dynamics (some examples in refs. 8, 18–21). Remarkably, only a handful of experimental studies have addressed the problem of characterizing the chromosomal structure from a physics viewpoint [5, 22–27].

In this chapter, we present an approach inspired by microrheology, where through the analysis of the movement of individual probes, it is possible to extract details on the local environment [28–32]. Particularly important in this respect is the pioneering work of Weber et al. [25–27, 33], where it is shown how the chromosomal markers exhibit a different dynamics than what is expected from free diffusion or standard polymer physics models [25]. They attributed this behavior to the viscoelastic properties of the cytoplasm, and in a subsequent work, they found that the amplitude of the markers vibrations is ATP dependent [26].

We describe in this chapter, the series of tools we developed to analyze the movement of the chromosomal markers. This includes the creation of a program to track each individual fluorescent focus with subpixel resolution, as well as an analysis of the different types of errors that could arise from it, and a series of strategies to correct for them. The outcomes in our lab were studies of the short-time dynamics in a collection of 27 strains, where each strain has a fluorescent marker in a different chromosomal position; The effect of three different growth media was also considered. The markers all share a similar subdiffusive behavior, but their mobility depends on (a) the chromosomal localization, (b) the subcellular position, and (c) the fluorescence intensity (which we have tested to be a GFP locus size effect as opposed to an error of localization) [1]. We also show how in a large dataset it is possible to dig for the existence of rare but ubiquitous subset of trajectories; we found a subset of tracks that exhibit near-ballistic dynamics. These movements are likely to be the result of segregation dynamics, either by active machinery or by stress–relaxation mechanics [2].

2 Materials

2.1 Bacteria Strains and Reagents

We studied a collection of 27 *E. coli* strains with the GFP-ParB/*parS* fluorescent label system (kindly provided by the Espeli and Boccard laboratories [19]). This collection of strains has a P1 *parS* inserted at 27 different positions around the chromosome; loci are assigned a name according to the macrodomain they belong to. The expression of the ParB-GFP fusion protein is driven by the pALA2705 plasmid; no IPTG induction is required to produce the ParB-GFP levels necessary to visualize loci in the cells [20]. As a control, IPTG can be added half an hour before visualization. All the chemical reagents were obtained from Sigma-Aldrich unless otherwise stated.

2.2 Microscopy

The *E. coli* cells on agar pads were imaged on a Nikon Eclipse Ti-E inverted microscope using a 60× oil immersion objective with NA 1.45. The images were further magnified with a 2.5× TV adapter before detection on an Andor iXon EM-CCD camera. The camera used in EM gain mode, capable of detecting single fluorophores, yields a high signal to noise ratio which in turn gives a high-loci localization precision. Field of view scanning and image acquisition were automated using custom-written software.

3 Methods

3.1 Sample Preparation

Strains were grown overnight in LB at 37 °C with Ampicillin 100 µg/mL. Cultures were diluted 200:1 into M9 minimal salts (Difco) supplemented with complementary salts ($MgSO_4$ 2 mM, $CaCl_2$ 100 µM, Tryptophan 4 µg/mL, and Tymidine 5 µg/mL), and a different carbon source: 0.4% glycerol, doubling time 150 min; 0.4% glucose (Surechem Products), 115 min doubling time; or 0.4% glucose and 0.5% casamino acids (Difco), 75 min doubling time.

For observations on agar pads, 10 µL of this culture were deposited on a pad swollen of the same medium used for the exponential growth and 1.5% of agarose. The pad was then sealed between two coverslips with silicone grease, preventing bacteria motility but allowing bacteria growth. The sample was kept on the microscope at 30 °C during the data acquisition for typically 40 min, waiting for 20 min before taking the first video.

3.2 Video Acquisition

During a typical experiment, up to 30 fields of view were chosen manually, then sequentially scanned automatically. Focus was maintained while scanning using the Nikon 'perfect focus' hardware autofocus system. Movies were taken for 45 s at frame rate of 9.6 fps with an exposure time of 104 ms producing approximately 425 frames. Agar experiments were performed at 30.0 °C.

3.3 Image Analysis

A variety of different algorithms have been developed to track individual particles. Due to the variety of the studied systems, there is not a single gold standard. However, independently of each individual implementation, it is possible to distinguish three required steps in all algorithms [35], each of them with its own challenges and potential sources of error:

1. Localization or identification of particles in individual frames. In the case of diffraction limited spots, the most important constrain is the signal to noise ratio, SNR, where the signal is the spot intensity, and the noise are the intensity fluctuations over the background. It was shown before that at SNR < 4 the tracking accuracy is drastically reduced [36].

2. Linking or connecting trajectories from individual frames. This step is relatively simple if there is a one to one correspondence between the identified particles in two contiguous frames. In real samples, especially if the sample is densely populated, it is

common that some particles disappear, that new particles appear, or that two trajectories merge because they approached to a distance below the resolution limit.

3. Interpretation or data extraction. This step consists in identifying the relevant features on the trajectory: the different types of movement, track velocity, mean-squared displacement, etc. It might be conceptually useful to think of each step as independent, but some approaches combine simultaneously some of them. For example, the detection in the next frame can be restricted to the neighborhood of a previously identified particle (localization and linking), or the knowledge on the expected kind of motion can be used to improve the linking [36] (linking and interpretation).

For the problem in hand the main challenge resides in determining accurately the particle position. This is achieved with sub-pixel resolution by fitting a two-dimensional Gaussian function to the diffraction-limited intensity distributions of each individual focus. At these timescales, the foci are typically well resolved, and there is one to one correspondence between frames. Therefore particle tracks are obtained by matching nearest objects in successive frames. Finally, the centre of mass motion of all the common foci in the image pair is subtracted (this removes collective motion that is due to microscope vibration or in some cases sample drifting). Additionally, the intensity of each focus and its local background is recorded in every frame; this information is required to characterize the expected static error as explained in the rest of the chapter, or to characterize how loci dynamics are effected by the fluorescent protein concentration.

The algorithm was implemented as a MATLAB code. Below are described the steps of localization (divided into identification of candidate particles and refinement of the position accuracy) and linking of trajectories.

A. *Localization of candidate particles.* The aim of this step is to obtain a rough estimate of the particle localization (Fig. 2). The processed images of part A are not used in subsequent steps. (*Note*: **Steps 4** and **5** use Matlab functions extracted from the supplementary material of Jaqaman et al. [36].)

A1. Obtain the average of three frames: the previous frame, the current frame, and the subsequent frame (Fig. 2b).

A2. Smooth by convolving with a 7×7 pixel Gaussian kernel with standard deviation of 1 pixel (Fig. 2c).

A3. Identify regions where cells are located (Fig. 2d). In order to decrease the number of false positives, the analysis is limited to regions of the images that contain cells. These regions have a slightly higher signal than the background due to the effect of cytoplasmic GFP-ParB and autofluorescence. Therefore, it is

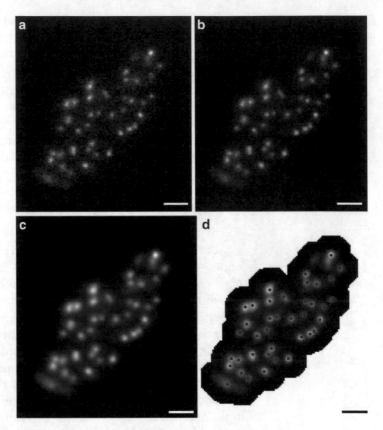

Fig. 2 Example of the different filters used by the tracking algorithm. (**a**) Original image. (**b**) Time average over three frames. (**c**) Convolution with a Gaussian kernel. (**d**) Final result: localized particles (*blue dots*), region with a background lower than cell autofluorescence (*white background*). Scale bar 2 μm. These images correspond to a cluster of approximately 20 cells

possible to identify these areas using Outsu thresholding followed by morphological dilation [37]. It is worth noting that this fluorescence signal is not large enough to segment individual cells.

A4. Calculate the regional mean and noise to estimate the background local intensity and its fluctuations. This information would be later used to test the probability that a given pixel value corresponds to a focus or to the background. In order to save computational time, the image is subdivided into blocks of 11×11 pixels that will be assigned the same mean and a standard deviation value. To calculate these parameters, we consider the pixel intensity values x n in a wider region of 31×31 pixels centred in each 11×11 pixel block. In order to obtain robust statistical parameters of the 31×31 region, first we need to remove the outliers that correspond mainly the foci pixels. To this purpose, we define a test value for each pixel *xn*, as

$$\varsigma_n^2 = \left(x_n - \text{Md}(x)\right)^2,$$

where $\text{Md}(x)$ refers to the median over all the *xn*. Then we take

$$\text{Test Value}_n = \varsigma^2{}_n / \left[\text{Md}(\varsigma^2) N_{\text{magic}}\right],$$

where $N_{\text{magic}} = 1.4826^2$. An *xn* with $\text{Test Value}_n > 9$ is considered an outlier, and will be excluded from the mean and standard deviation calculation. This step makes use of the Matlab function (spatialMovAveBG) developed by Jaqaman et al. [36].

A5. Identify the statistically meaningful local maxima. Considering 3×3 pixel neighborhoods, for each pixel of the original image, we select the ones for which the central pixel is a maximum. In order to determine if these local maxima have statistical significance, they are tested against the background mean and standard deviation (obtained at **step 4**) using the cumulative density function of a normal distribution. The local background intensity and noise are used as the μ and σ parameters of the distribution. Only maxima in the 90% tail of the distribution are considered as valid particles. This part of the procedure follows closely Jaqaman et al. [36] and makes use of the function (locmax2d) from that work.

B. *Subpixel resolution detection of the position.* Using the original unprocessed images, the regions around the candidate particles are fitted to a 2D Gaussian (Fig. 3).

B1. Using the raw images, a region of 5×5 pixels centred in the local maximum obtained above is selected. Each region is fitted to the function [35]

$$Z(x,y) = I_0 \exp\left[-\left[(x - \mu_x)^2 + (y - \mu_y)^2\right] / 2s^2\right] + B,$$

where

$$s = 0.21\lambda / (\text{NA} \times p),$$

λ is the wavelength, NA is the microscope numerical aperture, and p is the pixel size. In our experiments, $\lambda = 510\text{nm}$, NA 1.4 and $p = 106\text{nm}$.

B2. The difference between the local maxima position and the correction given by μy and μx is computed. The data are rejected as an artifact if $\mu^2{}_x + \mu^2{}_y > 2$.

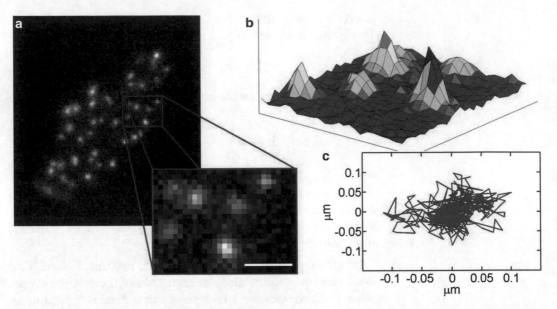

Fig. 3 Subpixel resolution detection of the position. (**a**) Raw image (scale bar 1 μm). (**b**) 3D representation of the zoomed region. In order to obtain subpixel resolution, each peak is fitted to a 2D gaussian. (**c**) Typical resulting trajectory for 430 frames

C. *Linking of the trajectories.* In this step the positions detected along the different time frames are assembled to reconstruct the trajectories.

C1. The closest neighbors between two consecutive frames are assigned to the same trajectory, except if their separation is larger than two pixels.

C2. Particles not assigned to any trajectory in the previous frame are considered as new trajectories.

C3. If the end of a trajectory is separated by less than two pixels and less than three frames from the beginning of another trajectory, the two trajectories are joined. The frames between the two original trajectories, where no particle was identified are considered as "not a number" (NaN). Displacements that require to include NaN data are excluded from the analysis.

3.4 Considerations on Precision and System-Specific Aspects of the Localization Data

The algorithm described above allowed us robust and unsupervised analysis of thousands of movies, proving hundreds of thousands of locus tracks. Of the many possible sources of error, it is worth focussing here just on the fundamental limit in the precision of localization that comes from the number of photons collected during an exposure. This was calculated in [38] as:

$$\varepsilon^2 = s^2 / N + a^2 / 12 / N + 4\sqrt{\pi}\, s^3 b^2 / \left(aN^2\right),$$

where ε^2 is the static error, s is the standard deviation of the point-spread function, a is the pixel size, N is the number of photons collected, and b is the background noise. For a given exposure

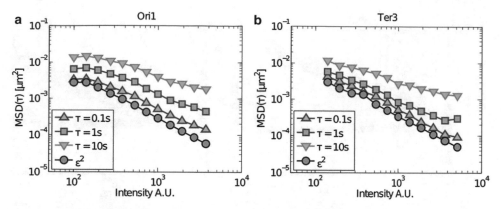

Fig. 4 The static error level is lower than the MSD (0.1 s) at every intensity range. The predicted levels of errors (*gray circle*) are smaller than the intensity binned ensemble average MSD at lag times of 0.1 s (*blue upward triangles*), but only at larger lag times (10 s, *green downward triangles*) the error is expected to be negligible (at least ten times smaller than the MSD). Data from either (**a**) Ori1 or (**b**). Ter3 locus

time, N is proportional to the intensity registered by the camera. The first term arises from the fluctuations in collected photons at a given time due to the Poissonian nature of photon emissions, the second term is consequence of the finite size of the pixels, and the third term considers the effect of background noise. This equation indicates that as the intensity decreases the static error drastically increases. With the ParB/*parS* system, there is typically a large distribution of intensities, and also under repeated imaging there is photobleaching. So the localization of some loci (increasing fraction during multiple acquisitions) will be subject to non-negligible "static error". An accurate statistics needs to take this variable error into account, and/or consider only loci above a threshold intensity for which the static error is negligible. This can easily be tested: we carried out tests by changing the intensity of the excitation illumination, ideally on the same field of view, and verifying the lower illumination threshold at which localization error becomes noticeable (Fig. 4). We also compared motility of loci in living cells with loci in fixed cells, and we generated artificial datasets as in silico "null-models" [1, 2].

The static error and the real displacement are independent, therefore it is possible to subtract the error from the observed MSD ("MSD_{raw}"). As reported in ref. 1, the loci in the Ter domain have a lower mobility, therefore similar levels of static error will have a larger effect on the MSD (Fig. 5a). MSDs from more mobile loci typically present a quite linear behavior in the log-log plots (Fig. 5b). However, once the static error is subtracted, the resulting MSD has a downturn at short lag times for Ori1, most likely a consequence of the dynamic error. The dynamic and static errors have opposite contributions. Since the exposure time and the lag time in our data are equal (movies are under continuous illumination), the dynamic error is not negligible, and can be masked under the effect of the static error.

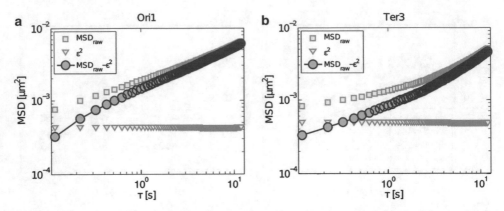

Fig. 5 Error subtraction increases the MSD slope and unmasks the effect of dynamic error. The graphs show the result (*blue circles*) of subtracting the predicted static error (*gray triangles*) from the raw MSD (*gray squares*). The MSDs are calculated using only data with narrow intensity window on data from Ori1 (**a**) and Ter3 (**b**) loci. In Ori1, after the error subtraction, the apparently linear curve shows a down turn at short lag times. The effect is likely to be the dynamic error previously hidden by the static error. In the Ter3 locus, that has lower motility, the effect of static error is still present suggesting that this locus could be close to the analysis limit, although the presence of a different mobility regime cannot be discarded

4   Notes

1. Broad intensity distributions that extend over one or two decades are typical in the analyzed samples. These distributions are observed under constant illumination even in individual experiments, and they seem to be a consequence of variation of GFP-ParB expression in individual cells. Therefore we expect to observe drastic differences in the level of static error between individual foci. A common procedure to determine the ε^2 is to apply the tracking algorithm to movies of immobile particles [39]. The recorded motion is then a measurement of the tracking precision of the experimental setup. Here, to avoid the effect of photobleaching, we used fluorescent beads dried over a coverslip. The processed signal is altered by inserting different neutral density filters into the fluorescent excitation path. As expected, the observed static error is drastically affected with the recorded intensity. While for the beads the effect can be entirely ascribed to changes in precision of the image-analysis procedure, the focus intensity has an important effect on its dynamics, *see* Fig. 4. This effect is independent of tracking errors and rather a consequence of "physics" of size, or binding to DNA of the GFP-ParB complex on the chromosome. Further work is ongoing in our lab investigating this aspect and relating to polymer physics models.

2. Each locus track is analyzed to extract an individual MSD, as a function of lag time τ, and all tracks from a given locus are averaged using both sliding and non-sliding means. Time- and

ensemble-averaged MSD(τ) data of each locus are fitted with the function

$$\mathrm{MSD}(\tau) = 4D_{\mathrm{app}}\tau^{\alpha},$$

where the fitted parameters are $4D_{\mathrm{app}}$ and α which characterize the amplitude and degree of sub-diffusivity of the motion.

3. Each movie contains a set of a minimum of ten moving loci, typically about 35. The typical tracks were composed of about 450 frames separated by 0.104 s intervals. To test the effect of finite track length, measurements were compared with simulations of fractional Brownian motion generated in order to obtain the same number of tracks and frames per track with similar D_{app} considering the two cases $\alpha = 0.4$ and $\alpha = 0.5$. Only loci whose trajectories are followed for at least 280 frames are used for averages (more than 80% of the tracks are 430 frames long). For each experimental run, 15–30 movies are recorded. Each set of movies (biological replicate) typically generates between 500 and 2000 individual loci tracks.

Acknowledgments

We are very grateful to K. Dorfman, V.G. Benza, B. Sclavi, A. Spakowitz, O. Espeli, P.A. Wiggins, N. Kleckner, L. Mirny, and G. Fraser for helpful discussions, Zhicheng Long, Eileen Nugent, Marco Grisi, Kamin Siriwatwetchakul, J. Kotar, and C. Saggioro for their help with the experimental setups and bacterial strains, and O. Espeli and F. Boccard for the gift of bacterial strains developed in their laboratory. This work was supported by the International Human Frontier Science Program Organization, grant RGY0070/2014, the EU ITN-Transpol, Royal Society International Joint Project, and Consejo Nacional de Ciencia y Tecnologia (CONACYT).

References

1. Javer A, Long Z, Nugent E, Grisi M, Siriwatwetchakul K, Dorfman KD, Cicuta P, Cosentino Lagomarsino M (2013) Short-time movement of E. coli chromosomal loci depends on coordinate and subcellular localization. Nat Commun 4:3003

2. Javer A, Kuwada NJ, Long Z, Benza VG, Dorfman KD, Wiggins PA, Cicuta P, Lagomarsino MC (2014) Persistent super-diffusive motion of Escherichia coli chromosomal loci. Nat Commun 5:3854

3. Valkenburg J, Woldringh C (1984) Phase separation between nucleoid and cytoplasm in

Escherichia coli as defined by immersive refractometry. J Bacteriol 160:1151–1157

4. Mondal J, Bratton BP, Li Y, Yethiraj A, Weisshaar JC (2011) Entropy-based mechanism of ribosome-nucleoid segregation in E. coli cells. Biophys J 100:2605–2613

5. Wiggins PA, Cheveralls KC, Martin JS, Lintner R, Kondev J (2010) Strong intranucleoid interactions organize the Escherichia coli chromosome into a nucleoid filament. Proc Natl Acad Sci U S A 107:4991–4995

6. Fisher JK, Bourniquel A, Witz G, Weiner B, Prentiss M, Kleckner N (2013) Four-dimensional

imaging of E. coli nucleoid organization and dynamics in living cells. Cell 153:882–895

7. Hadizadeh Yazdi N, Guet CC, Johnson RC, Marko JF (2012) Variation of the folding and dynamics of the Escherichia coli chromosome with growth conditions. Mol Microbiol 86: 1318–1333

8. Youngren B, Nielsen HJ, Jun S, Austin S, Jo H (2014) The multifork Escherichia coli chromosome is a self-duplicating and self-segregating thermodynamic ring polymer. Genes Dev 28: 71–84

9. Jun S, Wright A (2010) Entropy as the driver of chromosome segregation. Nat Rev Microbiol 8:600–607

10. Jun S, Mulder B (2006) Entropy-driven spatial organization of highly confined polymers: lessons for the bacterial chromosome. Proc Natl Acad Sci U S A 103:12388–12393

11. Lim HC, Surovtsev IV, Beltran BG, Huang F, Bewersdorf J, Jacobs-Wagner C (2014) Evidence for a DNA-relay mechanism in ParABS-mediated chromosome segregation. eLife 3, e02758

12. Jung Y, Jeon C, Kim J, Jeong H, Jun S, Ha B-Y (2012) Ring polymers as model bacterial chromosomes: confinement, chain topology, single chain statistics, and how they interact. Soft Matter 8:2095

13. Bryant JA, Sellars LE, Busby SJW, Lee DJ (2014) Chromosome position effects on gene expression in Escherichia coli K-12. Nucleic Acids Res 42(18):1–10

14. Cagliero C, Grand RS, Jones MB, Jin DJ, O'Sullivan JM (2013) Genome conformation capture reveals that the Escherichia coli chromosome is organized by replication and transcription. Nucleic Acids Res 41:6058–6071

15. Alberts B, Johnson A, Lewis J, Raff M, Roberts K, Walter P (2002) "Molecular" biology of the cell. Garland Science, New York, NY

16. Reyes-Lamothe R, Wang X, Sherratt D (2008) Escherichia coli and its chromosome. Trends Microbiol 16:238–245

17. Wang X, Montero Llopis P, Rudner DZ (2013) Organization and segregation of bacterial chromosomes. Nat Rev Genet 14:191–203

18. Joshi MC, Bourniquel A, Fisher J, Ho BT, Magnan D, Kleckner N, Bates D (2011) Escherichia coli sister chromosome separation includes an abrupt global transition with concomitant release of late-splitting intersister snaps. Proc Natl Acad Sci U S A 108:2765–2770

19. Espeli O, Mercier R, Boccard F, Espeli O (2008) DNA dynamics vary according to macrodomain topography in the E. coli chromosome. Mol Microbiol 68:1418–1427

20. Nielsen HJ, Li Y, Youngren B, Hansen FG, Austin S (2006) Progressive segregation of the Escherichia coli chromosome. Mol Microbiol 61:383–393

21. Wang XD, Liu X, Possoz C, Sherratt DJ (2006) The two Escherichia coli chromosome arms locate to separate cell halves. Genes Dev 20: 1727–1731

22. Kuwada NJ, Cheveralls KC, Traxler B, Wiggins PA (2013) Mapping the driving forces of chromosome structure and segregation in Escherichia coli. Nucleic Acids Res 41:1–8

23. Pelletier J, Halvorsen K, Ha B-Y, Paparcone R, Sandler SJ, Woldringh CL, Wong WP, Jun S (2012) Physical manipulation of the Escherichia coli chromosome reveals its soft nature. Proc Natl Acad Sci U S A 109:E2649–E2656

24. Hong S-H, Toro E, Mortensen KI, de la Rosa MAD, Doniach S, Shapiro L, Spakowitz AJ, McAdams HH (2013) Caulobacter chromosome in vivo configuration matches model predictions for a supercoiled polymer in a cell-like confinement. Proc Natl Acad Sci U S A 110: 1674–1679

25. Weber SC, Spakowitz AJ, Theriot JA (2010) Bacterial chromosomal loci move subdiffusively through a viscoelastic cytoplasm. Phys Rev Lett 104:1–4

26. Weber SC, Spakowitz AJ, Theriot JA (2012) Nonthermal ATP-dependent fluctuations contribute to the in vivo motion of chromosomal loci. Proc Natl Acad Sci U S A 109: 7338–7343

27. Weber SC, Thompson MA, Moerner WE, Spakowitz AJ, Theriot JA (2012) Analytical tools to distinguish the effects of localization error, confinement, and medium elasticity on the velocity autocorrelation function. Biophys J 102:2443–2450

28. Cicuta P, Donald AM (2007) Microrheology: a review of the method and applications. Soft Matter 3:1449

29. Saxton MJ (2009) Single-particle tracking. In: Jue T (ed) Fundamental concepts in biophysics, chap. 6. Humana, Totowa, NJ, pp 147–180

30. Levi V, Gratton E (2007) Exploring dynamics in living cells by tracking single particles. Cell Biochem Biophys 48:1–15

31. Meijering E, Dzyubachyk O, Smal I (2012) Methods for cell and particle tracking. Methods Enzymol 504:183–200

32. Crocker J (1996) Methods of digital video microscopy for colloidal studies. J Colloid Interface Sci 179:298–310

33. Weber SC, Theriot JA, Spakowitz AJ (2010) Subdiffusive motion of a polymer composed of subdiffusive monomers. Phys Rev E 82:1–11

34. Saxton M (2008) Single-particle tracking: connecting the dots. Nat Methods 5:671–672

35. Cheezum MK, Walker WF, Guilford WH (2001) Quantitative comparison of algorithms for tracking single fluorescent particles. Biophys J 81:2378–2388

36. Jaqaman K, Loerke D, Mettlen M, Kuwata H, Grinstein S, Schmid SL, Danuser G (2008) Robust single-particle tracking in live-cell time-lapse sequences. Nat Methods 5:695–702

37. Gonzalez RC, Woods RE (2006) Digital image processing, 3rd edn. Prentice-Hall, Inc., Upper Saddle River, NJ

38. Thompson RE, Larson DR, Webb WW (2002) Precise nanometer localization analysis for individual fluorescent probes. Biophys J 82: 2775–2783

39. Savin T, Doyle PS (2005) Static and dynamic errors in particle tracking microrheology. Biophys J 88:623–638

Chapter 14

Biophysical Characterization of Chromatin Remodeling Protein CHD4

Rosa Morra, Tomas Fessl, Yuchong Wang, Erika J. Mancini, and Roman Tuma

Abstract

Chromatin-remodeling ATPases modulate histones–DNA interactions within nucleosomes and regulate transcription. At the heart of remodeling, ATPase is a helicase-like motor flanked by a variety of conserved targeting domains. CHD4 is the core subunit of the nucleosome remodeling and deacetylase complex NuRD and harbors tandem plant homeo finger (tPHD) and chromo (tCHD) domains. We describe a multifaceted approach to link the domain structure with function, using quantitative assays for DNA and histone binding, ATPase activity, shape reconstruction from solution scattering data, and single molecule translocation assays. These approaches are complementary to high-resolution structure determination.

Key words Nucleosome, ATPase, Surface plasmon resonance, SAXS, TIRF, FRET

1 Introduction

Chromodomain helicase DNA-binding protein 4 (CHD4), which is sometimes referred to as Mi2β, is an SNF2-type chromatin remodeling motor [1] and the main subunit of the nucleosome remodeling and deacetylase (NuRD) [2–5]. The complex is involved in gene transcription regulation [6, 7] by mediating histone deacetylation. Unlike other remodelers, such as SWI/SNF, NuRD is thought to act as a transcriptional repressor [8] and achieves its function through the combination of a motor protein, CHD4, with other subunits such as the histone deacetylases HDAC1 and HDAC2 [6]. The key questions for any remodeling motor are how the ATPase is targeted to specific sites within the chromatin environment and how ATP hydrolysis is coupled to the remodeling activity. In order to answer these questions, it is important to dissect the domain structure and function of the protein.

In addition to the ATPase domain, CHD4 harbors two plant zinc finger homeodomains arranged in a tandem fashion (tPHD). These are common in nucleosome/histone-binding proteins

Mark C. Leake (ed.), *Chromosome Architecture: Methods and Protocols*, Methods in Molecular Biology, vol. 1431,
DOI 10.1007/978-1-4939-3631-1_14, © Springer Science+Business Media New York 2016

[9–11]. It also exhibits tandem chromodomains (tCHD) which have been shown to mediate chromatin interaction by binding directly to either DNA, RNA, or methylated histone H3 [12–15]. The combination of tPHD and tCHD is specific for the CHD family (CHD3, CHD4, and CHD5) [16], however simultaneous presence of several histone-binding modules is prevalent for many chromatin remodeling ATPases.

Here we describe biochemical and biophysical methods which were instrumental in shedding light on the mechanism by which these domains cooperate in the context of ATPase-driven nucleosome remodeling [17]. We describe cloning and purification of the individual tandem domains and various ATPase constructs and characterize their binding to nucleic acids and various modified histone tails using electrophoretic mobility shift assay (EMSA) and surface plasmon resonance (SPR), respectively. ATPase assay is used to demonstrate cooperation between the tPHD and tCHD domains and the ATPase module. We describe a novel single molecule assay to visualize CHD4 translocation along DNA.

2   Materials

2.1   Cloning and Expression

pTriEx2 vector (Novagen).

BL21 (DE3) supercompetent cells (Agilent).

XL1 supercompetent cells (Agilent).

DNA using miniprep kit (Qiagen).

1 M stock of isopropyl-thiogalactopyranoside (IPTG, Sigma).

Lysogeny broth (LB): 10 g bacto-tryptone, 5 g yeast extract, 10 g NaCl per 1 L media.

Terrific broth (TB): 12 g bacto-tryptone, 24 g yeast extract, 4 mL glycerol per 1 L media.

2.2   Protein Purification

Lysis buffer: 50 mM sodium phosphate pH 7.5, 500 mM NaCl, 5 mM imidazole, 0.2% Tween 20, protease inhibitor cocktail tablet (Roche).

Talon™ resin (Clontech).

Imidazole (Sigma).

HiTrap Chelating column 5 mL (GE Healthcare).

Superdex S200 10/30 (GE Healthcare).

S75 10/30 column (GE Heathcare).

SEC buffer: 20 mM Tris pH 7.5, 200 mM NaCl, 1 mM DTT.

Acryl amide 30% stock (Severn Biotec).

2.3 Nucleic Acid-Binding EMSA

MW marker Gene Ruler 100 bp Plus DNA ladder (Fermentas).

MW marker XIII 50-750 (Roche).

MW marker Gene Ruler 1 Kb and 100 bp Plus DNA ladder (Invitrogen).

Molecular biology grade agarose (Sigma).

DNA-binding buffer: 20 mM Tris pH 7.5, 200 mM NaCl.

TAE buffer: prepared from 10× TAE stock: 48.4 g Tris base, 11.4 mL glacial acetic acid, 3.7 g EDTA disodium salt per 1 L.

Ethidium bromide 1000× stock: 10 mg/mL.

2.4 ATPase Assay

EnzChek phosphate release assay (Life Technologies/Thermo-Fisher).

100 mM ATP stock solution, pH 7 (Jena Biosciences).

10× standard buffer: 400 mM Tris pH 7.5, 500 mM NaCl, 50 mM $MgCl_2$.

2.5 NCP Mobility Shift

NCP-binding buffer: 20 Tris–HCl pH 8, 200 mM NaCl, 10% sucrose.

λ-DNA (Stratagene).

Acryl amide 30% stock (Severn Biotec).

10% glycerol.

Native running buffer: 20 mM Hepes pH 8, 1 mM EDTA.

2.6 SPR

Streptavidin sensor chips (GE Healthcare).

0.05 M Sodium hydroxide activation and regeneration solution (GE Healthcare).

SPR buffer: 20 mM Tris pH 7.5, 200 mM NaCl, 0.05% (v/v) polysorbate 20 (GE Healthcare).

Biotinylated and differentially methylated (at Lys4 and Lys9) histone H3 peptides were custom synthesized by Millipore.

Wash solution 1: 0.05% SDS.

Wash solution 2: 0.9 M NaCl.

100 mM ATP stock solution, pH 7 (Jena Biosciences).

2.7 Labeling of Protein and DNA with Fluorescent Dyes

Plasmid pGEM-3z/601 (Addgene plasmid 26656).

Alexa Fluor 594 maleimide (Life Technologies/Thermo-Fisher).

Alexa Fluor 488-labeled forward primer (Life Technologies/Thermo-Fisher):

5′-AF 488-GCCCTGGAGAATCCCGGTGC-3′.

Biotinylated reverse:

5′-Biotin-CAGGTCGGGAGCTCGGAACACTATC-3′.

PCR kit (Promega).

SYBR Gold stain (Life Technologies/Thermo-Fisher).

BamHI restriction enzyme (New England Biolabs).

HindIII restriction enzyme (New England Biolabs).

Labeling reaction buffer: 20 mM Tris pH 7.5, 200 mM NaCl.

Dialysis buffer: 20 mM Tris pH 7.5, 200 mM NaCl, 1 mM DTT.

Molecular biology grade agarose (Sigma).

LB Amp agar plates.

2× TY-AC medium: 16 g bacto-tryptone, 10 g yeast extract, 5 g NaCl.

Ampicillin (Amp) 1000× stock solution 100 mg/mL.

2.8 Single Molecule Fluorescence Imaging

Glass cover slips (Thermo-Fisher).

Vectabond reagent (Vector Laboratories, Burlingame, USA).

Polyethyleneglycol succinimidyl ester (PEG-NHS, Rapp Polymere).

Biotinylated-PEG-NHS (Rapp Polymere).

0.1 M sodium bicarbonate buffer, pH 8.3 (SigmaUltra).

10 mM Tris, pH 7.4 (SigmaUltra).

Immunopure-streptavidin (Pierce Biotechnology).

Buffer A: 25 mM Tris acetate, pH 8.0 with 8 mM magnesium acetate (SigmaUltra), 100 mM KCl, 1 mM dithiothreitol, and 3.5 % (w/v) poly-ethylene glycol 6000 (SigmaUltra).

Anti-photobleaching cocktail; 1.25 mM propyl gallate, 5 mM DTT, 5 mM cysteamine, 1.5 mM β-mercaptoethanol (Fluka/SigmaAldrich).

3 Methods

3.1 Expression and Purification of CHD4 Constructs

The cloning and purification method is rather generic and is used for all the constructs generated here. However, it might need to be modified for different chromatin remodeling ATPases, which, as many nuclear proteins, are known to have solubility problems. For example it may not be possible to obtain the full-length protein in a soluble, active form and a suitable truncation will need to be devised, as shown here for CHD4 (Fig. 1).

1. Select domains based on predicted gene structure (GeneBank, Fig. 1). Generate C-terminal 8xHis-tagged construct by PCR using human CHD4 cDNA (Mammalian Gene Collection) as a template and appropriate sets of primers containing cloning sites compatible with the recipient plasmid (*see* **Note 1**).

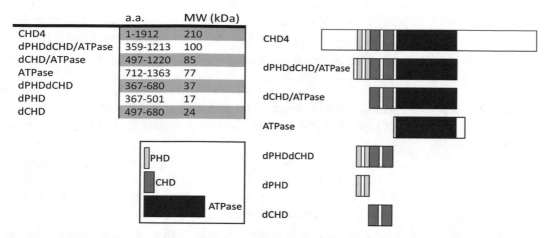

	a.a.	MW (kDa)
CHD4	1-1912	210
dPHDdCHD/ATPase	359-1213	100
dCHD/ATPase	497-1220	85
ATPase	712-1363	77
dPHDdCHD	367-680	37
dPHD	367-501	17
dCHD	497-680	24

Fig. 1 Domain constructs used in this study, relative molecular weights (*left*) and position within the full-length CHD4 (*right*)

2. Ligate the amplified PCR product into the expression vector (in this case pTriEx2) and transform XL1 cells using appropriate antibiotic (Amp) for selection.

3. Select colonies, grow overnight culture, and extract plasmid DNA using miniprep kit (Qiagen). Verify insert by sequencing.

4. Transform *E. coli* BL21 (DE3) supercompetent expression cells.

5. Select colonies and inoculate an overnight booster LB culture (100 mL).

6. Inoculate 6×0.5 L of TB with 10 mL of the booster and grow at 37 °C till $OD_{600} = 0.6$.

7. Chill to below 20 °C on ice or in cold room and induce with 0.7 mM IPTG (final concentration).

8. Grow culture overnight at 20 °C shaking (225 rpm).

9. Harvest cells by centrifugation at $3500 \times g$ for 15 min at 4 °C.

10. Resuspend cell pellets in 30 mL of the lysis buffer and lyse the cells using a French pressure cell (Aminco).

11. Clarify the lysate by centrifugation at $15,3446 \times g$ (SW32Ti rotor) for 1 h, 4 °C.

12. Collect supernatant and mix with Talon™ resin.

13. Elute with an imidazole gradient and check protein composition in fractions by 12% SDS-PAGE (10 μL samples mixed with 20 μL of 2× sample-loading buffer).

14. Inject up to 5 mL of the collected fractions onto S-200 (25/300) column and elute with flow rate 3 mL/min at room temperature.

15. Run SDS-PAGE gel on fractions and check the purity and integrity of proteins by mass spectrometry (*see* **Note 2**).

16. Determine the protein concentration using predicted extinction coefficient.

3.2 Multiple Angle Light Scattering (MALS)

MALS gives estimate of the native mass and thus can inform of the oligomeric status or non-covalent association between subunits or domains.

1. Configure the light-scattering instrumentation (DAWN HELEOS II, Wyatt Technology, Santa Barbara, CA) in a flow cell mode coupled to an analytical Superdex S200 or S75 10/300 column (flow rate 0.5 mL/min).

2. Line up a differential refractive index (RI, Optilab rEX, Wyatt Technology) and Agilent 1200 UV (Agilent Technologies) detectors after the exit from the light-scattering flow cell. If necessary adjust sensitivity of RI and UV/VIS detectors (*see* **Note 3**). Some light-scattering instruments allow adjusting the laser power, i.e. higher power for samples with low concentration (*see* **Note 4**).

3. Equilibrate the column in the desired buffer, flush the reference cell of the RI detector and zero both RI and UV/VIS detectors.

4. Inject 0.1–0.5 mL of BSA standard sample (*see* **Note 5**) (~2 mg/mL; *see* **Note 6**) and collect data for the duration of the HPLC run. This data will be used to calibrate the light-scattering detector. Analyze the data to determine the calibration constant.

5. Analyzed the data using the software provided with the instrument (ASTRA software package, Wyatt Technology). For the analysis you will need to specify the calibration constant (obtained in 3 above), temperature, an estimated dn/dc (refractive index increment, typical value 0.15) and/or molar extinction coefficient predicted from amino acid composition (http://web.expasy.org/protparam/).

3.3 Multiplexed DNA-Binding Assay

Electrophoretic gel mobility shift assays constitute a standard method to detect formation of stable nucleic acid protein complexes. Usually, these are done using a single-labeled probe with a defined length. However, chromatin remodeling complexes, which often have multiple DNA-binding domains, may discriminate between short and longer DNAs. Hence, it is desirable to probe association with multiple DNA fragments of various lengths. A simple way to implement this is to use a generic ladder DNA (Fig. 2). However, this approach is qualitative and, due to overlap of shifted bands, may not allow determination of dissociation constants.

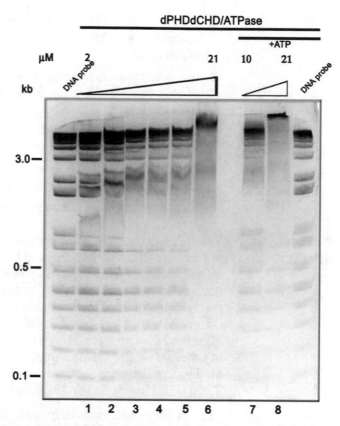

Fig. 2 Multiplexed variable length EMSA. Agarose gel image of ladder DNA in the absence (DNA probe) and presence of increasing concentration of CHD4 construct (*lanes 1–6*) and in the presence of 1 mM ATP (*lanes 7–8*)

1. Mix dsDNA MW marker (*see* **Note 7**) probe with increasing amounts of CHD4 (*see* **Note 8**) constructs in 20 µL of DNA-binding buffer and incubate for 5 min at room temperature (or any desired temperature).

2. Add 2 µL of loading buffer and load the sample onto a 2% agarose gel.

3. Run the gel in 1× TAE buffer at 20 mA for 40 min.

4. Stained for 10 min with 1× ethidium bromide and visualize DNA–protein complexes by UV light with long-pass filter.

5. If the bands are well resolved, quantification of the shifts can be attempted using imaging and analysis software.

3.4 Nucleosome Core Particle Mobility Shift Assay

Preparation of histones and reconstitution of nucleosomes (NC) is an art of its own and is beyond the scope of this chapter. We refer the reader to recent and classic publications on histone production [18, 19] and nucleosome core particle (NCP) reconstitution [20]. Only steps pertaining to the NC mobility shift assay are delineated below (*see* **Note 9**).

1. Reconstitute NCP (50 fmol) with radiolabeled (or fluorescently labeled) DNA (168 bp PCR fragment) by salt gradient dialysis [21].

2. Incubate with increasing amount of CHD4 construct for 15 min on ice in 10 μL of NCP-binding buffer.

3. For the chasing control experiment (*see* **Note 10**), after the incubation on ice, add 200× excess (by weight) of λ-DNA and incubate on ice for a further 10 min.

4. Run a native gel electrophoresis (5% polyacrylamide) containing 10% glycerol in the native running buffer at 15 mA for 3 h.

5. Visualize the gel by phosphorimager or autoradiography.

3.5 SPR Histone Tail Binding Studies

SPR is one of the most popular techniques to follow binding kinetics in vitro. It offers multiplexing and high-throughput in a fully automated format. Perhaps the only drawback is the requirement to immobilize one of the binding partners. Since the technique relies on the changes in refractive index close to the probed surface it is common that the smaller of the binding partners (ligand) is immobilized while the larger entity (receptor) is flown over the surface in order to produce large signal changes (*see* **Note 11**). Our SPR binding studies were performed using a Biacore 2000/3000 and T100 (GE Healthcare) at 25 °C in SPR buffer.

1. Check protein concentrations (*see* **Note 12**) by measuring absorbance at 280 nm using calculated molar extinction coefficients.

2. Unpack and insert the sensor and activate the surface with streptavidin following the manufacturer's recommendation (*see* **Note 13**).

3. Immobilize biotinylated histone peptides onto the sensor chip following manufacturer's instructions. Relatively low histone peptide immobilization levels (40–90 resonance units (*see* **Note 14**)) are desirable to minimize mass transport artifacts [22]. Prepare the surfaces of the three flow cells (Fc2, Fc3, Fc4) (*see* **Note 15**) and separately immobilize different peptides (flow rate of 20 μL/min) using Fc1 as the reference cell to gauge surface density (*see* **Note 16**).

4. Flow different concentrations of CHD4 construct through all chambers on the chip using a fast flow rate of 100 μL/min (*see* **Note 17**).

5. Between individual injections regenerate the chip by three repeated application of 0.05% SDS followed by a 0.9 M NaCl wash and then equilibrate in the binding buffer.

6. Repeat all measurements at least three times.

7. The signal from experimental flow cells is then corrected by subtraction of reference signal (flow cell Fc1).

8. When appropriate, the data can be globally fitted with a second-order association reaction model (approximated by a pseudo-first-order reaction with rate constant $k = k_{on}[\text{ligand}]$ for each ligand concentration) followed by a first-order dissociation with characteristic kinetic constants k_{on} and k_{off} (Fig 3b) (see **Note 18**).

9. In the case of fast binding/unbinding kinetics (Fig. 3a) the equilibrium dissociation constants K_d values can be obtained from the steady-state plateau values. These are simply fit to Langmuir binding isotherm (bound $= C^*\text{max}/(K_d + C)$, where C is analyte concentration and max is the saturation level, Fig. 3c).

10. Add ATP (1 mM final concentration) to the protein before injection onto the sensor chip to probe affinity modulation by ATPase domain (see **Note 19**).

3.6 ATPase Activity Assay

There are many ATPase assays available on the market. We have selected the EnzCheck (Thermo-Fisher) inorganic phosphate (P_i) release assay, which is a quantitative spectrophotometric assay based on coupled enzymatic reaction and chromogenic substrate. This assay supports steady-state kinetic measurements in real time without the need to quench and measure individual time points. The adaptation of the assay to a 96-well plate (see **Note 20**) is particularly useful for determination of kinetic parameters (k_{cat}, the turnover number; K_M, Michaelis constant) [23].

1. Calculate the mixing volumes for the desired conditions for each well. Use an optically transparent, flat bottom, 96-well plate.

2. Dilute the standard 10× buffer by adding 20 μL for 200 μL final volume per well, add 40 μL of MESG chromogenic substrate, 2 μL PnPase enzyme, suitable ATPase aliquot (final concentration 0.1 to 1 μM, depending on the expected activity). Add deionized water to top up to final volume (see **Note 21**).

3. Aliquot inorganic phosphate KH_2PO_4 standards (0, 20, 40, 60, and 100 μM final concentration) into positive control wells (see **Note 22**).

4. Mix wells and insert the plate into the plate reader equipped with absorption filter at 360 nm (or a monochromator tuned to that wavelength) and collect 5 min baseline read. Depending on number of wells read and the type of the plate, reader set the data collection to record each well at least every 30 s (see **Note 23**).

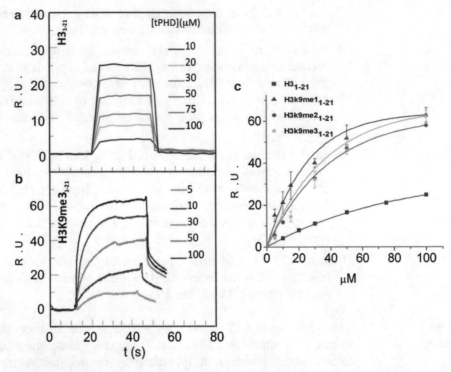

Fig. 3 SPR binding of tandem PHD domains to surface immobilized H3 unmethylated (**a**) and K9 trimethylated peptides (**b**) and the resulting Langmuir isotherm for equilibrium binding (**c**)

5. Add ATP alone without the ATPase as a background control (*see* **Note 24**). Another negative control is the assay mix including the ATPase but without ATP to check for presence of inorganic phosphate in the protein sample (*see* **Note 25**).

6. Add ATP to achieve the desired concentrations in the ATPase samples, mix wells and insert the plate, and record absorbance changes at 360 nm for 20 min.

7. To estimate the ATPase turnover rate, the initial, linear portion of the raw data is fitted by linear regression (*see* **Note 26**) (using e.g. GraphPad Prism or Origin software) and the amount of P_i released per second is obtained from the slope of the regression line normalized by the molarity of protein (concentrations determined from absorbance at 280 nm using calculated molar extinction coefficients).

3.7 SAXS Data Collection and Processing

SAXS provides information on oligomeric status and overall shape of macromolecular assemblies. Here, we describe how it can be used to delineate the spatial disposition of different functional domains within a large protein. This requires successful expression of the individual domains in a folded and biologically active form. The latter is underpinned by the array of biochemical data, such as DNA- and histone tail-binding assays and ATPase activity as discussed above. We only describe general sequence for data processing, leaving out much detail since that depends on the software package used. Our discourse is limited to the widely used ATSAS software package (http://www.embl-hamburg.de/biosaxs/software.html) developed by Dimtri Svergun and colleagues. Further technical intricacies of SAXS can be found in a recent excellent monograph [24].

1. Although SAXS data can be obtained on a modern laboratory X-ray source such a specialized equipment is not commonly found in labs and it is advisable to collect data at a synchrotron radiation facility such as ESRF (Grenoble, France), EMBL facility at the PETRA ring (Hamburg, Germany), or the Diamond Light Source (Harwell, U.K.). These facilities operate dedicated beamlines which are accessed via a rapid turnover proposal-based schemes. Collecting data for the work described here would need only one 8 h shift at present time. This might become even shorter with further automation of beamlines and remote access capacity.

2. This work employed ESRF beamline ID14-3 which uses a flow cell and automated sample loading system (*see* **Note 27**). A minimum of 10 μL of each sample is required to fill the scattering cell (*see* **Note 28**).

3. Confer with the beamline scientist to configure the system for the intended use, e.g. depending on the size of the complex and available amounts and concentrations.

4. Collect scattering from empty cell.

5. Collect scattering from water (*see* **Note 29**).

6. Collect scattering from buffer for the BSA standard (e.g. PBS).

7. Collect BSA standard of known concentration (2–5 g/L).

8. Each biomolecule sample is preceded and followed by collection of the matching buffer (*see* **Note 30**).

9. Ten or more successive frames (*see* **Note 31**) (10 s to 1 min duration) are collected and compared to check for radiation damage (*see* **Note 32**) and aggregation during each SAXS experiment.

10. The data are collected on 2D detectors and images are automatically integrated, averaged (*see* **Note 33**) and corrected to obtain 1D scattering intensities by the beamline software.

11. Further processing (manual background subtraction and averaging, data quality appraisal, Guinier plot) can be done with PRIMUS program package [25].

12. Draw the Guinier plot in PRIMUS to estimate molecular mass from the extrapolated intensity at zero angle (I_0) and radius of gyration (R_g) from the slope. Use BSA as standard (*see* **Note 34**) for estimating mass from I_0 (*see* **Note 35**).

13. Compute pair-wise distance distribution functions using indirect transformation method implemented in the GNOM program. The distribution is then used to estimate the maximum dimension (D_{max}) [26, 27] and refine R_g.

14. Use the output file from GNOM as input for ab initio shape determination by programs DAMMIN [28] or DAMMIF [29] (*see* **Note 36**).

15. Superimpose models using the SUPCOMB program [30] and average them using DAMAVER [31].

16. Use DAMFILT to trim the model to the desired volume derived either from SAXS or from hydrodynamic and light-scattering experiments (R_h and mass) [31].

17. After obtaining models of individual domains attempt to fit the component structures into larger entities, e.g. tCHD and tPHD models into the tPHDtCHD model and tPHD, tCHD, and ATPase models into the tPHDtCHD/ATPase model. An initial model can be arrived at by visual docking in CHIMERA using volume overlap correlation [32].

18. Perform multiphase ab initio modeling using the program MONSA [28] in which three phases correspond to tPHD, tCHD, and ATPase domains and are either pre-assigned on the basis of the manual fitting or randomized (*see* **Note 37**).

3.8 Labeling CHD4 with Fluorescent Dye

CHD4 is an ATPase and is thought to be a molecular motor which can move along nucleic acids and reposition nucleosomes. In order to probe short range motion, CHD4 tPHDtCHD/ATPase was labeled with acceptor dye Alexa Fluor 590 maleimide. Maleimide reacts with cysteines accessible on CHD4 surface. Cysteine is chosen, since it is the least abundant amino acid in CHD4 (22 Cys) only few of them are expected to be exposed on the surface (*see* **Note 38**). All steps below are performed to limit exposure to intense light, e.g. wrapping tubes with aluminium foil or using dark tinted tubes.

1. Mix protein stock (10 μM) with 10-fold molar excess of Alexa Fluor dye (10 mM DMSO stock) and incubate for 8 h at 4 °C (*see* **Note 39**).

2. Dialyze labeled protein overnight and store in dark at 4 °C (*see* **Note 40**).

3. Determine the degree of labeling by recording UV/VIS absorbance spectrum of the conjugated protein and computing the protein concentration from absorbance at 280 nm corrected for the dye contribution estimated from abs. maximum of the dye at 590 nm. The correction factor is dye-specific and is listed in manufacturer manual (*see* **Note 41**) (0.56 for AF594). The molar ratio of label to protein should ideally be 1 or slightly higher (*see* **Note 42**).

4. Check the ATPase activity and DNA binding of the conjugated protein using assays described above.

3.9 Preparation of Labeled 601 Sequence

1. The pGEM-3z/601 with 601 sequence insert (Fig. 4a) was transformed into XL-1 *E. coli* cells and selected on LB Amp agar plates.

2. Pick a single colony and inoculate 15 mL 2× TY-AC Amp media, grow overnight.

3. Harvest cells and extract the plasmid using a miniprep kit.

4. Digested with BamHI and HindIII.

5. Separate on 2 % agarose gel.

6. Extract band corresponding to 601 sequence.

7. Use the extracted 601 sequence as template with Alexa Fluor 488 and biotin-labeled primers (Fig. 4b) and perform PCR: 50 μl of PCR reaction prepared by adding of 37 μL water, 1 μL plasmid template, 1 μL of both primers, and 10 μL of 5× premixed PCR kit. PCR program: (5′ at 93 °C) and [(1′ at 93 °C and 1′ at 62 °C and 2′ at 72 °C)′ 30] and (10′ at 72 °C), product stored at 4 °C.

8. PCR product was separated on 2 % gel, excised and extracted by centrifugation and again purified on 2 % gel, stained with SYBR GOLD.

9. Check the degree of labeling and emission brightness of donor dye attached to DNA through recording UV/VIS absorption and fluorescence emission spectra.

3.10 DNA Immobilization

For TIRF imaging, DNA templates need to be immobilized onto a clean cover slip surface.

1. Prepare glass cover slip surfaces using the method presented by Rasnik and coworkers [33].

2. Incubate cover slips with Vectabond reagent according to the manufacturer instructions.

3. Coat with mixture of 25 % (w/v) PEG-NHS and 0.25 % (w/v) biotinylated-PEG-NHS in 0.1 M sodium bicarbonate (pH 8.3) for 3 h in order to eliminate non-specific adsorption of proteins.

4. Rinse with 10 mM Tris, pH 7.4 and incubate with 0.2 mg/mL Immunopure-streptavidin for 1 h then rinsed with 3 × 400 μL of buffer A. Excess buffer was blotted off and Alexa Fluor 488-labeled, biotinylated DNA in buffer A was applied to the surface and allowed to bind for 30 min.

5. Remove unbound DNA by blotting and rinsing using three times 400 μL of buffer A.

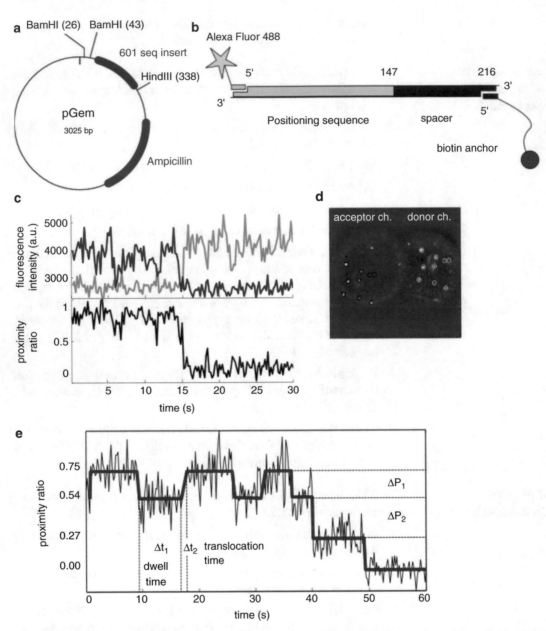

Fig. 4 Preparation of fluorescently labeled and biotinylated dsDNA and TIRF imaging. (**a**) Map of pGEM plasmid with Widom 601 sequence insert. (**b**) Schematics of linear PCR product created with AF488-labeled forward primer and biotinylated reverse primer. (**c**) Time traces of donor (*green*) and acceptor (*red*) and FRET signal (*black*) extracted from corresponding spots in a dual channel image (**d**). (**e**) Time resolved FRET changes observed upon addition of 1 mM ATP

3.11 Single Molecule Imaging

1. In order to avoid photo-destruction samples shall be imaged in anti-photobleaching cocktail: 1.25 mM propyl gallate, 5 mM DTT, 5 mM cysteamine, 1.5 mM β-mercaptoethanol (*see* **Note 43**).

2. Single molecule experiments performed on custom-build TIRFM FRET instrument [34] using imaging rate five frames per second.

3. Optimize protein concentration to minimize background from the bulk-labeled protein while observing enough association with the immobilized DNA (in our case 300 nM).

4. Briefly image immobilized-labeled DNA molecules alone and identify spots (*see* **Note 44**). Only these spots shall be used for further analysis. Image analysis can be done using free software developed by Ha's group: https://cplc.illinois.edu/software/ or simple Matlab scripts.

5. Add labeled protein and image again. Only spatially correlated spots in both channels shall be used (Fig. 4d).

6. Extract time traces and only retain those exhibiting single-step acceptor photobleaching (Fig. 4c).

7. Compute FRET efficiency (proximity ratio) using consecutive single-step acceptor–donor photobleaching sequence [34] or spot intensities corrected for channel sensitivity (Fig. 4c).

8. In steady state, histogram proximity ratios to obtain distributions [34].

9. Add ATP to observe time resolved changes, e.g. bidirectional stepping (Fig. 4e) until all spots photobleach.

4   Notes

1. Primers shall contain appropriate restriction sites for cloning into the desired vector.

2. May need further purifications steps, like ion exchange, to obtain certain proteins.

3. Consider loading concentration and about fivefold dilution on the column to set the sensitivity but the best is to run a test first.

4. Make sure the light scattering is not saturated at the peak maximum.

5. Spin (50 k for 1 h at 4 °C in tabletop ultracentrifuge) to remove as much aggregate as possible.

6. Concentration choice—needs to be high enough for the light-scattering detector to give decent signal while still being within the range.

7. Need to select the right ladder range for the expected length and spacing of putative binding sites, e.g. from less than a nucleosomal repeat (50 bp) to few repeats (1 kb).

8. Select suitable concentration range—usually between high nM to μM—since only relatively stable complexes with dissociation constant $K_d < 0.2$ μM produce discrete shift bands although retardation by transient binding is also possible.

9. NCPs shall be purified first for clean results.

10. The chase experiments are performed to rule out that NCPs are disrupted by CHD4 binding. If disrupted then NCP band would disappear.

11. However, modern instruments, such as GE Healthcare T100, are fully capable of detecting ligand binding in the reverse immobilization format.

12. This is important since K_d derives from the concentration.

13. This is specific for the type of chemistry and to some degree also depends on the vendor.

14. This depends on the instrument sensitivity, while higher density provides higher overall signal, mass transport would certainly be an issue for a large, 100 kDa protein such as CHD4.

15. New instruments have more channels.

16. In order to avoid overcoating this is often done in several steps while observing the R.I. signal.

17. Check flow rate dependence—it should not affect the kinetics. Otherwise there are transport effects and flow rate should be increased.

18. Note that at the beginning of association and dissociation there is an abrupt rise or drop due to so-called bulk contribution from slight buffer mismatch. This is taken into account during data processing.

19. Other nucleotide di/triphosphates and analogues can be used to probe changes in affinity.

20. This is done by scaling the reaction volume down to 200 μL which also saves on consumables having 500 assays instead only 100 per kit.

21. Account for ATP volume if present since it is added last.

22. Use 1:10 dilution of the provided 50 mM stock.

23. Collecting data faster is better but 5 s per well is more than sufficient. This is not an issue for camera-based imaging readers which read all wells at once. However, make sure that the camera-based system can be run in a kinetic mode.

24. Degraded ATP might pose high background and invalidate the assay.

25. This is important if the enzyme is inhibited by P_i—often the rate-limiting step is phosphate release.

26. Note the limits of the coupled reaction, e.g. there is a need to optimize ATPase concentration before doing Michaelis-Menten analysis. V_{max} must be within the rate limit by the coupled PnPase. This rate could be increased by higher PnPase concentration.

27. Similar system has been implemented at Bio-SAXS at Diamond.

28. For shape reconstruction a monodisperse sample is required, best obtained as a fraction from SEC. Some beamlines do have in-line HPLC capability to use with difficult (aggregative) samples.

29. These controls are important to evaluate cleanliness of the flow cell and check for any instrument problems.

30. It is imperative to use the same buffer since even small changes in salt concentration and composition can make subtraction of the baseline difficult or impossible. This is especially important for dilute samples, e.g. protein at or below 1 g/L (w/v) when most of the scattering comes from the solvent/buffer.

31. Now 20×10 s frames are common depending on flux.

32. Radiation damage is manifested by time dependence of the scattering curve and increase in I_0 due to aggregation.

33. However, although the software is smart enough to detect and deal with radiation damage it may not spot other problems. Always check!

34. Guinier plot also useful for extracting the radius of gyration, R_g, and checking for polydispersity (nonlinear Guinier region).

35. Rg for BSA should be ~3 nm, if it is significantly larger or the plot is nonlinear then BSA may be aggregated.

36. Also GASBOR can be used [35] for smaller proteins and takes into account a sequence and medium to wide angle scattering. However, modeling of internal structure is far from reliable.

37. Both fitting procedures should be performed but the latter is computationally intensive and may not yield a unique solution. However, if the data are robust then both solutions are roughly similar, which is reassuring.

38. This can be determined spectrophotometrically by Ellman's reagent or directly from degree of labeling.

39. The final fraction of DMSO needs to be below 5% to avoid protein aggregation.

40. We chose dialysis instead of LC to prevent further dilution of the sample but in some cases HPLC purification offers advantages of being faster and removing non-specifically attached dye which might leach from the sample later and introduce unwanted background.

41. Protein concentration $= (A_{280} - 0.56\,A_{590})/\varepsilon_M$, where ε_M is the molar extinction coefficient.

42. If the ratio is higher than 3 then labeling with less dye and for a shorter period might decrease the stoichiometry and preferentially label only the most accessible site(s).

43. Degassing all buffers and adding oxygen scavenging (catalase) mix may further prolong the life of the fluorophores.

44. Use shutter to control exposure and limit photobleaching.

Acknowledgements

Support of the U.K. MRC, Royal Society (E.M.J.) and Welcome Trust core facility (R.T.) is gratefully acknowledged.

References

1. Eisen JA, Sweder KS, Hanawalt PC (1995) Evolution of the SNF2 family of proteins: subfamilies with distinct sequences and functions. Nucleic Acids Res 23:2715–2723

2. Zhang Y, Ng HH, Erdjument-Bromage H, Tempst P, Bird A, Reinberg D (1999) Analysis of the NuRD subunits reveals a histone deacetylase core complex and a connection with DNA methylation. Genes Dev 13:1924–1935

3. Tong JK, Hassig CA, Schnitzler GR, Kingston RE, Schreiber SL (1998) Chromatin deacetylation by an ATP-dependent nucleosome remodelling complex. Nature 395:917–921

4. Xue Y, Wong J, Moreno GT, Young MK, Cote J, Wang W (1998) NURD, a novel complex with both ATP-dependent chromatin-remodeling and histone deacetylase activities. Mol Cell 2:851–861

5. Feng Q, Zhang Y (2003) The NuRD complex: linking histone modification to nucleosome remodeling. Curr Top Microbiol Immunol 274:269–290

6. Bowen NJ, Fujita N, Kajita M, Wade PA (2004) Mi-2/NuRD: multiple complexes for many purposes. Biochim Biophys Acta 1677:52–57

7. Denslow SA, Wade PA (2007) The human Mi-2/NuRD complex and gene regulation. Oncogene 26:5433–5438

8. Gao H, Lukin K, Ramirez J, Fields S, Lopez D, Hagman J (2009) Opposing effects of SWI/SNF and Mi-2/NuRD chromatin remodeling complexes on epigenetic reprogramming by EBF and Pax5. Proc Natl Acad Sci U S A 106:11258–11263

9. Bienz M (2006) The PHD finger, a nuclear protein-interaction domain. Trends Biochem Sci 31:35–40

10. Shi X, Kachirskaia I, Walter KL, Kuo JH, Lake A, Davrazou F, Chan SM, Martin DG, Fingerman IM, Briggs SD, Howe L, Utz PJ, Kutateladze TG, Lugovskoy AA, Bedford MT, Gozani O (2007) Proteome-wide analysis in Saccharomyces cerevisiae identifies several PHD fingers as novel direct and selective binding modules of histone H3 methylated at either lysine 4 or lysine 36. J Biol Chem 282:2450–2455

11. Pena PV, Davrazou F, Shi X, Walter KL, Verkhusha VV, Gozani O, Zhao R, Kutateladze TG (2006) Molecular mechanism of histone H3K4me3 recognition by plant homeodomain of ING2. Nature 442:100–103

12. Bouazoune K, Mitterweger A, Langst G, Imhof A, Akhtar A, Becker PB, Brehm A (2002) The dMi-2 chromodomains are DNA binding modules important for ATP-dependent nucleosome mobilization. EMBO J 21:2430–2440

13. Akhtar A, Zink D, Becker PB (2000) Chromodomains are protein-RNA interaction modules. Nature 407:405–409

14. Flanagan JF, Mi LZ, Chruszcz M, Cymborowski M, Clines KL, Kim Y, Minor W, Rastinejad F, Khorasanizadeh S (2005) Double chromodomains cooperate to recognize the methylated histone H3 tail. Nature 438:1181–1185

15. Flanagan JF, Blus BJ, Kim D, Clines KL, Rastinejad F, Khorasanizadeh S (2007) Molecular implications of evolutionary differences in CHD double chromodomains. J Mol Biol 369:334–342

16. Marfella CG, Imbalzano AN (2007) The Chd family of chromatin remodelers. Mutat Res 618:30–40

17. Morra R, Lee BM, Shaw H, Tuma R, Mancini EJ (2012) Concerted action of the PHD, chromo and motor domains regulates the human chromatin remodelling ATPase CHD4. FEBS Lett 586:2513–2521

18. Tanaka Y, Tawaramoto-Sasanuma M, Kawaguchi S, Ohta T, Yoda K, Kurumizaka H,

Yokoyama S (2004) Expression and purification of recombinant human histones. Methods 33:3–11

19. Klinker H, Haas C, Harrer N, Becker PB, Mueller-Planitz F (2014) Rapid purification of recombinant histones. PLoS One 9, e104029

20. Dyer PN, Edayathumangalam RS, White CL, Bao Y, Chakravarthy S, Muthurajan UM, Luger K (2004) Reconstitution of nucleosome core particles from recombinant histones and DNA. Methods Enzymol 375:23–44

21. Langst G, Bonte EJ, Corona DF, Becker PB (1999) Nucleosome movement by CHRAC and ISWI without disruption or trans-displacement of the histone octamer. Cell 97:843–852

22. Jonsson U, Fagerstam L, Ivarsson B, Johnsson B, Karlsson R, Lundh K, Lofas S, Persson B, Roos H, Ronnberg I et al (1991) Real-time biospecific interaction analysis using surface plasmon resonance and a sensor chip technology. Biotechniques 11:620–627

23. Lisal J, Tuma R (2005) Cooperative mechanism of RNA packaging motor. J Biol Chem 280:23157–23164

24. Svergun DI, Koch MHJ, Timmins PA, May RP (2013) Small angle X-ray and neutron scattering from solutions of biological macromolecules. International Union of Crystallography Texts on Crystallography, Oxford University Press, Oxford

25. Konarev PV, Volkov VV, Sokolova AV, Koch MHJ, Svergun DI (2003) PRIMUS: a Windows PC-based system for small-angle scattering data analysis. J Appl Crystallogr 36:1277–1282

26. Svergun DI (1991) Mathematical methods in small-angle scattering data analysis. J Appl Crystallogr 24

27. Svergun DI (1992) Determination of the regularization parameter in indirect-transform methods using perceptual criteria. J Appl Crystallogr 25:495–503

28. Svergun DI (1999) Restoring low resolution structure of biological macromolecules from solution scattering using simulated annealing. Biophys J 76:2879–2886

29. Franke D, Svergun DI (2009) DAMMIF, a program for rapid ab-initio shape determination in small-angle scattering. J Appl Crystallogr 42:342–346

30. Kozin MB, Svergun DI (2000) Automated matching of high- and low-resolution structural models. J Appl Crystallogr 34:33–41

31. Volkov VV, Svergun DI (2003) Uniqueness of ab initio shape determination in small-angle scattering. J Appl Crystallogr 36:860–864

32. Pettersen EF, Goddard TD, Huang CC, Couch GS, Greenblatt DM, Meng EC, Ferrin TE (2004) UCSF chimera—a visualization system for exploratory research and analysis. J Comput Chem 25:1605–1612

33. Ha T, Rasnik I, Cheng W, Babcock HP, Gauss GH, Lohman TM, Chu S (2002) Initiation and re-initiation of DNA unwinding by the Escherichia coli Rep helicase. Nature 419:638–641

34. Sharma A, Leach RN, Gell C, Zhang N, Burrows PC, Shepherd DA, Wigneshwararaj S, Smith DA, Zhang X, Buck M, Stockley PG, Tuma R (2014) Domain movements of the enhancer-dependent sigma factor drive DNA delivery into the RNA polymerase active site: insights from single molecule studies. Nucleic Acids Res 42:5177–5190

35. Svergun DI, Petoukhov MV, Koch MHJ (2001) Determination of domain structure of proteins from X-ray solution scattering. Biophys J 80:2946–2953

Chapter 15

Atomistic Molecular Dynamics Simulations of DNA Minicircle Topoisomers: A Practical Guide to Setup, Performance, and Analysis

Thana Sutthibutpong, Agnes Noy, and Sarah Harris

Abstract

While DNA supercoiling is ubiquitous in vivo, the structure of supercoiled DNA is more challenging to study experimentally than simple linear sequences because the DNA must have a closed topology in order to sustain superhelical stress. DNA minicircles, which are closed circular double-stranded DNA sequences typically containing between 60 and 500 base pairs, have proven to be useful biochemical tools for the study of supercoiled DNA mechanics. We present detailed protocols for constructing models of DNA minicircles in silico, for performing atomistic molecular dynamics (MD) simulations of supercoiled minicircle DNA, and for analyzing the results of the calculations. These simulations are computationally challenging due to the large system sizes. However, improvements in parallel computing software and hardware promise access to improve conformational sampling and simulation timescales. Given the concurrent improvements in the resolution of experimental techniques such as atomic force microscopy (AFM) and cryo-electron microscopy, the study of DNA minicircles will provide a more complete understanding of both the structure and the mechanics of supercoiled DNA.

Key words Atomistic molecular dynamics, DNA supercoiling

1 Introduction

DNA supercoiling is ubiquitous in vivo, and is implicated in both genome organization and gene regulation [1]. DNA packaging in both prokaryotic and eukaryotic chromosomes can be investigated by HiC experiments, which detect spatial proximity between pairs of genomic loci through chemical cross-linking [2], and alternatively, by optical techniques such as fluorescence in situ hybridization (FISH) which visualizes the spatial relationship of a few chosen genomic sites [3]. Simple polymer models including the supercoiling of DNA suggest that topology is a crucial factor

Mark C. Leake (ed.), *Chromosome Architecture: Methods and Protocols*, Methods in Molecular Biology, vol. 1431, DOI 10.1007/978-1-4939-3631-1_15, © Springer Science+Business Media New York 2016

to reproduce the experimental spatial contact maps [4]. Moreover, supercoiling directly induces strand separation [5, 6] for RNA polymerase binding [7] and altered the DNA geometry, which influences the regulatory protein binding and makes DNA able to direct its own metabolism by altering the level of supercoiling [8].

1.1 DNA Minicircles as Model Systems

While X-ray crystallography and NMR studies have provided atomistic resolution structural information for short (around 30 base pairs) linear DNA fragments, for protein–DNA complexes [9, 10], and even for nucleosomes [11], it has not been possible to visualize supercoiled DNA minicircles in atomistic detail because they are too structurally disordered to crystallize, they can contain kinks and defects in their structures due to the superhelical stress [12, 13], and they are too large for structural NMR. DNA minicircles have proven to be a more tractable model system for probing complex DNA topologies, because their smaller size significantly reduces the number of conformations. DNA minicircles have been studied experimentally using low-resolution structural techniques such as gel electrophoresis [14], atomic force microscopy (AFM) [15, 16], cryo-electron microscopy (cryo-EM) [13, 17, 18], and cryo-electron tomography (cryo-ET) [19]. While these techniques have provided information about the global shape of the DNA and how this changes in response to supercoiling, so far a fully atomistic description is only possible in computer simulation. Even the smallest DNA minicircles (around 60 base pairs [12]) produce a simulation box that is large in comparison with the linear sequences conventionally studied by the DNA simulation community (which are typically between 10 and 20 base pairs in length [20]), these calculations are nevertheless feasible, albeit with shorter simulation trajectories and poorer sampling. The fortuitous fact that minicircles are just large enough for low-resolution structural studies while being within the reach of atomistic simulation has enabled us to employ a combination of these complementary biophysical techniques to gain insight into the atomistic structure of supercoiled DNA [19, 21].

1.2 Overview of Simulation Protocols for DNA Minicircles

We have developed a bespoke series of protocols for simulating supercoiled DNA minicircles, that are summarized schematically in Fig. 1. Each numbered step within the protocols indicated in the flow diagram is described in detail in the Methods (Subheading 3).

Atomistic simulations of supercoiled DNA minicircles start from a simple planar circular structure constructed from the specific DNA sequence required (**step 1**). The chosen linking number is imposed by adjusting the DNA helical twist within this planar circle (*see* Fig. 2a). This then determines the superhelical density of the closed circular loop. After creating parameters and other essen-

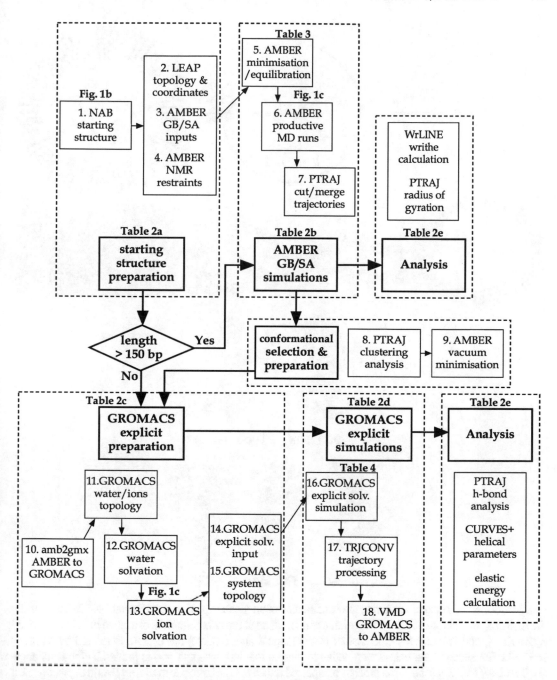

Fig. 1 Flow diagram providing an overview of DNA minicircle simulation protocols. The diagram shows (*top*) the preparation (*steps 1–4*) and running (*steps 5–7*) of AMBER GB/SA implicit solvent simulations for a ~300 bp supercoiled DNA minicircle, and (*bottom*) the preparation (*steps 8–15*) and running (*steps 16–18*) steps of GROMACS explicit solvent simulation of a ~300 bp supercoiled DNA minicircle. The flow diagram also shows the types of analysis performed on both the implicitly and explicitly solvated MD trajectories. A conditional statement is made for the size of DNA minicircle. If the minicircle sequence is shorter than 150 base pairs, the implicit solvent GB/SA simulations need not be performed (skip *steps 5–9*) as the DNA cannot writhe

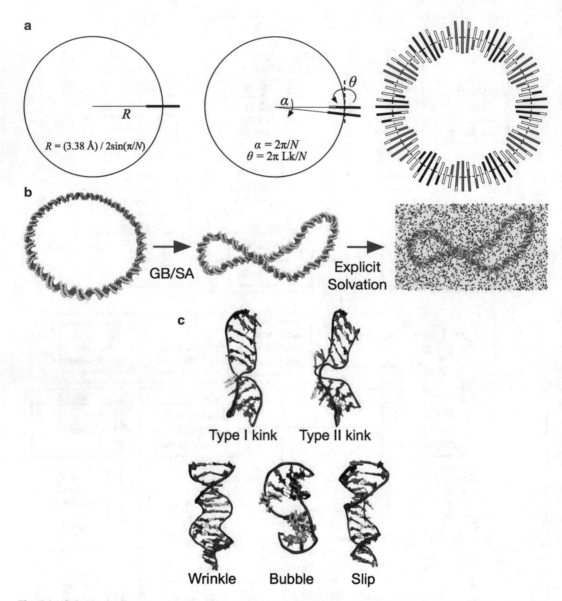

Fig. 2 (**a**) Schematic diagram showing the construction of an N-(base pair) planar circular DNA structure using the NAB program 'circ.nab': (*left*) the first base pair is placed at the circumference of a circle of radius $R = (3.38$ Å$)/2\sin(\pi/N)$, and is oriented perpendicular to the tangent line, (*middle*) the system is rotated by an angle $\alpha = 2\pi/N$. The second base pair is then added to replace the first base pair and is rotated by the twist angle $\theta = 2\pi \times Lk/N$ and (*right*) the same process is repeated until a full DNA circle is made. (**b**) Hybrid implicit/explicit solvation: (*left-middle*) A planar circular 336 bp DNA minicircle at $\Delta Lk = -2$ adopted a writhed conformation in AMBER GB/SA implicit solvent. (*right*) A selected writhed structure was then solvated in 0.1 M NaCl and TIP3P water box by using GROMACS. (**c**) Examples of DNA defects occurred when subjected to high bending and superhelical stress

tial input files (**steps 2–4**), we use a frictionless implicit solvent Generalized Born Surface Approximation (GB/SA) model, which attempts to reproduce the electrostatic screening effect of the high dielectric solvent environment (**steps 5–7**). Our estimates suggest that this speeds up conformational changes from the opened circular to the compacted, writhed structures by at least a factor of 10 [19]. However, the initial planar DNA conformation is highly artificial, and may place unphysical levels of conformational stress upon the duplex. Moreover, while in principle GB/SA simulations provide the same conformational ensemble for the DNA but in an accelerated timeframe, in practice, the neglect of discrete water molecules and solvent ions has a non-negligible effect on the structure of the DNA. Firstly, the duplex is marginally less stable in the implicitly solvated calculations, therefore, any kinks or denaturation we observe in the absence of explicit water cannot be ascribed to the levels of superhelical stress. We have also observed that the simple Debye-Huckel electrostatic screening approximation that is used to mimic the effect of salt is not as efficient at screening the repulsion within the DNA backbone as discrete counterions. Consequently, writhed structures in explicit water have a tendency to be more compact, particularly in the presence of divalent cations such as calcium. Moreover, we have occasionally observed unphysically narrow minor grooves with the implicit solvent model. To deal with these simulation artifacts, we gently equilibrate the DNA as it relaxes from the planar starting structure into a writhed configuration to ensure that the minicircles are not irreversibly distorted. The integrity of the duplex is maintained using restraints placed on the hydrogen-bonding interactions between complementary base pairs (this uses the facility for imposing NMR distance restraints implemented in AMBER) whenever we are using the GB/SA implicit solvent approximation, prior to solvation in explicit water.

During the implicitly solvated calculations, we commonly observe such large oscillations in the writhe (approximately ±0.3) that it is not possible to define a unique configuration. Instead, we use a conformational clustering analysis algorithm to select representative structures (**steps 8–9**), and subject as many configurations as is computationally feasible to explicit solvation to obtain a more reliable atomistic description (*see* Fig. 2b); typically we select three configurations, one from each of the most populated clusters [19]. These are then explicitly solvated within the GROMACS program (**steps 10–18**). A list of essential software tools, important source files, and careful simulation protocols are provided in Subheadings 2 and 3.

For the smaller DNA minicircles, the writhing transition is suppressed by the large bending energy necessary to maintain the circular form [22, 23]. Thus, for the simulations of DNA minicircles with the length <150 bp (the DNA persistence length), we skip **steps 5–9** (GB/SA MD runs and clustering analysis) and start preparing the system for explicit water and ions solvation using GROMACS from the starting structure of the planar minicircle.

1.3 Computer Hardware

Simulations of DNA minicircles require specialist high-performance computing facilities (HPC), such as the UK supercomputer ARCHER [24] or local HPC such as the University of Leeds supercomputers ARC1 and ARC2, where available. Running simulations in parallel over multiple CPU cores can effectively reduce the computing time. Within MD codes such as AMBER, GROMACS, and NAMD, parallelization is typically achieved through "domain decomposition". As a simulation progresses, partitioned spatial domains within the simulation box are assigned to each of the processors, and the Newtonian physics associated with the motion of the particles within each partitioned domain will be performed by its assigned processor [25], enabling multiple calculations to be performed concurrently. Table 1 compares the performance of parallel MD simulation processing performed by the University of Leeds ARC1/2 local HPC service and the UK ARCHER supercomputers on the implicitly and explicitly solvated DNA minicircles performed by our group.

1.4 Computer Software and MD Forcefields

To perform simulations at the fully atomistic level, the biomolecular simulation field has provided researchers with a wealth of tools for simulations and trajectory analysis for proteins and nucleic

Table 1
Comparison between implicit and explicit solvation of a 336 bp DNA minicircle system for the use of Generalized Born Surface Approximation (GB/SA), numbers of atoms, numbers of nucleotide residues, numbers of water residues, numbers of ionic residues, numbers of processors working in parallel, and simulation speed in ns/day

Simulations	108 bp Explicit	336 bp Implicit	336 bp Explicit
GB/SA	No	Yes	No
Number of atoms	~450,000	21,373	~2,100,000
Number of nucleotide residues	216	672	672
Number of water residues	~150,000	–	~700,000
Number of ionic residues	~750	–	~3200
HPC system	ARC1/ARC2	ARC1/ARC2	ARCHER
Number of processors used	32	32	256
Speed (ns/day)	~1	~1	~5

acids, which are fast and user friendly [24]. Among the most popular open-source MD packages are AMBER [26], GROMACS [25], and NAMD [27]. A choice of forcefields is also available; most commonly users must choose between the AMBER suite of forcefields [28–30] and those provided by the CHARMM community [31]. The parmbsc0 AMBER forcefield has become the default parameterization due to its capacity to produce stable MD simulations of DNA duplexes at the microsecond timescale [32] and to describe a variety of non-canonical DNA structures; for minicircles using a subsequent refinement of the gamma torsion, parameter from DNA backbone [29] allows a better description of severe distortions of the DNA duplex caused by strong mechanical stress. In parallel, CHARMM also provides good descriptions of DNA structure and dynamics [33] and has performed better for nanotechnology applications, such as, DNA origami [34]. Although further testing is required in simulating circular DNA, the most convenient parameter combination we have found so far is the AMBER parm99 + bsc0 + χ_{OL4} forcefield sets.

1.5 Comparison of DNA Minicircle Simulations with Experiments

While MD simulations are invaluable for the study of DNA minicircles because they are the only method capable of providing atomistically detailed information, it is always desirable to validate computer models against experiment wherever possible. For DNA minicircles, this can be achieved by comparing the results of the simulations with low-resolution structural studies and biochemical analysis.

One opportunity for validating the models arises because extreme bending and torsional stress can drive the DNA structures beyond their elastic regime, resulting in the formation of non-canonical DNA structures such as kinks and denaturation bubbles [5, 35] which can be detected biochemically using nuclease enzymes such as BAL-31 and S1 [12] which digest single-stranded DNA. DNA defects were firstly observed in minicircle simulations at the atomistic level by Lankas et al. [36], who reported that bending and torsional stress can give rise to type I kinks, in which the base stacking interactions are disrupted but all complementary hydrogen bonding interactions remain intact, and type II kinks, in which hydrogen bonding is disrupted. Subsequent simulations that explored higher superhelical densities also observed denaturation bubbles in which longer stretched of DNA melted into single-stranded regions [21, 22]. Examples of defects in DNA due to bending and superhelical stress are shown in Fig. 2c.

Direct visualization of minicircles in the size range of 100–400 base pairs has also been achieved with cryo-EM [13] and AFM [37], which has enabled the comparison of static experimental minicircle structures to be compared with simulations. A combination of gel electrophoresis, MD simulations, and cryo-ET has also been used to investigate the conformational diversity of supercoiled minicircle DNA [19]. Cryo-ET can provide 3D traces of the DNA minicircle helical axis for different topoisomerases, which can be compared with MD simulation trajectories. The cryo-ET shows that there is a diverse conformational ensemble for the minicircles, even for a single topoisomer. Similarly, MD simulations performed in implicit solvent show that the writhe of the minicircles is subjected to large fluctuations, however, when this more approximate solvation model is used, the conformational diversity of the DNA is restricted by the hydrogen bond restraints that are applied to maintain the stability of the duplex. Subsequent simulations for discrete conformers selected from this ensemble showed that the DNA becomes more compact in explicit water due to the inclusion of discrete counterions that facilitates the closer approach of the two strands at the crossing point. Also, the DNA forms kink and bubble defects at high superhelical densities that increase the local flexibility of the DNA. However, the global conformational flexibility of the DNA is severely curtailed by the huge viscosity of the surrounding solvent, which effectively "locks" the DNA into a given writhed conformation over the timescale accessible to explicit MD (~50 ns).

1.6 Analysis Tools for DNA Minicircle Simulations

The simulation community has access to a wide choice of sophisticated software for processing the velocity and coordinate data generated by MD simulations in order to both: (1) validate the simulation results by comparing the analyzed data with experiments and (2) obtain structural and dynamical data inaccessible by experiment alone.

Many of these tools are available as part of the MD simulation codes. The radius of gyration of the minicircles is a global structural parameter that quantifies the compactness of supercoiled DNA, and can be extracted using the PTRAJ module available within the AMBERTOOLS software (*see* Subheading 3.2). Figure 3a shows three types of supercoiled DNA structures. The 'open' circular conformation has the largest value of radius of gyration and is the least compact structure compared to the other two. Structural disruptions and defects within the minicircles that arise due to torsional or bending stress can also be detected and quantified by measuring the interatomic distances between complementary hydrogen bonding using PTRAJ, or using visualization software such as VMD [38]. VMD can also be used to convert GROMACS trajectories into AMBER trajectories, which are compatible with the conformational analysis performed by PTRAJ.

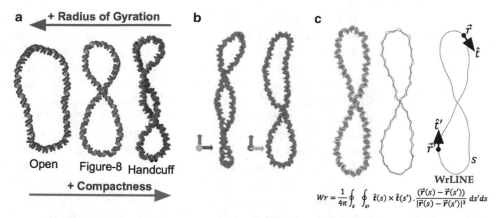

$$Wr = \frac{1}{4\pi} \oint_s \oint_{s'} \hat{t}(s) \times \hat{t}(s') \cdot \frac{(\vec{r}(s) - \vec{r}(s'))}{|\vec{r}(s) - \vec{r}(s')|^3} \, ds' ds$$

Fig. 3 (**a**) Three sample DNA minicircle structures of the 'opened', 'figure-8,' and 'handcuff' conformation. The 'opened' minicircle possesses the largest radius of gyration compared to the other two, while the 'handcuff' minicircle has the smallest radius of gyration and is the most compact structure. (**b**) A writhed DNA minicircle structure viewed from two different angles, showing the change in the number of apparent crossing points from different viewpoints. (**c**) DNA writhing calculation: a helical path (*blue*) is extracted from the atomistic structure of a minicircle DNA. The smoothed central helical axis (*red*) is then calculated by using 'WrLINE.py' python script. From this helical axis path *s*, writhe can be calculated by integration of the coiling of *s* about itself (*s'*)

However, other structural quantities that are specific to DNA require more specialized software. The DNA helical parameters that characterize the relative positions of the base pairs and base steps, such as twist, roll, tilt, etc., can be calculated using either the CURVES+ [39] or X3DNA [40] programs. In addition to the radius of gyration, the overall global shape and compactness of the DNA is determined by the writhe, which quantifies the number of crossings formed by the double helix in three dimensions. Quantifying the writhe is non-trivial because the number of times that the two DNA strands cross is extremely sensitive to the precise manner in which you view the structure, as shown in Fig. 3b. Mathematically, the writhe is defined by the Gauss integral calculated over the central helical axis (*see* Fig. 3c) [41]. However, defining an appropriate helical axis for a fully atomistic DNA structure is also non-trivial, because small local deviations from an ideal B-form helix can introduce artifacts into the writhe calculation. To eliminate these difficulties, we have developed a python script 'WrLINE.py', which performs a running average over each DNA helical turns [41], and is available online from the CCPForge website.

1.7 Future Developments and Perspectives

Improvements in the description of DNA minicircles at the atomistic level depend on two principal factors: improvements in the forcefields used to describe the DNA, and improvements in the simulation timescales and conformational sampling that can be achieved. In particular, the BSC0 forcefield is known to underestimate the twist of the DNA by approximately two degrees, although this has been partly corrected by the parmχ_{OL4} forcefield correction in which the average twist is increased from 33.2 to 33.5°/bp. This issue will likely be the main focus of future tests and developments for simulations of closed DNA topologies, since any discrepancy in the relaxed twist makes it difficult to make a direct comparison between the behaviors of simulated and experimental circles for a given superhelical density. However, it is not straightforward to obtain a precise comparison between twist at the atomistic level, and the global twist of the DNA (which is well established to be around 34°) because the MD forcefield has been parameterized through the interactions between atoms, not directly on the DNA helical twist itself, and DNA twist is highly sequence dependent. A consequence of this is that different sequences of the same size are likely to have significantly different superhelical densities, especially in the limit of small DNA loops.

Larger simulation timescales and improved conformational sampling will be achieved as computing technology continues to improve. For example, HPC resources continuously grow in terms of the number of processors available, which will, for example, allow for more conformations of writhed minicircle structures to be performed in explicit solvent. New computer technologies will also make a contribution to improving DNA minicircle simulations. Graphics processing units (GPUs) have already been adapted for biomolecular simulations, but as yet have not been applied to minicircles due to the limitations in systems sizes subjected to the memory constraints. GPUs have recently proven to be more cost effective than conventional computer clusters with the same number of cores [42], but require a re-engineering of the software. A GB/SA implicit solvent simulation routine has been created for GPU, which can produce a 1 μs MD trajectory for ubiquitin (containing 1231 atoms) within ~5 days [43]. Moreover, the recent development of a new GB/SA model that implements a charge hydration asymmetry (CHA) term has also improved the accuracy of the GB/SA model [44, 45]. The corrected water charge distribution may well eliminate the minor groove collapsing artifact seen in the GB/SA simulations of supercoiled DNA and may facilitate robust CHA-GB/SA simulations of supercoiled minicircles on GPU with a significantly reduced cost.

Another source of accelerated biomolecular simulations is the ANTON supercomputer, which is a special-purpose computer cluster built for molecular dynamics simulations [46] which have provided MD trajectories as long as 1.119 ms within 164 days (6.82 μs/day) using 128 nodes for the explicitly solvated small protein Fip35 WW domain (containing 10,000 atoms) [47].

While the first incarnation of ANTON was limited to simulations containing a maximum of 200,000 atoms, significantly less than is required for a DNA minicircle, the more recent ANTON2 machine is able to perform an MD simulation of a system containing 2,000,000 atoms and is approximately ten times faster than the original ANTON [48], which would in principle be able to simulate a DNA minicircle containing hundreds of base pairs over multiple microsecond timescales.

Atomistically detailed MD simulations of minicircles could assist in developing them as gene therapy vectors [49]. These DNA "minivectors" have already been shown to efficiently transfect lymphoma cells and have proven to be more resistant to hydrodynamic shear stress during the therapeutic gene delivery [50] than larger plasmids. Moreover, DNA minicircles of the same size (200–400 bp) have been detected in vivo where they have been excised from the chromosomes [51]. Understanding the dynamical properties of DNA minicircles would help to elucidate the occurrence and sequence specificity of chromosomal microdeletion processes.

2   Materials

2.1   MD Simulation, Analysis, and Visualization Software

1. *AMBER*: The molecular dynamics simulation software package, along with the forcefield ff99 + bsc0 + χ_{OL4} are the main tools we have used in the GB/SA implicit solvent simulation [52]. In an AMBER simulation, the module SANDER reads in a series of input parameter, topology, and coordinate files to output a *.mdcrd AMBER trajectory and restart coordinate files [53].

2. *GROMACS*: This MD software package currently has the reputation of being the most efficient at generating explicitly solvated simulations trajectories. Fast MD is extremely important for DNA minicircles, given that the simulation cell can contain more than 1,000,000 atoms. A similar forcefield (e.g. AMBER) as for the implicitly solvated calculations is used to maintain consistency between the two types of simulations. A perl script 'ambgmx.pl' is used to create GROMACS topology and coordinate files for AMBER forcefields [25].

3. *Specialized forcefield and ions parameters*: (a) Circular structures require a slight modification to the AMBER libraries (we call this parameter set 'ff99circ') in which the end residues are omitted to prevent the xleap module adding them automatically, (b) DNA simulations require the 'parmbsc0' modification for nucleic acid backbone dihedrals α and γ [28], (c) we

also use the 'OL4' modification for DNA backbone dihedral χ [29], and (d) the ion modification for Na and Cl counterions of Smith and Dang [54].

4. *Visual Molecular Dynamics* (*VMD*) [38]: This visualization software is fast and efficient, and is capable of reading molecular dynamics trajectory files of any format (e.g. NAMD, AMBER, GROMACS, etc.) and of rendering 3D images for dissemination in papers and in seminar presentations. For more complex tasks, '*.tcl' scripts can be written to control the program via the 'tk console'. We use a script that converts a GROMACS compressed trajectory into an AMBER trajectory that is compatible with PTRAJ for analysis of the conformations, while other researchers may prefer using VMD directly, or GROMACS analysis tools.

2.2   AMBERTOOLS Modules

1. *NAB* (*Nucleic Acid Builder*): This is a C-based high-level programming language, which performs specific operations on the starting coordinates of nucleic acid structures. NAB is capable of importing standard reference frames of coordinates of nucleotides from an AMBER library, performing coordinate transformations and creating a PDB file containing all the coordinates atomic types for a starting structure [53]. We use NAB to build minicircles; but knots and more complex topologies are also possible.

2. *LEAP*: This module generates topology files containing the interatomic connectivities and the associated forcefield parameters (e.g. stretching, bending and dihedral angles, and non-bonded interactions) from a PDB file created by NAB.

3. *PTRAJ*: This module is used for trajectory processing such as concatenation of MD trajectories and removing unwanted atoms or residues from the trajectories (e.g. stripping out the water molecules). This AMBER module also includes commands to measure distances between atoms or residues (e.g. for calculating distances between atoms that are engaged in complementary hydrogen bonds between base pairs), bending and dihedral angles, root mean square deviations between two structures, and the radius of gyration.

2.3   Source Files

Table 2 shows the list of input files used to prepare the start-up files for both the implicit and explicit solvent simulation protocols and the post-simulation analysis. To use these, AMBER, AMBERTOOLS, GROMACS, python (with NUMPY library), and perl software packages need to be installed.

Table 2
List of the files used in (a) preparing the minicircle DNA structures for GB/SA simulations, (b) running the AMBER GB/SA implicit solvent simulations, (c) preparing the GROMACS explicit solvent simulation, (d) running the GROMACS explicit solvent simulations, and (e) measuring writhe values by WrLINE

Categories	Files
(a) AMBER GB/SA preparation	• 'circ.nab': create a PDB file of DNA minicircle • 'leapscript_imp': generate AMBER topology and starting coordinate files • 'leaprc.ff99circ': a forcefield parameter set specially used for DNA minicircles (DNA with no ends) • 'all_nuc94bsc0_chiOL4.in', 'frcmod.parmbsc0' and 'frcmod.OL4.chi': forcefield modification files for the dihedral parameters • 'dangions.dat': a forcefield modification file for the ion electrostatic parameter
(b) AMBER GB/SA simulation	• 'molecule.prmtop' and 'molecule.inpcrd': AMBER topology and starting coordinate files • 'min1.in' and 'min2.in': input parameters for minimization in GB/SA implicit solvent • 'md1.in', 'md2.in' and 'md3.in': input parameters for equilibration in GB/SA implicit solvent with all atom coordinate restraints • 'md4.in': input parameters for a productive MD run in GB/SA implicit solvent with NMR distance restraints on hydrogen bonds • 'RST': all the information on the NMR restraints • 'gbsa.sh': shell commands to execute the minimization, equilibration and productive MD runs within AMBER GB/SA implicit solvent
(c) GROMACS explicit solvent preparation	• 'amb2gmx_dihe.pl': perl script to convert the AMBER topology and coordinate files into GROMACS format • 'ffbsc0.itp', 'tip3p.itp' and 'ions.itp': ff99bsc0 forcefield for DNA, TIP3P water and ion models in GROMACS topology file format • 'molecule.w.top', 'molecule.wp.top', and 'molecule.wnr.top': GROMACS topology files for the system with water, counter-ions and monovalent salt ions under no artificial restraints
(d) GROMACS explicit solvent simulation	• 'molecule.wpr.top': the GROMACS topology file for the system with water and ions under coordinate position restraints • 'em.mdp', 'eq.mdp,' and 'md.mdp': input parameter files for minimization, equilibration and productive MD runs • 'posre.itp': a topology file containing information of coordinate position restraints • 'gmxmd.sh': shell commands to execute the minimization, equilibration and productive MD runs within GRAMACS explicit solvent • 'xtc2crd.tcl': a tcl script for the VMD program to convert a GROMACS *.xtc compressed trajectory file into the AMBER *.mdcrd format
(e) WrLINE	• 'WrLINE.py': to run a package of PTRAJ and python scripts for the writhe measurement from AMBER topology and coordinate files

3   Methods

3.1   Molecular
Dynamics Simulations

1. *Build a circular DNA starting structure*: Run the NAB script 'circ.nab' to perform these operations: (a) Determine the radius of the circle and the average twist/base pair from the number of base pairs, the 'rise' parameter value (~3.38 Å), and the linking number. (b) Each base pair coordinate is imported and placed its centre at the circle circumference, normal to the tangent. (c) A coordinate transformation is performed to twist the base pair by the specified average twist angle per base pair relative to its predecessor. (d) The whole circle is rotated about its centre to create a space for the next base pair. Repeating this process will create a planar circular DNA with a uniform twist angle used at the MD starting structure, for which a PDB file will be created (*see* **Note 1**).

2. *Creating topology and coordinate files*: Run the prepared LEAP script to perform the following operations: (a) load the force-field parameter 'ff99circ' for circular DNA, all the preparation (all_nuc94bsc0_chiOL4.in [29]) and forcefield modification files for backbone dihedrals (frcmod.parmbsc0 [28] and frcmod.OL4.chi [29]), ions (dangion.dat [54]) and the modified DNA library (DNA_CI.lib) containing the updated version of DNA partial charges compatible with the 'bsc0' parameters [28]. (b) Map some of the atom names and types in the PDB files created by NAB to be compatible with LEAP by using the 'addPdbAtomMap' and 'addAtomTypes' LEAP commands (*see* **Note 2**). (c) Load the PDB file of the circular DNA created by NAB. (d) Manually create two covalent bonds to connect two backbone strands of the DNA ends by using the 'bond' LEAP command. (e) Use 'saveamberparm' LEAP command to export a .prmtop topology file and an .inpcrd coordinate file for an implicitly solvated simulation (*see* **Notes 3** and **4**).

3. *Prepare AMBER input files for GB/SA implicit solvent simulations*: (a) *two-stage minimization* 'min1.in' with all-atom coordinate restraints (ntr = 1) and 'min2.in' without coordinate restraints. (b) *Three-stage equilibration with all atom coordinate restraints* 'md1.in': system is heated from 100 K to the constant 300 K, 'md2.in' and 'md3.in': system is under the reduced restraint weight (*see* Table 2). (c) *Productive MD run* 'md4.in' the all-atom restraints have been removed and the system is restrained through its complementary base pair hydrogen bonds using the NMR distance restraints facility in SANDER (nmropt = 1, pencut = −0.001) (*see* **Note 5**).

4. *Prepare an AMBER NMR distance restraints file*: To prepare the NMR restraint file, run the python script 'genrst.py' to read the DNA sequence and to generate an input file for the

AMBER 'makeDIST_RST' command. This will create another file named 'RST' containing all the restraint information for the productive GB/SA MD run (*see* **Note 6**).

5. *AMBER GB/SA implicit solvent minimization and equilibration*: Run the first minimization stage from the prepared AMBER topology, starting coordinate, and 'min1.in' AMBER input files using the SANDER module. The final structure of 'min1' will be the starting structure for 'min2', for which the final structure will be the starting structure for 'md1'. This procedure will be repeated so that the final structure of 'md3' equilibration stage will be the starting structure for the productive MD run.

6. *AMBER GB/SA implicit solvent productive run*: From the final structure of 'md3', execute the 'md4' productive MD run in the GB/SA implicit solvent with all the hydrogen bonds restrained. If the simulation finishes before a sufficiently long trajectory has been obtained, it can be extended from the final structure using the AMBER restart and topology files (*see* **Note 7**).

7. *Cut and merge the trajectories of writhed DNA structures*: Use PTRAJ to concatenate the trajectories. Discard the first few nanoseconds (maybe 2–5 ns) of all the replicas, keeping only the snapshots where the writhe values become stable. If convenient, PTRAJ allows the user to merge all the replicas to create a single file containing the ensemble of writhed DNA structures of a given topoisomer for subsequent analysis.

8. *Clustering analysis and selection for the supercoiled DNA conformation to be explicitly solvated*: In PTRAJ, use the command 'cluster' with the option 'averagelinkage' to divide all the MD snapshots for each topoisomer into clusters (we typically generate around six clusters). Visualize the highly populated conformational clusters in VMD, and select a representative structure. Ensure that the chosen structure is free from structural disruptions, paying particular attention to the base stacking interactions (the hydrogen bond restraints prevent the formation of single-stranded regions, but do not maintain stacking).

9. *Vacuum minimization*: A representative structure of supercoiled DNA from a GB/SA simulation may contain regions where the minor groove is artificially narrow, especially at the plectoneme apices. This is an artifact of the approximate implicit solvent model, and therefore should be removed prior to adding counterions and water molecules. This minor groove compaction is relieved by a short minimization run in vacuum ($igb = 0$), as the electrostatic repulsion between backbone phosphate groups widens the minor groove.

10. *File conversion from AMBER to GROMACS*: the GROMACS topology (.top) and coordinate (.gro) files can be created using the *perl* script 'amb2gmx.pl' (which is available from the GROMACS website) along with AMBER topology and coordinate files of the starting structure (without solvent) (*see* **Notes 8** and **9**).

11. *Prepare the GROMACS topology files (*.top) from modular files (.itp)*: (a) 'ffbsc0.itp' specifies the type of forcefield to be chosen (e.g. AMBER, CHARMM, or GROMOS, we use AMBER [28]), (b) 'molecule.itp' contains all the forcefield parameters of the molecule to be studied, (c) 'tip3p.itp' contains the topology of a TIP3P water molecule, (d) 'ions.itp' contains the topology of the chosen model of ions (Dang and Smith in our case [54]), and (e) 'posre.itp' contains force constants for coordinate restraints used during the equilibration. The *.itp files will be specified as necessary inside the *.top files to build the final topology as structural modular parts.

12. *Explicit water solvation in GROMACS*: from the GROMACS topology and coordinate files created by 'amb2gmx.pl', the following commands should be executed to solvate the molecule in explicit water: (a) by using 'editconf', the structure is centred within a triclinic box and its principal axis is set to be parallel to the box axis (with the option '-princ'). (b) 'genbox' is used to generate a coordinate file of the molecule in a TIP3P water box 'molecule.w.gro' with the option to load the reference coordinates of water molecules (-cs spc216.gro) (*see* **Note 10**). (c) A run input file 'molecule.w.tpr' is generated from 'molecule.w.gro' and a topology file 'molecule.w.top' containing 'ffbsc0.itp', 'molecule.itp', 'tip3p.itp', 'ions.itp', and the exact number of water molecules is assigned using the 'grompp' command.

13. *Explicit ion solvation in GROMACS*: (a) The 'genion' command with the option '-norandom' (*not* included in GROMACS 5) is used to introduce a number of positive monovalent Na+ counterions, which replace water molecules around the negatively charged phosphate groups. This creates a coordinate file 'molecule.wp.gro', in which the system is electrically neutralized. (b) A run input file 'molecule.wp.tpr' is generated by the 'grompp' command from the files 'molecule.wp.gro' and the topology file 'molecule.wp.top'. This contains all the necessary .itp files and the number of water molecules and ions corresponding to 'molecule.wp.gro' (*see* **step 11**). (c) If a salt concentration higher than minimal is required, then additional positive and negative ions are introduced. This uses the options '-nn {number of negative ions}' and '-np {number of positive ions}' in the 'genion' command. The number of positive and negative ions required to emulate

Table 3
Force constants and time durations used in each stage of the AMBER GB/SA implicit solvent simulation protocols

Stages	Restraints	Durations
Minimization 1	$k = 50.0$ kCal/mol/Å²	10,000 cycles
Minimization 2	No restraints	10,000 cycles
Equilibration 1	$k = 50.0$ kCal/mol/Å², $T = 100$-300 K	10 ps
Equilibration 2	$k = 10.0$ kCal/mol/Å², $T = 300$ K	100 ps
Equilibration 3	$k = 1.0$ kCal/mol/Å², $T = 300$ K	200 ps
Productive Runs	NMR, $k = 1.0$ kCal/mol/Å²	10–100 ns

a specific salt concentration can be calculated from $0.0018 \times$ (salt concentration in molar) $\times$ (number of water molecules in the water box). The output coordinate file is named 'molecule. wnr.gro' (d) A new run input file 'molecule.wnr.tpr' is generated from 'molecule.wnr.gro' and the topology file 'molecule. wnr.top', which contains the final number of water molecules and ions.

14. *Prepare the .mdp input files for GROMACS explicit solvent simulations*: the parameters for the multistep equilibration protocols were designed based on the standard simulation protocols for relaxing DNA [55] (*see* Table 3), but with additional steps to relieve any additional conformational stress associated with the closed topology. This system undergoes a four-stage minimization and eight-stage equilibration prior to the production run.

15. *Prepare the topology files for GROMACS explicit solvent simulations*: The equilibration proceeds from the run input file 'molecule.wnr.tpr'. For each relaxation stage requiring all-atom coordinate restraints, a coordinate restraint file (e.g. 'posre. itp') needs to be generated using the 'genrestr' command. This will be included in the topology file corresponding to each minimization and equilibration (e.g. 'molecule.min1. top' for minimization stage 1) (*see* Table 4).

16. *Run GROMACS explicit solvent simulations*: For each minimization and equilibration stage the 'mdrun' command is executed, which produces the updated restart coordinate file (e.g. 'molecule.min1.gro' the minimization stage 1, etc). The command is then used to 'grompp' create a run input file (e.g. 'molecule.min2.tpr'), which is executed by 'mdrun' in the next stage. Minimization and equilibration continues through to the end of equilibration stage 8. Then, the productive MD run starts, in which all the coordinate restraints are lifted and

Table 4
Force constants and time durations used in each stage of the GROMACS explicit solvent simulation protocols

Stages	Restraints	Durations
Minimization 1	$k = 500.0$ kCal/mol/Å²	10,000 cycles
Minimization 2	$k = 50.0$ kCal/mol/Å²	10,000 cycles
Minimization 3	$k = 25.0$ kCal/mol/Å²	10,000 cycles
Minimization 4	No restraints	10,000 cycles
Equilibration 1	$k = 500.0$ kCal/mol/Å², $T = 100$ K	10 ps
Equilibration 2	$k = 50.0$ kCal/mol/Å², $T = 100$–300 K	10 ps
Equilibration 3	$k = 50.0$ kCal/mol/Å², $T = 300$ K	10 ps
Equilibration 4	$k = 25.0$ kCal/mol/Å², $T = 300$ K	10 ps
Equilibration 5	$k = 10.0$ kCal/mol/Å², $T = 300$ K	10 ps
Equilibration 6	$k = 5.0$ kCal/mol/Å², $T = 300$ K	10 ps
Equilibration 7	$k = 2.5$ kCal/mol/Å², $T = 300$ K	10 ps
Equilibration 8	$k = 1.0$ kCal/mol/Å², $T = 300$ K	10 ps
Productive Runs	(None)	10–100 ns

DNA is free to move under the explicit solvent environment. (*see* **Notes 11** and **12**).

17. *Processing the GROMACS MD trajectories*: After the productive MD simulation run finishes, we process the trajectory data by using 'trjconv' command. (a) It is often the case that it is only solute structure that is of interest. Fully solvated trajectory files are usually inconveniently large, which means they can be slow to transfer between the supercomputer and local workstations (where much of the visualization and analysis will be performed), they can be difficult to store, and can cause problems with memory during visualization. The water molecules and ions can be removed from the trajectory by specifying the atomic index numbers (turn on the option '-n' of 'trjconv') (*see* **Note 13**). (b) If required, it is also possible to reduce the time frames sampled in the trajectory using the option '-dt' (*see* **Note 14**). It is also possible to specify that only the solute molecules are output in the trajectories, however, as it is sometimes desirable to analyze the water molecule positions, particularly when structure defects are present, by default we save the water molecule coordinates and discard them only when we are sure they are not needed.

18. *Convert GROMACS trajectories back to AMBER *.mdcrd format*: To use PTRAJ for data analysis, is it first necessary to

convert the GROMACS trajectories into AMBER format. VMD is one of the software tools that is conveniently able to load most MD trajectory formats, and can interconvert between the different formats according to the preferences of the user.

19. *Repeat the process from stage 1 to run more simulations of other topoisomers or different minicircles sizes or sequences.*

3.2 Conformational Analysis

1. *Calculating the radius of gyration from the implicitly solvated trajectories:* The 'radgyr' command implemented in the AMBERTOOLS's PTRAJ module is able to calculate the radius of gyration from a series of MD trajectory snapshots. We use implicitly solvated trajectories to calculate this quantity, because the frictional term associated with inclusion of explicit water impedes conformational fluctuations of the minicircle, effectively freezing the DNA into a single writhed conformation. The radius of gyration calculated from implicitly solvated trajectories of different topoisomers is a useful physical parameter that can be compared with the experimentally measured mobilities of the corresponding supercoiled minicircle topoisomers within polyacrylamide gels (*see* Fig. 4a and **Note 15**).

2. *Calculation of the DNA minicircle writhe using by the python script WrLINE:* To calculate the writhe, the script takes as input the AMBER topology and trajectory files. The user needs to specify the number of base pairs and the number of MD snapshots within the 'WrLINE.py' script. The output consists of a time series of writhe values (*see* **Note 16**). Writhe calculated this way has been verified by the crossing vertical and horizontal dashed lines (*see* Fig. 4a.), as zero supercoiling corresponds to zero writhe.

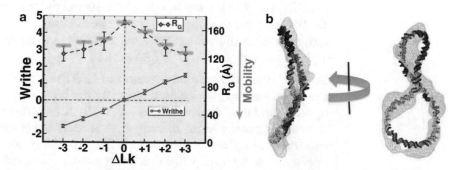

Fig. 4 (**a**) Time averages of writhe (*purple*) and radius of gyration (*maroon*) over the last 10 ns of the implicitly solvated DNA minicircles at seven different ΔLks. *Orange marks* indicate the relative mobility (down the vertical axis) of the seven minicircle topoisomers determined by gel electrophoresis experiments [19]. (**b**) An atomistic structure of a $\Delta Lk = -2$ DNA minicircle, obtained from an explicitly solvated MD simulations. The structure is superimposed into a cryo-ET density map and visualized by VMD

3. *Create traces from MD trajectories to be compared with cryo-EM/ET or AFM*: To create a 3D trace of the minicircle shape, use PTRAJ to strip all the atoms from the MD trajectory, except the 20 C1' carbon atoms that are approximately equally spaced from their neighbors, to represent the writhed structure (the number 20 is the arbitrary number of points used by our experimental collaborators to represent the cryo-ET computational trace) (*see* **Note 17**). While AFM and cryoEM give only 2D (not 3D) information, the trace is nevertheless useful for comparing with these experimental data.

4. *Calculate the RMSD between the explicitly solvated DNA to cryo-ET traces*: Given a set of computational traces obtained from cryo-ET density maps, it is possible to quantify the level of agreement between the experiments and the simulations by using the 'rms' command in PTRAJ to calculate the root mean square deviation (RMSD) values for all pairs of the discrete points that constitute the MD and cryo-ET traces. We assign the MD trace that gives the smallest RMSD value with any of the cryo-ET traces to be the 'best representative' atomistic structure for the supercoiled DNA (*see* Fig. 4b).

4   Notes

1. To build a DNA starting structure, a script containing commands and operations on the coordinates of DNA base pairs can be written by using the NAB scripting language, which is implemented in AMBERTOOLS. This is then compiled as an executable file. Given the required number of base pairs, the radius of the DNA circle can be specified (this is calculated from the rise), a circle can be drawn from that point and the average local twist angle can be given. For example, for a 336 bp DNA, with the linking number $Lk = 30$ and the 'rise' parameter (the optimal stacking distance between base pairs) of 3.38 Å, the circle has the average twist angle between two neighboring base pairs of $(30 \times 360°)/336 = 32.14°$.

2. Either XLEAP (the graphical version of LEAP) or TLEAP (the text-based version) can be used to create the basic start-up files topology and coordinate files for an AMBER MD simulation. To ensure that the atom naming conventions are compatible with the output from NAB, the 'addPdbAtomMap' command should be used to map the following atomic nomenclatures: {{OP1 O1P}{OP2 O2P}{H5′ H5′1}{H5″ H5′2}{H2′ H2′1}{H2″ H2′2}}, and two additional ringed carbon atom types "C1" and "C2" are defined by 'addAtomTypes {{"C1" "C" "sp2"}{"C2" "C" "sp2"}}'.

3. The coordinate file (.inpcrd in AMBER7 or later) contains all of the position and velocity information for the system necessary to restart the simulation and continue a dynamics run. The topology file (.mdcrd in AMBER7 or later) contains all the necessary physical, chemical information for describing each atom and its interactions (mass, radius, partial charge, etc.) and covalent bonding (e.g. stretching, bending, and dihedral force constants).

4. With the information from topology and coordinate (restart) files, a PDB file of a molecule can be reconstructed using the AMBER utility script 'ambpdb'. This operation can be useful for visualizing the molecule to quickly check the starting coordinates, or to check progress during the simulation (as restart files are continuously output as the MD progresses), or as a way of identifying problems if a simulation crashes.

5. In the absence of friction from the hydrodynamic interactions associated with explicit water molecules, we use either all-atom or NMR distance restraints between complementary base pairs to prevent structural disruptions within the DNA, which could be due to approximated solvent model, as this generally destabilizes the DNA. All of the restraints are removed only when explicit solvent is used, which is the only time that we can observe defects involving broken hydrogen bonds. The option 'pencut = −0.001' is set to have a negative value in order to print out all the energy associated with the distance deviation from the NMR restraints.

6. The input file for NMR restraint generation contains eight columns for each line representing a distance restraint: '1 ADE N1 8 THY H3 1.70 2.10,' the first six columns identify residue numbers, residue types and atomic types of a pair of restrained atoms, and the last two columns describe the restraint boundaries.

7. To obtain replica trajectories to improve conformational sampling, simply run 'md4' but assigning a new set of velocities to the DNA from the restart file (irest = 1, ntx = 5). Running dynamics using an independent set of initial starting velocities will cause the trajectories to diverge in conformational space, even if the initial atomic coordinates are the same.

8. In order to explicitly solvate the 336 bp supercoiled DNA minicircles, a large water box containing around 700,000 water molecules (over 2,000,000 atoms) is required. AMBER is not currently capable of simulating systems containing more than 1,000,000 atoms. Thus, GROMACS is used to carry out these large systems. On our supercomputer resources, GROMACS is currently the most efficient MD engine for explicitly solvated calculations.

9. For smaller systems (e.g. minicircles containing around 100 base pairs), we are able to carry out the explicitly solvated MD simulations in AMBER. Additional LEAP commands are added to solvate the circular starting DNA structure in an explicit solution: (a) including a TIP3P water box by using 'solvatebox' command, (b) neutralizing the system by a number of positive monovalent counterions (Na+, K+, etc.) by using 'addions' command, (c) adding further ions to emulate a specified salt concentration.

10. For a short explicit solvent simulation (10–20 ns) of a 336 bp supercoiled minicircle that involves no major changes in DNA writhe, a triclinic or rectangular waterbox with 30–40 Å solution buffer is an optimal choice to prevent clashing of a pair of DNA segments from neighboring periodic box.

11. In productive MD runs within GROMACS, the trajectory files with full precision produced by 'mdrun' are in the '*.trr' format (option '-o'). Alternatively, to significantly reduce the file size, the option '-x' can be used to output the compressed MD trajectory in the '*.xtc' format.

12. Many supercomputing systems have their own time limit for running a job, which is typically between 12 and 48 h. Therefore, if one needs to produce a long MD trajectory (e.g. 100 ns), simulations need to be conducted by continuously resubmitting the job from the restart files produced by a previous run. When the trajectory reaches the length required (or the user runs out of patience!), all the separate trajectories can be catenated using the GROMACS command 'trjcat'.

13. The GROMACS module 'make_ndx' is a tool for obtaining the atomic index numbers of any specified groups (e.g. DNA, water, ions, non-water), corresponding to the index numbers in the *.gro coordinate files. Indices produced by 'make_ndx' serve as input files for any GROMACS commands performed on specific groups of atoms.

14. In the frequent instance when sections of the solute "jump out" of the primary periodic water box, this can spoil the visualization and create errors in conformational analysis. Using 'trjconv' with the option '-pbc' can repair this problem. (For further details, please consult GROMACS manual.)

15. Errors can occur when comparing the radius of gyration calculated from the ensemble of implicitly solvated MD snapshots of supercoiled DNA minicircles with experimental data due to the need to impose hydrogen bond restraints when using approximate solvent models. The artificial hydrogen bonding restraints prevent the DNA relieving torsional or bending stress through structural disruptions and defect formation. These errors are most severe for highly supercoiled minicircles

that are under the most torsional stress. Therefore, it is most important to perform explicitly solvated calculations for topoisomers at higher superhelical densities.

16. The PTRAJ module and the NUMPY python library are required in order to run the 'WrLINE.py' script.

17. To pick 20 representative atoms from MD trajectories to be compared with the cryo-ET traces of 336 bp minicircles (1 point represents 16.8 base pairs), for example, C1′ atoms can be picked from the base pair 17, 34, 51, 68, 84, ..., 336.

Specimen input files and scripts to build the DNA structures and perform the simulations, and analysis described are provided as Supplementary Materials in the file "Source.zip".

References

1. Bates AD, Maxwell A (2005) DNA topology. Oxford University Press, Oxford

2. Dekker J, Marti-Renom M, Mirny L (2013) Exploring the three-dimensional organization of genomes: interpreting chromatin interaction data. Nat Rev Genet 14:390–403

3. Williamson I, Berlivet S, Eskeland R et al (2014) Spatial genome organization: contrasting views from chromosome conformation capture and fluorescence in situ hybridization. Genes Dev 28:2778–2791

4. Benedetti F, Japaridze A, Dorier J et al (2015) Effects of physiological self-crowding of DNA on shape and biological properties of DNA molecules with various levels of supercoiling. Nucleic Acids Res 43:2390–2399

5. Drew HR, Weeks JR, Travers AA (1985) Negative supercoiling induces spontaneous unwinding of a bacterial promoter. EMBO J 4:1025–1032

6. Kouzine F, Levens D, Baranello L (2014) DNA topology and transcription. Nucleus 5:195–202

7. Pemberton IK, Muskhelishvili G, Travers AA et al (2002) FIS modulates the kinetics of successive interactions of RNA polymerase with the core and upstream regions of the tyrT promoter. J Mol Biol 318:651–663

8. Fogg JM, Randall GL, Pettitt BM et al (2012) Bullied no more: when and how DNA shoves proteins around. Q Rev Biophys 45:257–299

9. Olson WK, Gorin AA, Lu X-J et al (1998) DNA sequence-dependent deformability deduced from protein–DNA crystal complexes. Proc Natl Acad Sci U S A 95:11163–11168

10. Luscombe NM, Austin SE, Berman HM et al (2000) An overview of the structures of protein-DNA complexes. Genome Biol 1:1

11. Richmond TJ, Davey CA (2003) The structure of DNA in the nucleosome core. Nature 423:145–150

12. Du Q, Kotlyar A, Vologodskii A (2008) Kinking the double helix by bending deformation. Nucleic Acids Res 36:1120–1128

13. Lionberger TA, Demurtas D, Witz G et al (2011) Cooperative kinking at distant sites in mechanically stressed DNA. Nucleic Acids Res 39:9820–9832

14. Fogg JM, Kolmakova N, Rees I et al (2006) Exploring writhe in supercoiled minicircle DNA. J Phys Condens Matter 18:S145–S159

15. Shlyakhtenko LS, Potaman VN, Sinden RR et al (1998) Structure and dynamics of supercoil-stabilized DNA cruciforms. J Mol Biol 280:61–72

16. Schmatko T, Muller P, Maaloum M (2014) Surface charge effects on the 2D conformation of supercoiled DNA. Soft Matter 10:2520–2529

17. Bednar J, Furrer P, Stasiak A et al (1994) The Twist Writhe and overall shape of supercoiled DNA change during counterion-induced transition from a loosely to a tightly interwound superhelix. J Mol Biol 235:825–847

18. Amzallag A, Vaillant C, Jacob M et al (2006) 3D reconstruction and comparison of shapes of DNA minicircles observed by cryo-electron microscopy. Nucleic Acids Res 34:e125

19. Irobalieva RN, Fogg JM, Catanese DJ et al (2015) Structural diversity of supercoiled DNA. Nat Commun 6:8440

20. Beveridge DL, Cheatham TE, Mezei M (2012) The ABCs of molecular dynamics simulations on B-DNA, circa 2012. J Biosci 37:379–397

21. Mitchell JS, Laughton CA, Harris SA (2011) Atomistic simulations reveal bubbles, kinks and wrinkles in supercoiled DNA. Nucleic Acids Res 39:3928–3938

22. Harris SA, Laughton CA, Liverpool TB (2008) Mapping the phase diagram of the writhe of DNA nanocircles using atomistic molecular dynamics simulations. Nucleic Acids Res 36:21–29

23. Liverpool TB, Harris SA, Laughton CA (2008) Supercoiling and denaturation of DNA loops. Phys Rev Lett 100:238103

24. Gray A, Harlen OG, Harris SA et al (2015) In pursuit of an accurate spatial and temporal model of biomolecules at the atomistic level: a perspective on computer simulation. Acta Crystallogr D D71:162–172

25. Pronk S, Páll S, Schulz R et al (2013) GROMACS 4.5: a high-throughput and highly parallel open source molecular simulation toolkit. Bioinformatics 29:845–854

26. Case DA, Cheatham TE, Darden T et al (2005) The Amber biomolecular simulation programs. J Comput Chem 26:1668–1688

27. Phillips JC, Braun R, Wang W et al (2005) Scalable molecular dynamics with NAMD. J Comput Chem 26:1781–1802

28. Pérez A, Marchán I, Svozil D et al (2007) Refinement of the AMBER force field for nucleic acids: improving the description of alpha/gamma conformers. Biophys J 92: 3817–3829

29. Krepl M, Zgarbová M, Stadlbauer P et al (2012) Reference simulations of noncanonical nucleic acids with different χ variants of the AMBER forcefield: quadruplex DNA, quadruplex RNA, and Z-DNA. J Chem Theor Comput 8:2506–2520

30. Zgarbova M, Luque FJ, Jir S et al (2013) Toward improved description of DNA backbone: revisiting epsilon and zeta torsion force field parameters. J Chem Theor Comput 9:2339–2354

31. Vanommeslaeghe K, Hatcher E, Acharya C et al (2009) CHARMM general force field: a force field for drug-like molecules compatible with the CHARMM all-atom additive biological force fields. J Comput Chem 31:671–690

32. Pérez A, Luque FJ, Orozco M (2007) Dynamics of B-DNA on the microsecond time scale. J Am Chem Soc 129:14739–14745

33. Hart K, Foloppe N, Baker CM et al (2012) Optimization of the CHARMM additive force field for DNA: improved treatment of the BI/BII conformational equilibrium. J Chem Theor Comput 8:348–362

34. Yoo J, Aksimentiev A (2013) In situ structure and dynamics of DNA origami determined through molecular dynamics simulations. Proc Natl Acad Sci U S A 110:20099–20104

35. Crick FHC, Klug A (1975) Kinky helix. Nature 255:530–533

36. Lankas F, Lavery R, Maddocks JH (2006) Kinking occurs during molecular dynamics simulations of small DNA minicircles. Structure (London 1993) 14:1527–1534

37. Ackermann D, Rasched G, Verma S et al (2010) Assembly of dsDNA nanocircles into dimeric and oligomeric aggregates. Chem Commun (Camb) 46:4154–4156

38. Humphrey W, Dalke A, Schulten K (1996) VMD: visual molecular dynamics. J Mol Graph 14:33–38

39. Lavery R, Moakher M, Maddocks JH et al (2009) Conformational analysis of nucleic acids revisited: Curves+. Nucleic Acids Res 37:5917–5929

40. Lu X-J, Olson WK (2008) 3DNA: a versatile, integrated software system for the analysis, rebuilding and visualization of three-dimensional nucleic-acid structures. Nat Protoc 3:1213–1227

41. Sutthibutpong T, Harris SA, Noy A (2015) Comparison of molecular contours for measuring writhe in atomistic supercoiled DNA. J Chem Theor Comput 11(6):2768–2775

42. Dror RO, Dirks RM, Grossman JP et al (2012) Biomolecular simulation: a computational microscope for molecular biology. Annu Rev Biophys 41:429–452

43. Goetz AW, Williamson MJ, Xu D et al (2012) Routine microsecond molecular dynamics simulations with amber – part I: generalized born. J Chem Theor Comput 8:1542–1555

44. Mukhopadhyay A, Fenley AT, Tolokh IS et al (2012) Charge hydration asymmetry : the basic principle and how to use it to test and improve water models charge hydration asymmetry: the basic principle and how to use it to test and improve water models. J Phys Chem B 116:9776–9783

45. Mukhopadhyay A, Aguilar BH, Tolokh IS et al (2014) Introducing charge hydration asymmetry into the generalized born model. J Chem Theor Comput 10:1788–1794

46. Shaw DE, Deneroff MM, Dror RO et al (2008) Anton, a special-purpose machine for molecular dynamics simulation. Commun ACM 51:91–97

47. Piana S, Lindorff-Larsen K, Shaw DE (2012) Protein folding kinetics and thermodynamics

from atomistic simulation. Proc Natl Acad Sci 109:17845–17850

48. Shaw DE, Grossman JP, Bank JA et al (2014) Anton 2: raising the bar for performance and programmability in a special-purpose molecular dynamics supercomputer, SC14: international conference for high performance computing, networking, storage and analysis, pp 41–53

49. Zhao N, Fogg JM, Zechiedrich L et al (2011) Transfection of shRNA-encoding Minivector DNA of a few hundred base pairs to regulate gene expression in lymphoma cells. Gene Ther 18:220–224

50. Catanese DJ, Fogg JM, Schrock DE et al (2012) Supercoiled Minivector DNA resists shear forces associated with gene therapy delivery. Gene Ther 19:94–100

51. Shibata Y, Kumar P, Layer R et al (2012) Extrachromosomal microDNAs and chromosomal microdeletions in normal tissues. Science (New York) 336:82–86

52. Tsui V, Case DA (2000) Theory and applications of the generalized born solvation model in. Biopolymers 56:275–291

53. Case DA, Darden TA, Cheatham TE III et al (2010) Amber 11. University of California, San Francisco, CA

54. Smith DE, Dang LX (1994) Computer simulations of NaCl association in polarizable water. J Chem Phys 100:3757

55. Shields GC, Laughton CA, Orozco M (1997) Molecular dynamics simulations of the d(T·A·T) triple helix. J Am Chem Soc 119: 7463–7469

Chapter 16

Super-Resolution Microscopy and Tracking of DNA-Binding Proteins in Bacterial Cells

Stephan Uphoff

Abstract

The ability to detect individual fluorescent molecules inside living cells has enabled a range of powerful microscopy techniques that resolve biological processes on the molecular scale. These methods have also transformed the study of bacterial cell biology, which was previously obstructed by the limited spatial resolution of conventional microscopy. In the case of DNA-binding proteins, super-resolution microscopy can visualize the detailed spatial organization of DNA replication, transcription, and repair processes by reconstructing a map of single-molecule localizations. Furthermore, DNA-binding activities can be observed directly by tracking protein movement in real time. This allows identifying subpopulations of DNA-bound and diffusing proteins, and can be used to measure DNA-binding times *in vivo*. This chapter provides a detailed protocol for super-resolution microscopy and tracking of DNA-binding proteins in *Escherichia coli* cells. The protocol covers the construction of cell strains and describes data acquisition and analysis procedures, such as super-resolution image reconstruction, mapping single-molecule tracks, computing diffusion coefficients to identify molecular subpopulations with different mobility, and analysis of DNA-binding kinetics. While the focus is on the study of bacterial chromosome biology, these approaches are generally applicable to other molecular processes and cell types.

Key words Super-resolution fluorescence microscopy, Single-molecule imaging, Single-particle tracking, DNA-binding proteins, DNA repair, Lambda red recombination, *Escherichia coli*

1 Introduction

Super-resolution fluorescence microscopy [1] has matured as a technique and is now widely applied in fundamental research. Photoactivated localization microscopy (PALM) [2] and stochastic optical reconstruction microscopy (STORM) [3] reach image resolution below the diffraction limit of light by localizing individual spatially isolated fluorophores. This is achieved by optically switching fluorophores from a non-fluorescent state to a fluorescent state such that only a sparse subset of fluorophores is visible at any time. Automated computer analysis detects fluorescent spots and determines their centroid positions. A super-resolution image can then

Mark C. Leake (ed.), *Chromosome Architecture: Methods and Protocols*, Methods in Molecular Biology, vol. 1431,
DOI 10.1007/978-1-4939-3631-1_16, © Springer Science+Business Media New York 2016

be reconstructed from the list of molecule localizations that have been recorded sequentially over a series of images.

The study of microorganisms particularly benefits from the ~10-fold increase in image resolution, allowing the visual examination of subcellular molecular structures, such as cell wall components, cell division machinery, and chromosomes [4–15]. Here, we focus on the application of PALM and photoactivated single-molecule tracking to study DNA-binding proteins in *Escherichia coli*. Conventional fluorescence microscopy obscures the measurement of most of these proteins because they bind DNA transiently and are distributed throughout the bacterial nucleoid. By imaging single molecules, unsynchronized reaction events and small molecular subpopulations can be observed without population averaging.

Beyond recording static structures, the ability to determine precise localizations of single fluorescent molecules has enabled tracking proteins in live cells [16]. With the super-resolution microscopy concept, this approach can now be applied for arbitrary densities of labeled molecules [17]: each photoactivation event gives a glimpse into the function of a single protein. Reaction events, such as the binding of a DNA repair enzyme to a DNA damage site, are marked by a change in the diffusion characteristics [9]. Progress has also been made in the application of live-cell super-resolution microscopy to study DNA-binding proteins in eukaryotic cells [18, 19].

This chapter provides a detailed protocol covering the sample preparation for PALM imaging and data analysis procedures. Similar general principles also apply to other super-resolution microscopy modalities such as STORM. First, the protocol describes the construction of *E. coli* strains carrying an endogenous photoactivatable fluorescent fusion protein using lambda Red recombination [20]. As opposed to exogenous plasmid expression systems, this approach maintains native expression levels and permits complete replacement of the native gene with the fluorescent version. The following steps in the protocol include the preparation of cell cultures for microscopy, PALM data acquisition, and data processing to obtain single-molecule localizations and tracks. Once localizations and tracks have been recorded, there are many options for further analysis. Here, the most common and general approaches are presented, such as reconstruction of super-resolution images, mapping single-molecule tracks, computing diffusion coefficients to identify molecular subpopulations with different mobility, and analysis of DNA-binding kinetics.

The protocol is illustrated using data of DNA polymerase I (Pol1), a typical DNA-binding protein with key functions in DNA replication and DNA repair in *E. coli*. Photoactivated single-molecule tracking has been applied to directly visualize binding events of single Pol1 enzymes at DNA repair sites following DNA alkylation damage [9].

2 Materials

2.1 Lambda Red Recombination

1. *E. coli* AB1157 background strain (other *E. coli* K12 strains such as MC4100 or MG1655 can also be used).

2. Plasmid pKD46 [20], encoding the lambda Red integration proteins under an arabinose-inducible promoter. pKD46 carries an ampicillin resistance marker and the temperature sensitive origin of replication repA101ts (to be grown at 30 °C).

3. Plasmid encoding the photoactivatable fluorescent protein PAmCherry [21] with an N-terminal flexible linker and an antibiotic resistance marker (e.g. *see* [9, 22]).

4. PCR primers to amplify the PAmCherry insertion fragment from the template plasmid. The protocol provides guidance on primer design.

5. PCR kit with a high-fidelity polymerase.

6. Dpn1 enzyme.

7. LB medium and LB agarose plates.

8. Antibiotics as required for pKD46 plasmid and selection of the PAmCherry insertion (e.g. ampicillin, kanamycin).

9. 10 % arabinose solution: freshly dissolved in dH₂O and sterilized using a 0.2 μm filter.

10. PCR primers to verify the PAmCherry insertion.

2.2 Cell Culture and Slide Preparation

1. LB medium and LB agarose plates.

2. Supplemented M9 medium. Recipe for 500 ml medium: 100 ml 5× M9 salts, 1 ml 1 M MgSO₄, 500 μl 100 mM CaCl₂, 10 ml 50× MEM amino acids, 5 ml 100 μg/ml l-proline, 50 μl 0.5 % thiamine, 5 ml 20 % glucose, dH₂O up to 500 ml. Sterilize with 0.2 μm filter.

3. Microscope coverslips (no 1.5 thickness) burnt in a furnace at 500 °C for 1 h to remove fluorescent background contamination.

4. Low-fluorescence molecular biology grade agarose (e.g. BioRad).

2.3 Microscope

Detailed descriptions of how to design and assemble a custom total internal reflection fluorescence (TIRF) microscope for single-molecule imaging can be found in refs. 2, 13, 23, 24. Suitable commercial instruments are also available from different manufacturers. The essential components are:

1. 100× NA1.4 oil immersion objective.

2. Electron multiplying CCD camera.

3. 405 nm laser with at least 20 mW output power.

4. 561 nm laser with at least 50 mW output power.

5. TIRF excitation module.

6. Transmitted light illumination.

2.4 Data Analysis

1. Automated data processing can be performed in MATLAB (Mathworks). Optional toolboxes with useful functions include:

   (a) Image processing toolbox, containing functions to read and write image files, as well as image filtering, registration, and segmentation tools.

   (b) Statistics toolbox, containing tools for plotting data histograms and performing statistical tests.

   (c) Optimization toolbox, containing curve fitting functions (e.g. lsqcurvefit).

3 Methods

3.1 Lambda Red Integration to Generate an Endogenous PAmCherry Fusion

This protocol follows the method developed by Datsenko and Wanner [20] that employs the phage lambda Red recombinase to generate an endogenous C-terminal PAmCherry fusion with a protein of interest in *E. coli*. The gene encoding PAmCherry with a flexible N-terminal linker is PCR amplified from a template plasmid together with an antibiotic resistance gene that allows for selection of the chromosomal integration.

1. Transform the target *E. coli* strain with plasmid pKD46. This plasmid encodes the lambda Red integration factors and an ampicillin resistance marker. The transformed strain needs to be grown at 30 °C to maintain the temperature-sensitive plasmid.

2. Find the gene sequence of the protein you wish to tag with PAmCherry using the online *E. coli* Genome Browser: http://microbes.ucsc.edu/cgi-bin/hgGateway?db=eschColi_K12.

3. Design lambda Red PCR primers flanking the PAmCherry and antibiotic resistance genes on the template plasmid and add overhangs with homology to the chromosomal insertion site. For the forward PCR primer, use 40–50 nt of homology at the 3′ terminal end of the gene just upstream of the stop codon and add a primer sequence at the 5′ terminus of the fusion linker on the template plasmid. For the reverse PCR primer, use 40–50 nt of homology immediately downstream of the stop codon of the gene and add a primer sequence downstream of the antibiotic resistance gene on the template plasmid.

4. Run a 50 μl PCR to amplify the insertion fragment from the template plasmid using a high-fidelity DNA polymerase.

5. Add 1 μl of Dpn1 enzyme to the PCR product and incubate for at least 2 h at 37 °C. This digests the template plasmid.

6. Run the PCR product on a 1 % agarose gel (e.g. 100 V for 1 h). Cut out the 2.7 kb DNA band and extract the DNA, e.g. using the Qiagen gel extraction kit. Elute the DNA in a small volume of dH$_2$O (e.g. 30 μl) to obtain a concentrated solution.

7. Grow a 5 ml culture of the target strain carrying plasmid pKD46 in LB medium with 50 μg/ml ampicillin at 30 °C overnight.

8. Dilute 500 μl of the culture in 50 ml LB medium containing 50 μg/ml ampicillin and 0.2 % arabinose. Grow the culture at 30 °C until it reaches an OD$_{600}$ of 0.6.

9. Place the culture on ice for 10 min and swirl to chill it abruptly.

10. Spin down the culture in a chilled 50 ml tube for 10 min in a centrifuge at 2900×g, cooled to 4 °C.

11. Repeat multiple cycles of centrifugation and resuspension of the culture in decreasing volumes of ice-cold dH$_2$O: 50 ml, 35 ml, 2 ml, 500 μl. The last two resuspensions are in dH$_2$O with 10 % glycerol. Keep the culture on ice between steps and centrifuge at 4 °C.

12. Add 1–6 μl of DNA (typically 30–200 ng/μl concentration) to 60 μl of cell suspension and incubate on ice for 15 min.

13. Electroporate the cells with DNA in a pre-chilled cuvette. Following electroporation, immediately add 1 ml of LB medium (at room temperature) and mix gently.

14. Recover the cells at 37 °C for 1 h and plate on LB agarose containing the appropriate antibiotic to select for insertions. Incubate plates at 37 °C overnight to promote the loss of the temperature sensitive plasmid pKD46.

15. Plates typically show a few up to several tens of cell colonies. Pick several colonies and streak again to isolate single colonies. Replica plate on LB agar with 50 μg/ml ampicillin to confirm the loss of plasmid pKD46.

16. Verify correct lambda Red insertion by colony PCR and sequencing using primers flanking the insertion site.

17. Use P1 transduction [25] to move the PAmCherry fusion allele to a strain which had not been transformed with plasmid pKD46.

18. Functionality of the fusion protein should be assessed by comparing the growth rate of the generated strain to the wild-type strain and using other appropriate assays (e.g. sensitivity to DNA damage for a strain carrying a fusion of a DNA repair protein). *See* **Note 1** for more information.

3.2 Cell Culture

The following protocol is for the culture of *E. coli* AB1157 strains exhibiting wild-type phenotypes. Mutant strains may require different growth conditions.

1. Two days before a microscopy session: Streak cells from a frozen glycerol stock onto an LB agar plate containing the appropriate antibiotic for the PAmCherry fusion strain.

2. The next day, inoculate an LB culture from a single cell colony and grow for 3–5 h at 37 °C.

3. Add 1 μl of LB culture to 5 ml of supplemented M9 medium and grow overnight at 37 °C.

4. The next morning, dilute 25 μl of the culture in 5 ml of supplemented M9 medium and grow for 2 h at 37 °C so that cells are imaged during early exponential growth phase (~OD 0.05–0.1).

5. Pellet cells in a benchtop centrifuge at $3300 \times g$ for 3 min.

6. Thoroughly resuspend the cell pellet in a small volume (e.g. 10 μl) of supernatant medium.

7. Microscopy should be performed immediately after preparation of the concentrated cell suspension.

3.3 Microscopy

1. Prepare 5 ml of a 1 % low-fluorescence agarose solution in supplemented M9 medium.

2. Spread 1 ml of melted agarose solution on a microscope coverslip and place a burnt coverslip onto the solidifying gel to create a flat pad.

3. Remove the burnt coverslip from the gel pad and drop 1 μl of concentrated cell suspension onto it. Place a new burnt coverslip on top to sandwich the cells.

4. Place the sample on the microscope and bring cells into focus using transmitted light illumination.

5. Activate the electron multiplying gain of the EMCCD camera and display the live camera data. Only background noise should be visible. Typical frame acquisition rates for single-molecule imaging in live cells are between 10 and 100 frames/s.

6. Switch on the 561 nm laser for excitation of PAmCherry and the 405 nm laser for photoactivation. Wait for individual fluorescent spots to appear inside cells and adjust the TIRF illumination angle to maximize the brightness of the spots.

7. Record a short movie, examine the saved images, and optimize the acquisition settings (frame rates and laser intensities) as explained in **Note 2**.

8. For data acquisition, first expose cells to 561 nm excitation for a few seconds to bleach the autofluorescence background, then start recording a movie. Switch on the 405 nm laser for

PAmCherry photoactivation. For tracking experiments, activated molecules should be visible for a few frames until photobleaching. Gradually increase the 405 nm intensity over the course of the movie while the pool of pre-activated molecules depletes. Keep the density of activated molecules sparse at less than one spot per cell in each frame. Record a movie of several thousand frames until most molecules have been activated (Fig. 1).

9. Several movies of different cells can be recorded for approximately 45 min before the agarose gel starts to dry out.

3.4 Reconstructing a Super-Resolution Map of Localizations

1. Use a localization algorithm to identify fluorescent spots and determine their centroid with high precision. Several algorithms have been developed for this purpose, e.g. [26–28]. *See* **Note 3** for guidance.

2. Display the resulting localizations as a scatter plot (Fig. 2a, b).

3. Generate a super-resolution image by binning localizations into a two-dimensional color-coded histogram (Fig. 2c). Alternatively, each localization can be rendered as a Gaussian spot with a width corresponding to the estimated localization error. The super-resolution image is then reconstructed as the super-position of all Gaussian spots (Fig. 2d).

4. The super-resolution image can be used to analyze protein structures [7, 12, 13], foci [8, 10], or partitioning of molecules between different cellular compartments [15, 29].

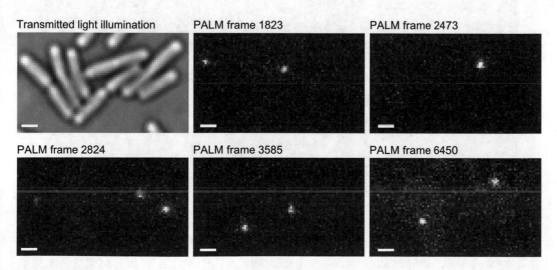

Fig. 1 Example images of a PALM recording. The transmitted light image shows live *E. coli* cells immobilized on an agarose pad. Cells are expressing a fusion of DNA polymerase 1 (Pol1) with PAmCherry. Example frames of a PALM movie show isolated fluorescent spots of single Pol1-PAmCherry molecules. Different molecules become photoactivated in different frames such that their precise positions can be recorded over time. Scale bars: 1 μm

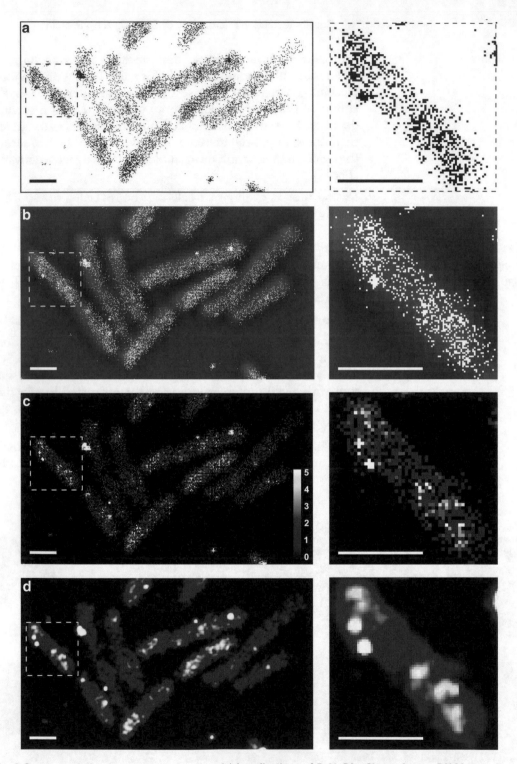

Fig. 2 Super-resolution image reconstruction. (**a**) Localizations of Pol1-PAmCherry from a PALM recording of 7500 frames (example frames in Fig. 1) are displayed as a scatter plot. (**b**) Localizations are mapped onto the transmitted light image of cells. (**c**) Histogram visualization: Localizations are binned into a two-dimensional grid of subpixels (38 nm × 38 nm, i.e. 4 × 4 subpixels per original pixel). The number of localizations per bin is represented according to the colors in the scale bar. (**d**) Gaussian kernel visualization: The image is reconstructed by summing normalized Gaussian kernels with 40 nm standard deviation (equivalent to the localization precision) centred on the localizations. The boxed regions are shown magnified. Scale bars: 1 μm

3.5 Short Exposure Times to Quantify Diffusion

In live cells, protein movement can be measured by recording a PALM movie at high frame rates and short exposure times (e.g. 15 ms/frame) and using an automated tracking algorithm.

1. Determine molecule tracks by linking localizations that appear nearby in consecutive frames. Simple algorithms use a fixed tracking window within which localizations get connected [30], while other methods apply global tracking analysis [31]. *See* **Note 4** for more information on the following analysis procedure.

2. Compute the mean-squared displacement (MSD) from the (x,y) localizations for each track with at least $N = 5$ localizations: $\text{MSD} = 1/(N-1) \sum_{N-1}^{i=1}(x_{i+1}\ x_i)^2 + (y_{i+1}\ y_i)^2$.

3. Compute the apparent diffusion coefficient (D^*) per track using the mean-squared displacement: $D^* = \text{MSD}/(4\ \Delta t)$. Here, Δt is the time interval between frames.

4. Plot a histogram to examine the distribution of diffusion coefficients. Molecule subpopulations with different mobility (e.g. mobile and bound molecules) can be identified as distinct species in the histogram (Fig. 3).

5. In the case of a bound and a mobile population of molecules, the fraction of molecules in the bound state can be quantified using a threshold on the apparent diffusion coefficient (Fig. 3b, c).

6. An alternative approach to quantify subpopulations with different mobility is to fit the distributions using an analytical equation [5, 11, 15].

3.6 Long Exposures to Quantify Binding Kinetics

The time a single photoactivated molecule can be observed for is limited by irreversible photobleaching. This duration is typically only a few frames for PAmCherry, which complicates quantification of binding kinetics from tracking data recorded at high temporal resolution. A simple solution to this problem is to reduce laser intensities—which extends the photobleaching lifetime — while equally increasing exposure times to circumvent the loss of signal due to the reduced emission intensities. At long exposure times, mobile molecules will appear as blurred spots, while bound molecules result in diffraction-limited spots. A spot finding algorithm can be used to extract diffraction-limited spots only, and the average binding time corresponds to the average number of frames a diffraction-limited spot is visible for. It is important to correct for the residual effect of photobleaching on the apparent binding time by measuring photobleaching rates under identical illumination conditions using fixed cells or a sample for which binding times are very long compared to the average bleaching time. Crucially, photobleaching should not be faster than the

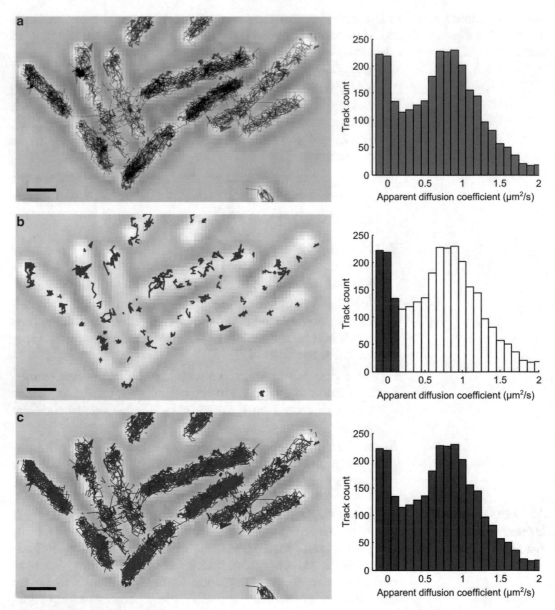

Fig. 3 Photoactivated single-molecule tracking analysis. Tracks of Pol1-PAmCherry molecules were generated from the localization data in Fig. 2 and shown on a transmitted light image of cells. The *histograms* show the distribution of apparent diffusion coefficients. Live cells were treated with the DNA-damaging agent methyl methanesulfonate (100 mM MMS) for 20 min before imaging. Base-excision repair of MMS damage creates gapped DNA substrates to which Pol1 binds for DNA repair synthesis. Single-molecule tracking of Pol1 allows identifying such events by the low apparent diffusion coefficient of DNA-bound proteins. (**a**) Data for all tracks with at least five localizations. (**b**) Detecting individual bound molecules by plotting only tracks with an apparent diffusion coefficient below 0.15 μm²/s. (**c**) All observed tracks, color coded by their classification as bound or mobile, in *red* and *blue*, respectively. Apparent diffusion coefficients were corrected for localization error (*see* **Note 4**). Scale bars: 1 μm

average binding time because small errors in the estimation of the photobleaching rate will cause very large errors in the estimation of the binding time constant. More information on this type of analysis can be found in reference [9].

3.7 Clustering Analysis

Clustering algorithms identify foci of localizations that might represent a spatial organization of proteins performing their function in cells. Methods to quantify clustering include k-means, nearest-neighbour clustering, and point-correlation analysis. These algorithms report the size and number of localizations per cluster. k-Means assigns all observed localizations to a fixed number of clusters. This number has to be defined prior to the analysis. Nearest-neighbour clustering groups localizations that are within a user-defined distance threshold [8]. Point-correlation analysis examines the spatial correlation between localizations, and compares the observed distribution to a random homogenous distribution of points [32, 33].

4 Notes

1. Protein functionality can be affected by the fusion to a fluorescent protein. Therefore, care should be taken to closely compare growth characteristics and specific phenotypes of the strain carrying the fluorescent fusion protein to the wild-type strain. For nonessential proteins, functionality of the fusion can also be evaluated by comparison with a strain in which the gene is deleted [34]. Additional control experiments can be performed that abolish specific activities of the protein (e.g. by introducing point mutations, drug treatments, or deletion of protein interaction partners).

   Furthermore, many fluorescent proteins are prone to dimerize or multimerize which can cause aggregation artifacts of fusion proteins [35, 36]. Localization clusters may therefore represent protein aggregates instead of a genuine spatial organization of the native protein. Moreover, photoactivatable fluorescent proteins typically blink, i.e. they randomly convert between bright and dark states once they have been photoactivated by 405 nm light [37, 38]. Each fusion protein may therefore be observed several times, which can result in apparent clustering of tracks and complicates counting molecule numbers. Conventional fluorescence imaging with a monomeric fluorescent protein fusion can be performed to evaluate the genuine presence of clusters [35].

2. Before data acquisition it is important to identify appropriate imaging conditions. To this end, record a short movie, examine the images, and change the microscope settings as required.

For example: (a) increase the 561 nm laser power or use a longer camera exposure time if the fluorescent spots are too dim against the background noise. (b) Decrease the 561 nm laser power or use faster camera exposures if the spots are very clear but appear to bleach very quickly. Estimation of diffusion coefficients requires observing the same molecule for multiple frames. (c) Shorten the camera exposure time if the fluorescent spots appear blurry due to fast movement of the fusion protein during each frame. Appropriate laser intensities and exposure times will vary between instruments due to differences in the alignment and quality of optical components.

3. Microscopy images are subject to several factors that complicate the precise localization of single fluorophores. These factors include image pixelation, camera read noise, electron multiplying noise, background noise, and photon shot noise. Background noise can be reduced by TIRF excitation, while photon shot noise is dictated by the fluorophore brightness. Once all experimental factors have been optimized, the localization algorithm is key to maximize the localization precision [39]. Most localization algorithms either use least-squares [26, 40] or maximum likelihood parameter estimation [27, 28].

In addition to minimizing localization error, a key metric for the performance of localization algorithms is the recall, i.e. the fraction of successfully detected spots. The recall fraction decreases with increasing density of fluorescent spots per image. However, high densities are often desired because the time required to record a PALM movie that represents the majority of labeled molecules in the sample is limited by the number of accurate localizations per frame. Moreover, the total density of all localizations dictates the resolution of the reconstructed image according to Shannon's sampling theorem. Several algorithms have been developed that substantially improve the localization recall in images of densely overlapping fluorescent spots [41, 42].

4. Because of photobleaching, the number of localizations per track is usually small, which causes large statistical uncertainty in the estimation of the diffusion coefficient of a single molecule. For this reason, only tracks with a certain minimum number of steps should be included in the analysis (e.g. at least five localizations or four steps). The term *apparent* diffusion coefficient is used because this measurement of the diffusion coefficient includes several biases: Confinement of molecules within the cell volume or cellular compartments leads to an underestimation of the diffusion coefficient. Furthermore, molecule movement during the exposure time reduces the apparent diffusion coefficient because the localizations represent time-averaged positions. The localization error, on the other hand,

effectively adds a random step to each true position, which causes an overestimation of the diffusion coefficient. This error can be corrected by measuring the average localization error σ_{loc} using a sample with immobile molecules and applying the equation: $D^* = \text{MSD}/(4\,\Delta t) - \sigma_{loc}^2/\Delta t$.

Acknowledgments

Rodrigo Reyes-Lamothe, David J. Sherratt, and Achillefs N. Kapanidis helped with the original development of this protocol. Katarzyna Ginda and David J. Sherratt are thanked for their comments on the manuscript. Stephan Uphoff was funded by a Sir Henry Wellcome Postdoctoral Fellowship by the Wellcome Trust (101636/Z/13/Z) and a Junior Research Fellowship at St. John's College, Oxford. Microscopy at Micron Oxford was supported by a Wellcome Trust Strategic Award (091911) and MRC grant (MR/K01577X/1).

References

1. Hell SW (2007) Far-field optical nanoscopy. Science 316:1153–1158

2. Betzig E, Patterson GH, Sougrat R et al (2006) Imaging intracellular fluorescent proteins at nanometer resolution. Science 313:1642–5

3. Rust MJ, Bates M, Zhuang X (2006) Sub-diffraction-limit imaging by stochastic optical reconstruction microscopy (STORM). Nat Methods 3:793–795

4. Biteen JS, Thompson MA, Tselentis NK et al (2008) Super-resolution imaging in live Caulobacter crescentus cells using photo-switchable EYFP. Nat Methods 5:947–949

5. English BP, Hauryliuk V, Sanamrad A et al (2011) Single-molecule investigations of the stringent response machinery in living bacterial cells. Proc Natl Acad Sci U S A 108:E365–373

6. Garner EC, Bernard R, Wang W et al (2011) Coupled, circumferential motions of the cell wall synthesis machinery and MreB filaments in B. subtilis. Science 333:222–225

7. Greenfield D, McEvoy AL, Shroff H et al (2009) Self-organization of the Escherichia coli chemotaxis network imaged with super-resolution light microscopy. PLoS Biol 7, e1000137

8. Badrinarayanan A, Reyes-Lamothe R, Uphoff S et al (2012) In vivo architecture and action of bacterial structural maintenance of chromosome proteins. Science 338:528–531

9. Uphoff S, Reyes-Lamothe R, de Leon FG et al (2013) Single-molecule DNA repair in live bacteria. Proc Natl Acad Sci U S A 110:8063–8068

10. Endesfelder U, Finan K, Holden SJ et al (2013) Multiscale spatial organization of RNA polymerase in Escherichia coli. Biophys J 105:172–181

11. Bakshi S, Dalrymple RM, Li W et al (2013) Partitioning of RNA polymerase activity in live Escherichia coli from analysis of single-molecule diffusive trajectories. Biophys J 105:2676–2686

12. Fiche J-B, Cattoni DI, Diekmann N et al (2013) Recruitment, assembly, and molecular architecture of the SpoIIIE DNA pump revealed by superresolution microscopy. PLoS Biol 11, e1001557

13. Holden SJ, Pengo T, Meibom KL et al (2014) High throughput 3D super-resolution microscopy reveals Caulobacter crescentus in vivo Z-ring organization. Proc Natl Acad Sci U S A 111:4566–4571

14. Diepold A, Kudryashev M, Delalez NJ et al (2015) Composition, formation, and regulation of the cytosolic c-ring, a dynamic component of the type III secretion injectisome. PLoS Biol 13, e1002039

15. Stracy M, Lesterlin C, de Leon FG et al (2015) Live-cell superresolution microscopy reveals the organization of RNA polymerase in the bacterial nucleoid. Proc Natl Acad Sci U S A 201507592

16. Saxton MJ, Jacobson K (1997) Single-particle tracking: applications to membrane dynamics. Annu Rev Biophys Biomol Struct 26:373–399

17. Manley S, Gillette JM, Patterson GH et al (2008) High-density mapping of single-molecule trajectories with photoactivated localization microscopy. Nat Methods 5:155–157

18. Gebhardt JCM, Suter DM, Roy R et al (2013) Single-molecule imaging of transcription factor binding to DNA in live mammalian cells. Nat Methods 10:421–426

19. Etheridge TJ, Boulineau RL, Herbert A et al (2014) Quantification of DNA-associated proteins inside eukaryotic cells using single-molecule localization microscopy. Nucleic Acids Res 42:e146–e146

20. Datsenko KA, Wanner BL (2000) One-step inactivation of chromosomal genes in Escherichia coli K-12 using PCR products. Proc Natl Acad Sci U S A 97:6640–6645

21. Subach FV, Patterson GH, Manley S et al (2009) Photoactivatable mCherry for high-resolution two-color fluorescence microscopy. Nat Meth 6:153–159

22. Reyes-Lamothe R, Possoz C, Danilova O et al (2008) Independent positioning and action of Escherichia coli replisomes in live cells. Cell 133:90–102

23. Roy R, Hohng S, Ha T (2008) A practical guide to single-molecule FRET. Nat Methods 5:507–516

24. Uphoff S, Sherratt DJ, Kapanidis AN (2014) Visualizing protein-DNA interactions in live bacterial cells using photoactivated single-molecule tracking. J Vis Exp 85:24638084

25. Thomason LC, Costantino N, Court DL (2007) E. coli genome manipulation by P1 transduction. Curr Protoc Mol Biol Chapter 1:Unit 1.17

26. Holden SJ, Uphoff S, Hohlbein J et al (2010) Defining the limits of single-molecule FRET resolution in TIRF microscopy. Biophys J 99:3102–3111

27. Mortensen KI, Churchman LS, Spudich JA et al (2010) Optimized localization analysis for single-molecule tracking and super-resolution microscopy. Nat Methods 7:377–381

28. Smith CS, Joseph N, Rieger B et al (2010) Fast, single-molecule localization that achieves theoretically minimum uncertainty. Nat Methods 7:373–375

29. Bakshi S, Siryaporn A, Goulian M et al (2012) Superresolution imaging of ribosomes and RNA polymerase in live Escherichia coli cells. Mol Microbiol 85:21–38

30. Crocker JC, Grier DG (1996) Methods of digital video microscopy for colloidal studies. J Colloid Interface Sci 179:298–310

31. Persson F, Lindén M, Unoson C et al (2013) Extracting intracellular diffusive states and transition rates from single-molecule tracking data. Nat Methods 10:265–269

32. Veatch SL, Machta BB, Shelby SA et al (2012) Correlation functions quantify super-resolution images and estimate apparent clustering due to over-counting. PLoS One 7, e31457

33. Sengupta P, Jovanovic-Talisman T, Lippincott-Schwartz J (2013) Quantifying spatial organization in point-localization superresolution images using pair correlation analysis. Nat Protoc 8:345–354

34. Baba T, Ara T, Hasegawa M et al (2006) Construction of Escherichia coli K-12 in-frame, single-gene knockout mutants: the Keio collection. Mol Syst Biol 2:2006.0008

35. Landgraf D, Okumus B, Chien P et al (2012) Segregation of molecules at cell division reveals native protein localization. Nat Methods 9:480–482

36. Wang S, Moffitt JR, Dempsey GT et al (2014) Characterization and development of photoactivatable fluorescent proteins for single-molecule-based superresolution imaging. Proc Natl Acad Sci U S A 111:8452–8457

37. Lee S-H, Shin JY, Lee A et al (2012) Counting single photoactivatable fluorescent molecules by photoactivated localization microscopy (PALM). Proc Natl Acad Sci U S A 109:17436–17441

38. Durisic N, Laparra-Cuervo L, Sandoval-Álvarez Á et al (2014) Single-molecule evaluation of fluorescent protein photoactivation efficiency using an in vivo nanotemplate. Nat Methods 11:156–162

39. Small A, Stahlheber S (2014) Fluorophore localization algorithms for super-resolution microscopy. Nat Methods 11:267–279

40. Thompson RE, Larson DR, Webb WW (2002) Precise nanometer localization analysis for individual fluorescent probes. Biophys J 82:2775–2783

41. Holden SJ, Uphoff S, Kapanidis AN (2011) DAOSTORM: an algorithm for high-density super-resolution microscopy. Nat Methods 8:279–280

42. Zhu L, Zhang W, Elnatan D et al (2012) Faster STORM using compressed sensing. Nat Methods 9:721–723

Chapter 17

Studying the Dynamics of Chromatin-Binding Proteins in Mammalian Cells Using Single-Molecule Localisation Microscopy

Srinjan Basu, Yi Lei Tan, Edward J.R. Taylor, Ernest D. Laue, and Steven F. Lee

Abstract

Single-molecule localisation microscopy (SMLM) allows the super-resolved imaging of proteins within mammalian nuclei at spatial resolutions comparable to that of a nucleosome itself (~20 nm). The technique is therefore well suited to the study of chromatin structure. Fixed-cell SMLM has already allowed temporal 'snapshots' of how proteins are arranged on chromatin within mammalian nuclei. In this chapter, we focus on how recent developments, for example in selective plane illumination and protein labelling, have led to a range of live-cell SMLM studies. We describe how to carry out single-particle tracking (SPT) of single proteins and, by analysing their diffusion parameters, how to determine whether proteins interact with chromatin, diffuse freely or do both. We can study the numbers of proteins that interact with chromatin and also determine their residence time on chromatin. We can determine whether these proteins form functional clusters within the nucleus as well as whether they form specific nuclear structures.

Key words Chromatin, Super-resolution microscopy, PALM, STORM, SPT, Fluorescence imaging, SPIM, Mean squared displacement, Jump distance, Residence time, Diffusion coefficient

1 Introduction to Role of Live-Cell Single-Molecule Localisation Microscopy

Understanding protein/chromosome dynamics is critical to understanding chromosome architecture [1]. Recent advances have led to the imaging of live cells well below the diffraction limit of light, allowing us to now dissect previously inaccessible dynamics critical to chromosome function [2–4].

The relevant imaging approach generally depends on the spatial scale at which chromosome function is being studied (Fig. 1a). The mammalian nucleus is ~10–30 μm in size. Chromosomes are known to occupy discrete regions of ~3 μm within the mammalian nucleus called 'chromosome territories' [5], although intermingling between adjacent chromosomes does occur [6]. Most of the DNA within chromosomes is

Mark C. Leake (ed.), *Chromosome Architecture: Methods and Protocols*, Methods in Molecular Biology, vol. 1431,
DOI 10.1007/978-1-4939-3631-1_17, © Springer Science+Business Media New York 2016

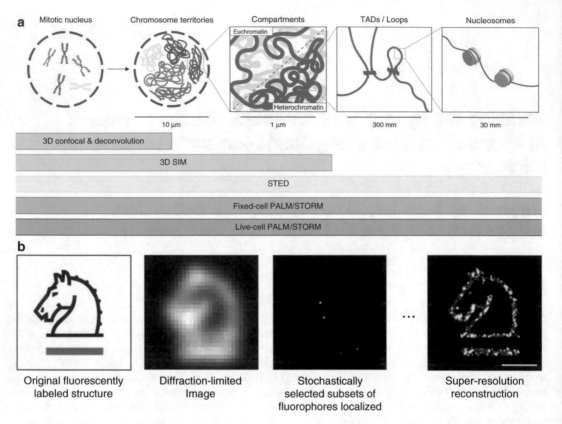

Fig. 1 (**a**) Length scales at which live-cell single-molecule localisation microscopy (SMLM) is currently used to study chromatin structure. This is compared to other common microscopy approaches. (**b**) Schematic of single-molecule localisation microscopy (SMLM) adapted from Horrocks et al. [4]. Conventional imaging is diffraction limited. By turning one molecule at a time to the 'on' state, it is possible to precisely localise them at higher resolution (~20 nm)

packaged into nucleosomes of around 20 nm but these nucleosomes are not uniformly compacted into chromosomes. Genome-wide chromosome conformation capture (3C) assays such as Hi-C [7–9], that highlight physical proximity between DNA sequences within the genome, have confirmed physical 'megadomains' of active and inactive genes at the 5–20 Mb scale, thought to be less densely packed euchromatin and more condensed heterochromatin [10, 11]. Traditional imaging approaches have focussed on studies at this magnification. However, Hi-C studies have also revealed smaller sub-compartments ('topologically associating domains' or TADs) ranging in size from 40 kb to 3 Mb [12–15]. Little is known about the dynamics of proteins that act at these smaller levels of compaction and this has driven the development of several higher resolution imaging approaches.

The main three live-cell imaging approaches developed for studying chromosome dynamics at high resolution are the following:

1. 3D confocal microscopy (usually with deconvolution): This approach has been used, for example, to monitor detailed changes in DNA compaction during M phase [16].

2. Microscopy approaches that pattern the illumination light such as stimulated emission depletion (STED) [17], reversible saturable optical fluorescence transition (RESOLFT) microscopy [18] and structured illumination microscopy (SIM) [19]. SIM halves the resolution limit to ~100 nm and has been used, for example, to study nuclear membrane invaginations during M phase [20] and changes in the structure of the X chromosome during X inactivation [21].

3. Single-molecule localisation microscopy (SMLM) approaches detect and localise single molecules with a localisation precision of 10–20 nm including stochastic optical reconstruction microscopy (STORM) [22], photoactivated localisation microscopy (PALM) [23] and fluorescence photoactivation localisation microscopy (fPALM) [24]. SMLM approaches take advantage of photoswitchable fluorophores that can modulate their fluorescence between an emissive 'on' state and a non-emissive 'off' state to separate molecules temporally such that their point spread functions (PSFs) do not overlap spatially during the image acquisition (Fig. 1b). The resolution is then no longer determined by the diffraction limit [25] but instead by the uncertainty at which a single molecule can be super-localised and detected, the density at which it is labelled and the size of the probe use to label the molecule. Photoswitchable fluorescent proteins and dyes have been used as both switch between this 'on' and 'off' state.

Live-cell SMLM approaches can address dynamics that occur at the level of nucleosomes as well as larger structures that require a resolution of ~20 nm. It has allowed single-particle tracking (SPT) of proteins on chromatin. Such studies have been used to extract information on the diffusion coefficients of proteins, their residence time on DNA as well as the search time of a protein for its specific site on DNA [26–31]. In addition, live-cell SMLM has allowed us to study the dynamics of proteins that cluster in the nucleus such as RNA polymerase II and nucleosomes [32, 33]. It has even been used to study more complex structures such as heterochromatin fibres [34].

In this chapter, we describe how live-cell SMLM can be used to acquire these parameters for your protein of choice.

2 Materials

2.1 SMLM Microscope Configuration

The SMLM microscope requires collimated excitation lasers (and activation lasers for photoswitchable proteins/dyes) for the relevant wavelengths aligned and focussed at the back aperture of a

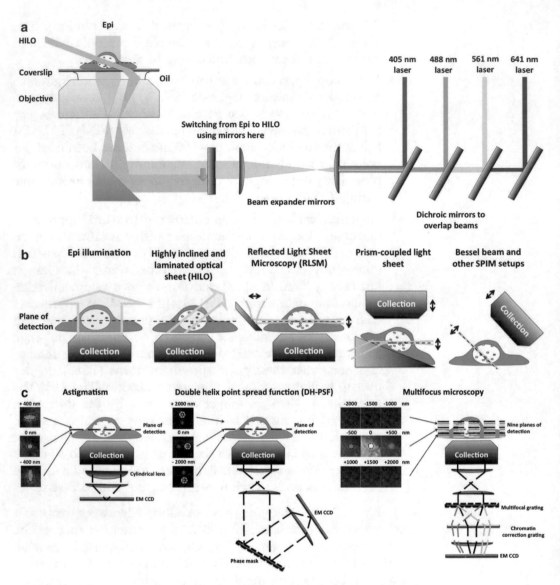

Fig. 2 Typical microscope set-up for single-particle tracking. (**a**) Beam path and lasers common to a micro-scope set-up also showing how HILO is typically set up. (**b**) Comparison of wide-field, partial illumination and selective plane illumination microscopy (SPIM) set-ups. (**c**) Schematic of common 3D detection approaches

high N.A. objective mounted, typically, on an inverted microscope frame. An example set-up for imaging of a photoswitchable protein called mEos (see Subheading 2.2.1 later) is shown below (Fig. 2a) and includes the following components:

- Optical table, vibration isolated (e.g. Thorlabs/Newport).
- High numerical aperture objective lens (e.g. Olympus Apo TIRF 60X N.A. = 1.49 Oil).
- Inverted optical microscope (e.g. Olympus IX71/73).

- Excitation laser, 488 nm—to image green form of mEos before photoactivation (e.g. Toptica, iBeam Smart 488).

- Excitation laser, 561 nm—to image red form of mEos after photoactivation (e.g. Cobolt, Jive 200).

- Activation laser, 405 nm—to photoconvert mEos (e.g. Oxxius, LaserBoxx 405).

- Laser power meter (e.g. Thorlabs PM100D).

- Mechanical shutters for pulsing of lasers (e.g. Uniblitz/Prior).

- An electron-multiplying charge-coupled device (EMCCD) camera for detection of individual fluorophores with high quantum efficiency (e.g. Photometrics Evolve/Delta 512, Andor iXon3 897).

- High-efficiency optical filters and dichroics (e.g. Semrock, USA):

  - Multi-band dichroic (e.g. Semrock, Di01-R405/ 488/561/635).

  - 488 long-pass filter (e.g. Semrock, BLP01-488R).

  - 561 long-pass filter (e.g. Semrock, BLP01-561R) and band-pass filter (Semrock, FF01-587/35).

2.1.1 Sample Illumination

The sample may be illuminated using wide-field illumination; however this is most appropriate in mammalian cells for 3D detection where it is necessary to excite molecules in all the axial planes of interest simultaneously. A common technique employed to increase the signal-to-background of a fluorophore is to confine the excitation geometry by reducing the volume of the nucleus that is illuminated by the excitation source and therefore reducing the background noise generated by cellular autofluorescence and laser scattering. These can be implemented in software via smart filtering of existing datasets [35], or more commonly experimentally using one of several selective plane illumination microscopy (SPIM) approaches (Fig. 2b). Common ways to illuminate the sample usually involve partial illumination of the nucleus:

1. Highly inclined and laminated optical sheet or HILO microscopy [36] simply involves the use of a high N.A. objective and is therefore the simplest technique to implement for SPT of molecules within a mammalian nucleus. Whereas in total internal reflection fluorescence (TIRF) microscopy the beam is reflected off the top surface of the imaging coverslip by the incident light being directed above the critical angle, HILO brings in the light beam at a subcritical angle such that it refracts through the glass but at an oblique angle that creates a light sheet illuminating only part of the nucleus. TIRF itself is rarely used as it only illuminates the bottom surface of the cell

(~100 nm) and so usually misses most of the nucleus, only really allowing the study of nuclear membrane-associated proteins.

2. Reflected light sheet microscopy (RLSM) [28] and single-objective SPIM (soSPIM) [37] are approaches based on the reflection of a light beam across the cell at the detection plane. The first requires an excitation objective from above and detection from below whereas the second excites and detects from below. Both require some skill to assemble. For example, the first requires the positioning of a disposable tipless atomic force microscopy (AFM) cantilever (e.g. fHYDRA2R-100N-TL-10, Nanoscience) next to the cell being imaged. The cantilever is coated with a 1 nm titanium layer followed by a 40 nm aluminium layer by thermal evaporation so it can act as a mirror to reflect a light sheet coming from above across the cell. The light sheet illumination is thinner (~1 μm) and so this leads to lower background fluorescence than HILO. At a low density, the signal-to-background improvement is only 1.5-fold but it can be as much as 5-fold at high densities [28]. This approach is therefore particularly appropriate if there is a high density of fluorophores in the focal plane of detection either because the molecules are not photoactivatable or because large numbers of molecules must be activated quickly (for example, to visualise structures).

3. Prism-coupled light sheet illumination [34]: This is where the illumination is from below through a prism and it follows the same principle as RLSM in that the light sheet is in the detection plane.

4. Bessel beam illumination [38] is more difficult to experimentally implement but is useful if a thinner sheet or more even illumination is required over larger distances, e.g. when imaging several cells at the same time or when imaging thicker samples. Bessel beams are propagation invariant because the transverse profile of the beam remains unaltered during free-space propagation, leading to properties such as a tight (<0.5 μm), self-healing beam that does not diffract or spread out.

2.1.2 Sample Detection

The fluorescent signal is then filtered using a dichroic mirror and a set of relevant emission filters, and projected by an infinity-corrected tube lens onto an EMCCD camera [39] in the image plane. For 3D detection, different methods have been developed to gain information about the axial positions of biomolecules [4]:

1. PSF shaping methods involve manipulation of fluorescent puncta as a function of the axial position of the single molecule relative to the focal plane of the objective lens. The easiest approach uses astigmatism [40] and involves placing a cylindrical lens in the emission path. This will result in the fluorescence emission forming an ellipse above and below the detection

plane in different orientations. The z range of this approach is ~600 nm, which is enough to track a chromatin-bound molecule but not suitable to track over a larger range. Another approach that has a much larger z range (~4 μm) is called double-helix point spread function (DH-PSF) [41] and involves placing a reflective phase mask in 4-f imaging system in the emission path (Fourier optics) such that each molecule appears as two puncta such that the centre of the two spots form the lateral (x.y) position of the molecule and the angle subtended between the spots corresponds to the axial (z) position.

2. Multifocal plane detection methods involve imaging more than one lateral plane at defined spacing to infer axial position. This can be implemented with biplane imaging that enables 3D single-molecule super-resolution imaging by acquiring two focal places simultaneously in a photon-limited environment [42], or by super-localising bright foci over many (nine) planes simultaneously to cover a much larger z range (4 μm) named aberration-corrected multifocus microscopy [43]. It is implemented by a diffractive multifocus grating (Fourier optics) in the emission path to form a multifocus image, corresponding to nine detection planes separated by 500 nm each. The aberration correction is carried out using a chromatic correction grating (custom made by Tessera) and prism (custom made by Rocky Mountain Instruments).

3. Light property detection methods involve detecting parameters of the fluorescent puncta such as their phase as in interferometric PALM (iPALM) [44, 45] or their angle of detection as in supercritical angle localisation microscopy (SALM) [46]. In iPALM, two objectives collect the emitted light, interfere it through dichroic mirrors and then detect using multiple CCD cameras. The intensity ratios between these cameras are used to determine the phase of the puncta observed. This approach is demanding to implement and also limited to twice the working distance of the two objectives used and has therefore been limited in imaging live mammalian nuclei. SALM involves splitting the beam and using a ring aperture to block out the undercritical angle emission in one image. By comparing the supercritical angle emission with the undercritical angle emission, it is possible to determine the 3D position of a fluorescent puncta.

The first two types of approach are more common in 3D live-cell single-molecule localisation studies and are shown in Fig. 2c.

2.2 Labelled Mammalian Cells

The labelling of mammalian cells requires the basics of mammalian cell culture imaging such as:

1. Cell culture incubator (37 °C, 5 % CO_2).

2. Phenol-red-free cell growth medium especially if detecting fluorescence in the red part of the spectrum (>600 nm).

3. No. 1.5 glass coverslip-bottomed dishes, e.g. from Mat-tek or Nunc Lab-Tek II dishes.

4. Fixation buffers: Methanol, ethanol, formaldehyde, phosphate-buffered saline (PBS).

2.2.1 Fluorophore Choice

When considering which fluorescent protein/organic dye to use for a specific experiment, it is important to consider their properties. Here are a few critical properties that affect which fluorophore to choose for a given experiment (a–c for single-molecule tracking and d–e also for switching experiments) [47, 48]:

(a) Photostability or photobleaching quantum yield—if a fluorophore is more photostable, it can be imaged for longer before irreversible photobleaching. These long track lengths are ideal for determining the residence time of proteins bound to chromatin. Dyes generally have greater photostability than fluorescent proteins.

(b) Fluorescence quantum yield—if a fluorophore has a high fluorescence quantum yield, more photons are emitted for a given number of photons absorbed. Higher photon counts give rise to greater localisation precision and therefore a better characterisation of diffusion.

(c) Switching cycles/dye molecule—when used in photoswitching experiments, the number of switching cycles can vary from fluorophore to fluorophore but is generally higher for dyes than for fluorescent proteins. A high number of switching cycles allows the structure to be imaged repetitively over a longer time frame.

(d) 'On'/'off' ratio (or duty cycle) during switching cycle—fluorophores with a lower 'on'/'off' duty cycle may be useful when studying denser structures that have a higher likelihood of fluorophores overlapping during their blinking cycles whereas a greater 'on'/'off' duty cycle allows the structure to be imaged quicker.

There are six major types of fluorophore to choose from:

1. Fluorescent proteins with high photostability and fluorescence quantum yield such as YPet or TagRFP can be used [28, 49–51]. However, this approach requires that the density of fluorophores in the illuminated region is low enough to prevent overlap of the PSFs. This can be achieved by having low expression levels of the protein of interest or by reducing the illumination volume, e.g. by using RLSM, soSPIM or Bessel beam illumination.

2. Photoswitchable fluorescent proteins [52] such as photoactivatable green fluorescent protein (PA-GFP) [53], Dronpa [55], PA-mCherry [54], mEos2/3 [55, 56] and Dendra/

Dendra2 [57] are commonly used in SMLM. These are fluorophores that can be activated into a fluorescent 'on' state using an activation laser (often 405 nm). The power of the activation laser determines the number of molecules in the 'on' state. When choosing which photoswitchable protein to use for a specific experiment, several of its properties are usually considered [47]. When designing counting experiments, it is important to take into account that photoswitchable fluorescent proteins vary considerably in the number of times they can be activated. Some can only be activated once or twice, such as PA-mCherry and mEos2/3, respectively, whereas others can be reversibly switched to the 'on' state many times (e.g. Dronpa). In addition, some photoswitchable proteins may not fold and mature as well as others and so have a smaller percentage of their molecules actually able to switch to the fluorescent 'on' state. When studying whether proteins cluster together, it is also important to take into account that some of these proteins have dimerisation tendencies. When studying structures over time, molecules that photoswitch reversibly (i.e. can undergo many switching cycles between the 'on' and 'off' states) such as Dronpa are ideal as they can then be imaged multiple times, allowing for time-lapse imaging.

3. HaloTag®/SNAP-/eDHFR-tagged proteins [30, 32] are enzymes recently developed to specifically label proteins with organic dyes that are introduced to cells. At low laser powers, dyes do not photoswitch and can be used to track molecules at high spatial resolution for longer than is possible with fluorescent proteins (ideal for determining residence time) since dyes generally emit more photons. However, in such conditions, one must be careful that PSFs of the dyes do not overlap and so either fewer proteins must be labelled per cell (low concentrations of dye added) or you must control the active emitter concentration. At high laser powers, dyes can be used to image structures over time since they reversibly photoswitch. To image structures, high concentrations of dye should be added to ensure efficient labelling of enough molecules to visualise the structure. When choosing a dye, it is of course important to consider factors such as quantum yield and the number of switching cycles as described above [18]. In addition, it is important to consider dye permeability as dyes that are not permeable may need to be electroporated or injected into the cell. Some actually become permeable after addition of the HaloTag® ligand [58]. The major disadvantage of dye labelling is that it requires longer than photoswitchable fluorescent proteins to prepare and label the sample, especially given that the concentration of dye to be added needs to be optimised given the concentration of tagged proteins per cell. Common dyes to use are tetramethylrhoda-

mine (TMR), Atto 655 as well as some more recently derived rhodamine-based dyes [60] since they are cell permeable, have high photostability and quantum yield and also reversibly photoswitch at high laser powers. If a dye is needed that is not available, it can be prepared. For example, new HaloTag® dyes require the following to prepare:

- Relevant dye: Alexa Fluor 647/Atto 655 NHS ester (4 mM in DMSO).

- Relevant ligand: HaloTag® O2/O4 amine (10 mM in DMSO).

- Labelling buffer: $NaHCO_3/Na_2CO_3$ (100 mM) pH~8.5.

- Reverse-phase high-performance liquid chromatography (HPLC) C18 column.

- HPLC buffers: Acetonitrile, trifluoroacetic acid.

- Mass spectrometry (MALDI TOF).

4. Dyes can also be used to directly label proteins before they are injected into the cell if a specific dye is required [26] but this approach is less common given the enzymes described above as the protein will then need to be expressed, purified and labelled in vitro.

5. Unnatural amino acids with side groups that can react with dyes introduced to cells [61]: This approach, although very promising, has yet to be widely adopted by the community.

2.2.2 Designing Expression Vectors

There are several common ways to express your tagged protein and the preferred method is dependent on the question being asked:

1. Transient transfection of a tagged protein expressed from a promoter of choice is the easiest but least favoured approach. It does not label every cell and shows cell-to-cell variation in the percentage of fluorescent molecules labelled. Analysis of data like this can be difficult as expression-level differences can often affect binding of proteins to chromatin and to other chromatin-binding proteins. However, it is still possible to interpret changes in binding that arise from mutations as long as the expression level is not too high. Transient transfection is usually used to verify expression and localisation of a construct prior to making a stable cell line.

2. Stable expression of the tagged protein is usually important when characterising the binding dynamics of a protein since association rates are concentration dependent. It means that there is a consistent expression level between cells. Stable expression can be achieved using the same expression vector as above but transfection is followed by selection using an antibiotic-resistant gene (also on the vector) and expansion of a colony with a given expression level arising from a single cell.

However, over time these expression constructs are often silenced and so more recently Piggybac vectors that insert genes at specific transposon sites are becoming popular as they exhibit less silencing [62].

3. Knock-in cell line generation is the preferred approach as then all the proteins are labelled at close to the endogenous levels of the protein. However, this approach is time consuming and involves recombining the fluorophore sequence into the relevant genomic site. Recent advances in RNA-guided genome editing based on clustered, regularly interspaced, short palindromic repeat (CRISPR) technology can significantly increase the speed at which such cell lines can be made [63]. If carrying out counting/clustering experiments, it means that there are no untagged proteins to worry about. If proteins associate with other proteins before binding to DNA, maintaining expression levels similar to the endogenous protein in this way allows a better mimic of the endogenous interactions being studied. It is worth noting that the chosen tag can actually affect protein degradation and so its actual expression level should still be checked by Western blotting.

Other considerations when designing an expression construct are:

1. Promoter choice—the expression level of a promoter and its likelihood of being silenced are cell line dependent [63] and so this should be considered for the specific cell line being used.

2. Antibiotic-resistance gene—this allows the cells to be selected. There are a range of antibiotic resistance genes and some take longer than others to select. For example, puromycin is often quicker than geneticin selection.

3. Does tagging affect protein function? It is critical to check the function of the protein after tagging through a functional study. Sometimes tagging of the N- but not the C-terminus can affect the function of the protein or vice versa. Also, adding amino acid linkers between the protein and its tag can sometimes rescue protein function.

3 Methods

3.1 Sample Preparation

1. Cells should be grown on coverslip-bottomed dishes in phenol-red-free medium (*see* **Notes 1** and **2**). Keep away from short-wavelength light (typically 350–450 nm) as much as possible if working with photoswitchable proteins to prevent prior photoactivation.

2. Proteins tagged with photoswitchable proteins can proceed straight to imaging. HaloTag®/SNAP-tagged proteins must, however, be labelled in the cells using the following protocol:

(a) Replace medium of cells with dye for 15 min (can increase to 30 min if labelling is inefficient). Incubate cells in normal culture incubator conditions.

(b) Wash cells three times with medium to remove dye and then incubate in normal culture incubator conditions for another 30 min (*see* **Notes 3** and **4**).

(c) Finally replace medium for imaging.

The concentration of the dye depends on the type of experiment. For single-molecule tracking, low concentrations of dye should be added to prevent overlap of molecules (typically ~5 nM). For imaging of structures using blinking dyes where the intention is to label all the protein, higher concentrations are required (typically ~10 µM). The exact dye concentration depends on the cellular protein concentration and so should be determined by finding the concentration at which there is no further increase in the number of labelled molecules.

To make the relevant HaloTag® dye for a specific experiment, an example labelling reaction is given (Fig. 3) (*see* **Notes 5** and **6**).

1. Mix relevant components:

   (a) 8 µl of 10 mM HaloTag® amine ligand.

   (b) 20 µl of 4 mM *N*-hydroxysuccinimidyl ester Alexa Fluor 647 dye.

   (c) 72 µl of labelling buffer.

2. Incubate at room temperature for >4 h.

3. Run reaction onto a C18 reversed-phase HPLC column with a gradient of 0–50% acetonitrile for 30 min, then 50–100% for 10 min, and finally 100–0% for 5 min.

4. The reacted ligand peak can be purified from the unreacted or hydrolysed dye peaks and verified using mass spectrometry.

3.2 Microscope Set-Up

There are changes in the microscope set-up depending on the fluorophore of choice, so here we describe the imaging of mEos3-tagged proteins to give an idea of the steps involved.

1. Measure the laser power densities at the sample plane and make sure that they are as follows:

   (a) 561 nm laser ~1–10 kW cm^{-2}

   (b) 488 nm laser ~1 kW cm^{-2}

   (c) 405 nm laser ~10–100 W cm^{-2}

2. Prepare a fixed cell sample for setting up the imaging:

   (a) Methanol:ethanol (1:1), 6 min at −20 °C.

   (b) 4% Formaldehyde in PBS, 20 min at room temperature.

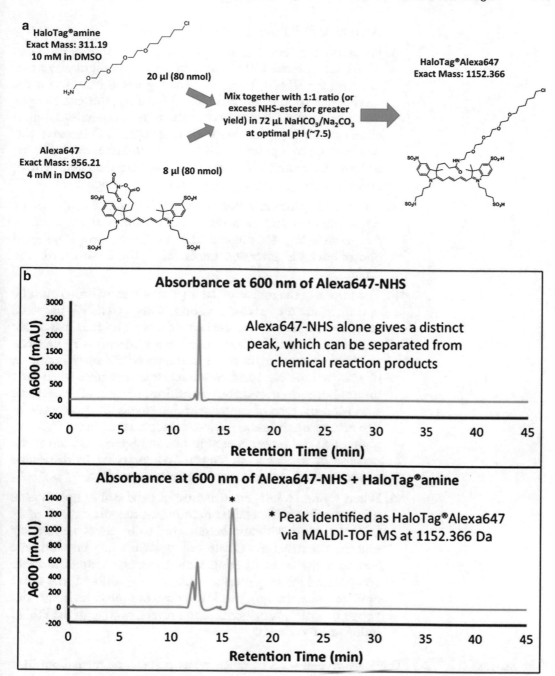

Fig. 3 A schematic representation of HaloTag®dye synthesis using reverse-phase high-performance liquid chromatography (RP-HPLC). (**a**) An example reaction using HaloTag® amine and Alexa Fluor 647. (**b**) The separation of the reaction products using an RP-HPLC gradient from 0 to 100 % acetonitrile in 0.1 % trifluoroacetic acid into distinct peaks, which allows product identification by mass spectrometry

Wash with PBS three times before imaging.

3. Focus on the centre of nucleus using the white light. Then adjust the optimal HILO angle or set up the light sheet (for example, for RLSM) to achieve the highest excitation for the specific detection plane. For mEos3 imaging, this can be optimised using the 488 nm laser as the non-photoactivated molecule emits in the green part of the spectrum. Otherwise, this can be done by a pulse of 405 nm laser and imaging using the 561 nm laser until the single molecules are detected with an optimised signal-to-background fluorescence signal.

4. The power of the activation laser (in this case 405 nm) must be optimised to ensure the activation of isolated single molecules. As shown in Fig. 4b, single molecules should show single-step photobleaching intensity traces with time with 561 nm excitation.

5. The power of the excitation laser (in this case 561 nm) must be optimised for the specific question being asked. We use fixed cells here to prevent the analysis of molecules that may move out of the detection plane. There is a trade-off here between precision (a measure of the uncertainty of the spatial position of a single molecule) and bleaching time (the time taken for a fluorophore to irreversibly transition to a non-fluorescent state) and the type of experiment determines the powers used. For measuring diffusion parameters such as the jump distance, higher 561 nm power is used to obtain higher precision at the expense of smaller track lengths. When trying to determine residence time, longer track lengths are useful.

6. When trying to image a structure, a fixed cell sample can be used to estimate the emitter density and therefore the number of molecules that should be detected to be able to effectively visualise the structure. Clusters of molecules may take less time and so allow faster imaging than molecules that form more complicated spatial patterns, e.g. fibres. In addition, the active emitter concentration, that is the ratio of molecules in the 'on' versus the 'off' state, is critical to prevent overlap of the PSF of individual molecules.

3.3 Imaging for Single-Molecule Tracking

There are several types of experiments that can be carried out here based on the questions outlined in the introduction. For ease of discussion, we will predominantly discuss the concepts behind these experiments using the mEos tag. However, the principles apply to any other fluorophore being imaged.

3.3.1 Tracking of Single Proteins

SPT is used to determine the diffusion parameters or residence times of single proteins.

Fixed cells can readily be used to determine the relevant 405 nm laser power densities for photoactivation and the 561 nm laser power densities for imaging. The 405 nm laser can be either

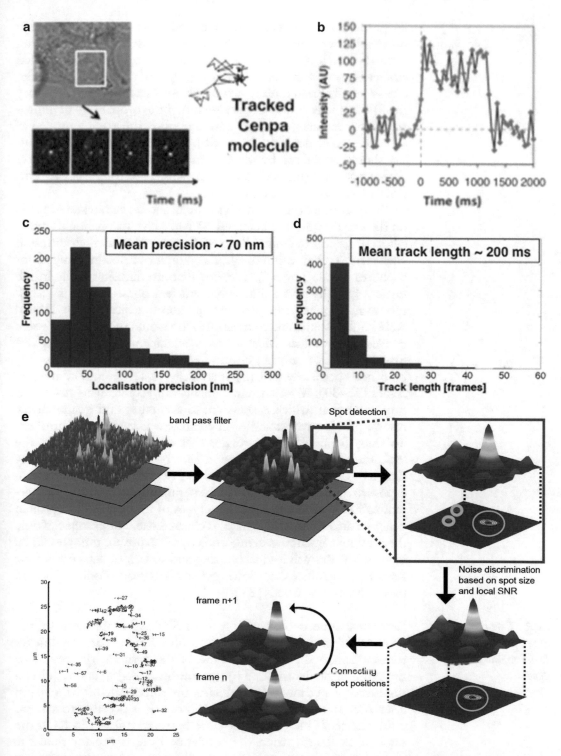

Fig. 4 Typical single-molecule data parameters demonstrated using mouse embryonic stem cells labelled with mEos3-tagged CENPA, a centromeric histone variant [35]. (**a**) Bright-field image of a cell in which single mEos3-CENPA molecules are imaged using the 561 nm laser and tracked. (**b**) The single molecules show single-step photobleaching in fixed cells. A *typical precision histogram* (**c**) and *track length histogram* (**d**) are shown. (**e**) The details of a typical spot finding and tracking program are also provided [67]

left at low power and thus mEos will undergo continuous activation or at a higher power but with desynchronised alternate pulsing such that each pulse is spaced in time to avoid the unintended stochastic activation of two overlapping PSFs from single molecules spatially located near each other. Another approach is to vary the 405 nm laser power density such that the probability of photoactivation remains constant and therefore the total number of activated molecules is the same [56]. The 561 nm laser power density should be chosen by whether the specific experiment requires higher precision (higher laser power density) or long track lengths (lower laser power density).

The exposure time at which a protein should be tracked depends on the specific question being asked. Most chromatin-bound molecules appear mostly immobile in SPT experiments as their diffusion coefficient is often within the precision limit of detecting single fluorophores (<0.05 μm^2 s^{-1}). Proteins that are diffusing freely in the nucleus typically have a diffusion coefficient of 10–20 μm^2 s^{-1} [29]. However, proteins can also interact non-specifically with DNA/RNA/nucleosomes and so their diffusion would then be somewhere between these values. Most proteins exhibit multiple modes of diffusion—they not only (1) diffuse freely in the nucleus but also (2) bind non-specifically and (3) specifically to DNA and/or nucleosomes [26–30]. Most current cameras can acquire data at <33 ms time resolution, which is adequate to accurately and quantitatively resolve proteins whose diffusion coefficient is less than ~5 μm^2 s^{-1}. To study freely diffusing proteins that diffuse faster than this, the exposure time must go lower to ~10 ms by reducing the area being imaged to less than 100×100 pixels [29]. When choosing which exposure time to use in a specific experiment, it is therefore important to first decide which of these types of diffusion of the protein being studied is most important to characterise. For example, if only the immobile fraction is being studied, the exposure time should be increased as this will lead to blurring and so lack of detection of the faster moving molecules, allowing characterisation of only the bound molecules in the nucleus [31].

3.3.2 Time-Lapse Experiments for Determining Residence Time

Residence time determination from SPT is complicated by the problem of photobleaching. If photobleaching occurs at a quicker timescale than the residence time of the protein, the residence time cannot be determined by continuous imaging and requires a time-lapse experiment. By reducing the duty cycle of the 561 nm laser after an activation pulse of 405 nm, it is possible to achieve a time lapse. If increasing the time between pulses results in the same track length, then the residence time is greater than the pulse length. If the track length decreases, then the residence time can be determined. Therefore the experiment involves several imaging experiments in which the time between pulses is increased (Fig. 5d).

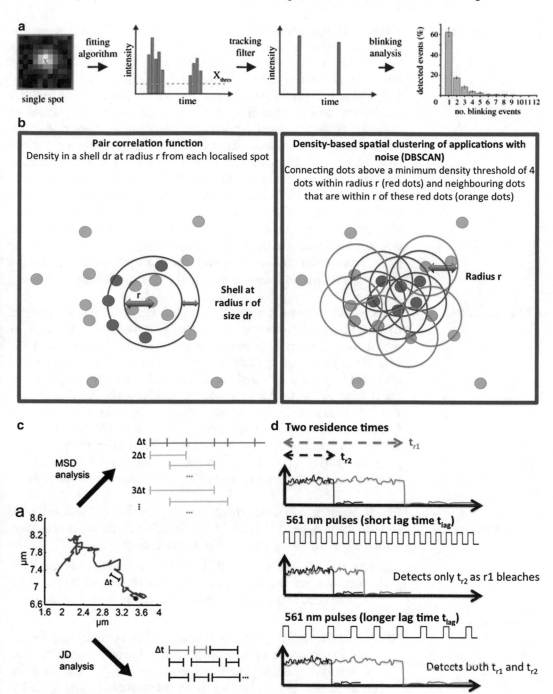

Fig. 5 Analytical tools for single-particle tracking experiments. (**a**) Counting experiments use a tracking filter to count single-molecule spots localised within a given precision over subsequent frames. Blinking analysis is then carried out to help correct for this when calculating the actual number of molecules [72]. (**b**) The two common clustering algorithms are called the pair correlation function (PCF) and the density-based clustering of applications with noise (DBSCAN) is schematically described. (**c**) Diffusion coefficient parameters—jump distance (JD) refers to the distances moved at Δt whereas the mean squared displacement (MSD) calculates for each molecule the distances moved in Δt, $2\Delta t$, $3\Delta t$ and so on [68]. (**d**) Residence time—By varying the lag time between exposure pulses, longer residence times can be detected as shown [28]

3.3.3 Structural Imaging   Live-cell imaging of a structure depends on its size and complexity. By imaging the structure in fixed cells, the number of localisations required to accurately reconstruct a super-resolved image of the structure of interest can be determined. In super-resolution imaging, temporal resolution is often traded off for increased spatial resolution, so for dynamic biological structures it is important to consider these temporal constraints. To visualise how the structures change over time, a sliding window analysis can be applied [32, 64, 65]. So for example, if it takes 10 s to resolve the structure but the single molecules are imaged at 33 ms time resolution, the structure generated from every 10 s of localisation data can then be used to generate frames of a movie at 33 ms time resolution. However it is often the case that the structure moves slower than this in which case to prevent bleaching of the fluorophores, a time-lapse experiment can be designed, for example, such that a 10-s pulse of continuous imaging is carried out every 5 min.

3.4 Data Analysis

For this section, we focus on 2D data but the analysis is the same in 3D. Data analysis software like ImageJ/Fiji is usually required, as well as the need for fluorescent puncta localisation programs [66–68]. Such programs typically apply a band-pass filter (since noise occurs at high frequency and background at low frequency) to accurately identify the initial fluorescence localisations, followed by fitting of the raw data above a user-defined threshold that (1) have a high signal-to-noise ratio (typically 5–15 for mEos3) and (2) have a PSF width predicted by theory (to avoid fitting of noise or overlapping molecules) (Fig. 4e). Blurring that occurs when molecules move quickly during an exposure can also be accounted for [29].

3.4.1 Quantifying Numbers of Molecules   Much progress has been made recently in the quantification of SMLM approaches [69]. Here we describe three main considerations when analysing this kind of experiment:

1. Are all the proteins tagged? If a knock-in cell line has not been generated and the untagged endogenous protein is still present, the ratio of tagged to untagged protein must be accounted for.

2. Are all the tagged proteins fluorescent? Even if all the proteins are tagged (e.g. in a knock-in cell line), dye labelling in the case of HaloTag®/SNAP tag is often protein dependent and for endogenous fluorophores, their maturation is rarely 100% (e.g. GFP is ~80% and mEos2 is ~50%) [70, 71]. The percentage of expressed fluorophores that are fluorescent can be calculated by comparing the concentration predicted by fluorescence against the actual protein concentration calculated from the absorbance at 280 nm (either using the purified tagged protein or by quantitative Western blot from a known number of cells).

3. Does the molecule undergo fluorescence intermittency or 'blinking'? Many photoactivatable fluorophores go to a recov-

erable/reversible dark state rather than via the photobleaching pathway, which can result in systematic overcounting. For example, mEos2 molecules blink an average of two times before bleaching [72]. Recent work has shown that these blinking events can be separated temporally and spatially [73], that is, they occur within a specific time frame after the first localisation. By applying a filter to take into account the precision of the detected molecule (count as one molecule if tracked in successive frames) and by calculating the number of expected blinking events for a specific fluorophore, it is possible to determine the number of molecules [72].

To summarise:

$$\text{Protein count} = \frac{\text{Number of molecules counted}}{(\text{Blinks} / \text{fluorophore}) \times (\text{Fraction of fluorophores fluorescent})}$$

3.4.2 Extracting Clustering Parameters

Clustering algorithms are used to study whether molecules form functional clusters either in time or space within the mammalian nucleus. There are two major types of clustering algorithm commonly used (Fig. 5b). The first approach gives one average number and one cluster size, whereas the second assigns individual localisations to clusters that can have varying shape and size.

The first approach is based on the spatial point statistics tools such as Ripley's function or others such as the pair correlation function (PCF) and analyses the numbers of molecules within a given radius [33, 74]. The PCF approach has given rise to two analytical SMLM tools called pair-correlative pcPALM and time-correlative tcPALM. pcPALM determines if molecules are likely to be clustered in space and tcPALM determines if they are clustered in time. To be clustered in space could imply a functional structure and to be clustered in time suggests a transient structure. Both of these approaches have been developed because even randomly distributed photoswitchable proteins and dyes will always show clustering in the spatial and temporal domains because they both undergo fluorescence intermittency, or 'blinking', giving rise to multiple localisations per molecule. A brief description of the steps involved in this kind of analysis is as follows:

1. Filtering is first applied as in Subheading 3.4.1 to deal with localisations from the same molecule.

2. The PCF takes a circle of radius r from a localised spot and adds a shell of thickness dr. The PCF of the protein peaks, $g(r)$, is used to determine whether the density of molecules present in this shell are greater than the expected protein density ρ^{protein}:

$$g(r)^{\text{peaks}} = \frac{\text{Density of molecules in } dr}{\text{Expected density}} = \frac{\left(\text{Spots counted in } dr \middle/ 2\pi r dr \right)}{\rho^{\text{protein}}}.$$

In this equation, $g(r)$ equals 1 if there is no cluster. However, in SMLM images, a localised molecule will usually appear as a cluster since each molecule has usually photoswitched/blinked several times. Therefore, the function $g(r)$ must also take into account the precision of the detected molecule, σ_s, as shown below:

$$g(r)^{\text{peaks}} = 1 + \frac{1}{4\pi\sigma_s^2\rho^{\text{protein}}}\exp\left(\frac{-r^2}{4\sigma_s^2}\right)$$

3. If it fits this curve within ±25 % of the measured values for σ_s and ρ^{protein}, then the protein is randomly distributed. Otherwise, the proteins are likely clustered and must be fit to this new equation to find the values A and ξ:

$$g(r)^{\text{peaks}} = \frac{1}{4\pi\sigma_s^2\rho^{\text{protein}}}\exp\left(\frac{-r^2}{4\sigma_s^2}\right) + \left(\left(1 + A\exp\left(\frac{-r}{\xi}\right)\right)\times\left(\frac{1}{4\pi\sigma_s^2}\exp\left(\frac{-r^2}{4\sigma_s^2}\right)\right)\right)$$

4. This allows us to determine the mean size of the cluster (ξ) and also the number of molecules per cluster (N) using this equation:

$$N \approx 2A\pi\xi^2\rho^{\text{protein}}$$

The final step is to take this number and adjust to the actual number of molecules as described in Subheading 3.4.1.

The second approach works very differently and is called density-based spatial clustering of applications with noise or DBSCAN [75]. It first identifies localisations that are above a density threshold and then connects them and neighbouring edge-of-cluster localisations to identify clusters of any shape or size. These regions can then be analysed to find their size and the average number of molecules within these regions. The DBSCAN approach is advantageous in that it does not assume clusters of a specific shape. However, given the noise of traditional PALM images, DBSCAN assignments can sometimes be inaccurate, leading to the development of simulation-aided DBSCAN (SAD) in which a simulated number of clusters of varying size are used to train the assignment [76, 77]. A brief description of the steps involved is as follows:

1. DBSCAN starts by defining whether points are above or below a specific density threshold. The minimum density is defined as

$$\text{Minimum cluster density} = \frac{\text{MinPts}}{\pi r^2}$$

where MinPts is the minimum number of neighbours (usually 4) and r is the radius. If r is too small, real clusters will be missed. If it is too big, then noise will be seen as a cluster. r is usually defined by using a control unclustered sample or a simulated sample.

2. A cluster is then defined by connecting points above this threshold into clusters if the points are mutually less than r from each other.

3. Any points below this threshold but within r of these clustered points are also included in the defined cluster.

4. The density-connected clusters are then analysed for number and size, for example by fitting them to Gaussian distributions.

Building on the principles of the PCF and DBSCAN approaches, more sophisticated clustering algorithms have been developed that are now more commonly used (REF). It is also worth noting that clustering analysis can be affected by whether or not the entire structure is in the plane, so it may be important to only count molecules within the plane by analysing the shape and intensity of the localised spot [35] or by using 3D detection methods described previously.

3.4.3 Extracting Diffusion Parameters

There are two parameters traditionally used to study the diffusion of a protein in the nucleus (Fig. 5c): the mean-squared displacement (MSD) and the jump distance (JD) [78].

MSD analysis obtains diffusion coefficients for individual tracked molecules by monitoring the mean squared displacement from their original location over different time lapses. It cannot be used easily for molecules that spend part of their trajectory bound to chromatin and part unbound as MSD analysis obscures transitions between diffusion modes. In addition, if the trajectory length is small (<32 steps), it can be difficult using MSD analysis to determine the diffusion coefficients of molecules that move short distances (relative to the precision of the tracked molecule) [79] such as proteins bound to chromatin.

The equation of classical MSD for motion in *two dimensions* is as follows:

$$\text{MSD} = \frac{\sum \left(x^2 + y^2\right)}{n} = 4Dt^\alpha$$

where D refers to the effective diffusion coefficient, α refers to the anomalous diffusion exponent and $t =$ (camera exposure time) × (number of frames between the exposures). Theoretically $\alpha = 1$ indicates random Brownian motion, $0 < \alpha < 1$ indicates subdiffusion (or constrained diffusion), while $\alpha > 1$ is observed for processes involving superdiffusion (or active motion).

However, the actual measured MSD is affected by the precision at which the molecule is detected ('static error') as well as the movement of the molecule ('dynamic error'). Static error is usually dealt with using the following equation:

$$\mathrm{MSD}_{measured} = 4Dt^{\alpha} + 4\sigma^2$$

In most cases, this equation is sufficient but for superdiffusive molecules (less common for chromatin-binding proteins), it may be necessary to account for dynamic error too [80, 81].

MSD analysis is not appropriate if molecules cannot be tracked for >100 frames (most fluorophores do not last this long) or if they exhibit changes in diffusion mode during a trajectory. Changes in diffusion mode can arise from a molecule interacting dynamically with chromatin or because the DNA itself to which it is bound has more than one type of motion [32, 82]. Previous studies have demonstrated that chromatin exhibits motion ranging from 1 to 10 nm/s interrupted by ATP-dependent jumps of about 150 nm lasting for 0.3–2 s. Longer time scales show that this motion is also confined to a region (chromosome territory) with radii of constraint ranging from 0.5 to 1 μm.

For single-fluorophore tracking where the fluorophore has changing diffusion parameters and rarely lasts long enough for MSD analysis (<100 frames), JD analysis may be more reliable [68]. For JD analysis, jump distances within intervals $[r, r+dr]$ travelled by single particles in Δt were counted to calculate the probability that a particle starting at $r_1 = 0$ will be encountered within a shell of radius r and width dr at time Δt. The integrated probability distribution is fitted to experimental data:

$$P\left(r^2, \Delta t\right) = \int_{r^2}^{0} p\left(r^2\right) dr^2 = 1 - e^{-\frac{r^2}{4D\Delta t}}$$

If m species are present, an integrated distribution for a sum of m terms is used:

$$P\left(r^2, \Delta t\right) = \sum_{m}^{j=1} \frac{f_j}{4D_j \Delta t} e^{-\frac{r^2}{4D_j \Delta t}} dr^2$$

with f_j denoting respective fraction of particles in mobility mode j and D_j the respective diffusion coefficient.

The residual is inspected to evaluate the goodness of the fit. The simplest model whose fit result shows no systematic deviation is usually chosen to prevent over-fitting. It is important when using jump distance data to take into account the jump distance that corresponds to the precision of the imaging data as this is the lower limit that can be measured. This can often be attained from fixed cell imaging (see Note 7). In addition, when 2D imaging is carried out, it is important to account for the fact that molecules that diffuse quickly (>5 μm^2 s^{-1}) are less likely to have as many jumps recorded as jumps are more likely to occur out of the detection plane [29].

More recent approaches have used Bayesian modelling to determine not only how many types of diffusion occur for molecules but also how often the molecules transition from one state to another by assigning a jump distance to each diffusion mode [83].

3.4.4 Residence Time [28]

If the residence time (t_r) is smaller than the bleaching time, the residence time can be determined by the number of frames a molecule is observed in its 'on' state before it turns 'off' (k_{off}). However, as the residence time increases relative to the bleaching time, this measured k_{off} parameter ($k_{measured}$) is affected more and more by the bleaching rate (k_b) (Fig. 5d) as described by this equation:

$$k_{measured} = k_{off} + k_b.$$

However, if we now pulse the excitation at different lag times T_{lag}, since the bleaching rate is related to the number of exposures rather than the total time T_{total}, the equation can be written as follows:

$$k_{measured} = k_{off} + k_b \times T_{total} / T_{lag}.$$

If we presume two off rates ($k_{off,1}$ and $k_{off,2}$), the data can then be fit to the following equation, where B is the fraction of molecules with $k_{off,1}$:

$$f(t) = A \left(Be^{-\left(k_b \frac{T_{total}}{T_{lag}} + k_{off,1}\right)} + (1-B)e^{-\left(k_b \frac{T_{total}}{T_{lag}} + k_{off,2}\right)} \right)$$

For dyes that bleach slowly, it is possible that the residence time is considerably shorter than the bleaching time and so this kind of analysis is often ignored. However, it may still be useful if only to prove that there are no longer residence times unaccounted for.

3.4.5 Analysing Images with High Density of Localisations

The data analysis for images of structures depends on the density of the fluorophores being imaged. Clearly by imaging more molecules in a given time frame, the time resolution of imaging a structure can be improved but fitting overlapping molecules can reduce the overall resolution. In order to deal with this problem, approaches have been developed to deal with multi-emitter fitting [84, 85]. Other approaches include iterative deconvolution [86], presuming that the emitters in the high-density image are far enough apart in any given image to deconvolute them, and another called compressed sensing, a sparse-signal recovery technique that deals with the problem of always getting enough photoactivations to reconstruct a structure [87]. The final approach

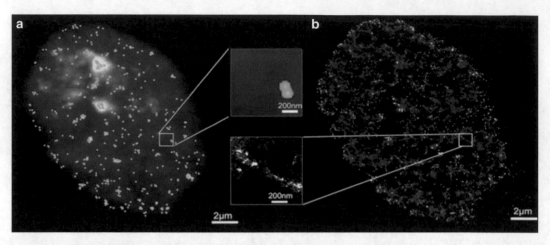

Fig. 6 Comparison of traditional single-emitter localisation algorithms with Bayesian-based method (3B) [34]. Using prism-coupled light sheet illumination, mEos3-tagged HP1α were imaged in human embryonic stem cells (**a**). Heterochromatin fibres can only be seen after the Bayesian analysis (**b**) whereas traditional algorithms have lower resolution and so only show localised clusters (*green spots* highlighted in (**a**))

called 3B analysis produces a map of the statistical likelihood of an emitter being in a given position through Bayesian-based fitting of an emitter that blinks and bleaches (Fig. 6) [88]. This approach allows much more emitter overlap but is limited by its data processing time.

4   Notes

1. Adding 2 M glycine to clean slides before adding the cells is useful when adding dyes for Halo-/SNAP-tagged proteins that would otherwise stick to the coverslip.

2. One should grow cell in phenol-red-free media for a few days as we have noticed that changes in media prior to an experiment can result in higher background and also some initial stress of the cells.

3. This protocol can be very dye dependent. Some dyes take longer to get out. Some dyes also clump, so must vortex before adding.

4. When the dye of interest is not cell permeable, electroporation of the cells is attempted followed by replating of the cells to allow for recovery (1–4 h depending on cell line).

5. Dye can be attached to either the O2 or O4 ligand. We sometimes find that the O4 ligand is better for labelling certain proteins due to its slightly longer linker.

6. Sometimes there is a need to alter pH subtly in range 7.0–9.0 to optimise reaction for a specific dye as dye could affect pH.

7. It is worth bearing in mind that even fixed cells show some movement of proteins bound to chromatin presumably as the chromatin still moves a little even in fixed conditions. To fix the chromatin further, you may want to add 0.1 % glutaraldehyde to the formaldehyde fixation mix followed by a 7-min wash with 0.1 % sodium borohydride.

Acknowledgements

We would like to thank the Royal Society for the University Research Fellowship of Steven F. Lee (UF120277) and the Medical Research Council for the Research Fellowship of Srinjan Basu (MR/M010082/1). We would like to thank Brian Hendrich and David Klenerman for generous use of the cell culture facilities used to grow the mouse embryonic stem cells imaged here. The figures shown were made by Srinjan Basu with the help of Yi Lei Tan, Thomas A. Drury, Edward J.R. Taylor and Steven F. Lee. I would like to thank Ulrike Endesfelder, Kai Wohlfahrt, Melike Lakadamyali and David Lando for discussion and for critical reading of the manuscript.

References

1. Misteli T (2001) Protein dynamics: implications for nuclear architecture and gene expression. Science 291:843–847
2. Lakadamyali M, Cosma MP (2015) Advanced microscopy methods for visualizing chromatin structure. FEBS Lett 589(20 Pt A):3023–3030
3. Cattoni DI, Valeri A, Le Gall A, Nollmann M (2015) A matter of scale: how emerging technologies are redefining our view of chromosome architecture. Trends Genet 31(8):454–464
4. Horrocks MH, Palayret M, Klenerman D, Lee SF (2014) The changing point-spread function: single-molecule-based super-resolution imaging. Histochem Cell Biol 141:577–585
5. Cremer T, Kurz A, Zirbel R, Dietzel S, Rinke B, Schröck E, Speicher MR, Mathieu U, Jauch A, Emmerich P, Scherthan H, Ried T, Cremer C, Lichter P (1993) Role of chromosome territories in the functional compartmentalization of the cell nucleus. Cold Spring Harb Symp Quant Biol 58:777–792
6. Branco MR, Pombo A (2006) Intermingling of chromosome territories in interphase suggests role in translocations and transcription-dependent associations. PLoS Biol 4, e138
7. Dekker J, Rippe K, Dekker M, Kleckner N (2002) Capturing chromosome conformation. Science 295:1306–1311
8. Lieberman-Aiden E, van Berkum NL, Williams L, Imakaev M, Ragoczy T, Telling A, Amit I, Lajoie BR, Sabo PJ, Dorschner MO, Sandstrom R, Bernstein B, Bender MA, Groudine M, Gnirke A, Stamatoyannopoulos J, Mirny LA, Lander ES, Dekker J (2009) Comprehensive mapping of long-range interactions reveals folding principles of the human genome. Science 326:289–293
9. Rao SS, Huntley MH, Durand NC, Stamenova EK, Bochkov ID, Robinson JT, Sanborn AL, Machol I, Omer AD, Lander ES, Aiden EL (2014) A 3D map of the human genome at kilobase resolution reveals principles of chromatin looping. Cell 159:1665–1680
10. Bickmore WA, van Steensel B (2013) Genome architecture: domain organization of interphase chromosomes. Cell 152:1270–1284
11. Gibcus JH, Dekker J (2013) The hierarchy of the 3D genome. Mol Cell 49:773–782

12. Dixon JR, Selvaraj S, Yue F, Kim A, Li Y, Shen Y, Hu M, Liu JS, Ren B (2012) Topological domains in mammalian genomes identified by analysis of chromatin interactions. Nature 485:376–380

13. Hou C, Li L, Qin ZS, Corces VG (2012) Gene density, transcription, and insulators contribute to the partition of the Drosophila genome into physical domains. Mol Cell 48:471–484

14. Nora EP, Lajoie BR, Schulz EG, Giorgetti L, Okamoto I, Servant N, Piolot T, van Berkum NL, Meisig J, Sedat J, Gribnau J, Barillot E, Blüthgen N, Dekker J, Heard E (2012) Spatial partitioning of the regulatory landscape of the X-inactivation centre. Nature 485:381–385

15. Sexton T, Yaffe E, Kenigsberg E, Bantignies F, Leblanc B, Hoichman M, Parrinello H, Tanay A, Cavalli G (2012) Three-dimensional folding and functional organization principles of the Drosophila genome. Cell 148:458–472

16. Liang Z, Zickler D, Prentiss M, Chang FS, Witz G, Maeshima K, Kleckner N (2015) Chromosomes progress to metaphase in multiple discrete steps via global compaction/expansion cycles. Cell 161:1124–1137

17. Klar TA, Jakobs S, Dyba M, Egner A, Hell SW (2000) Fluorescence microscopy with diffraction resolution barrier broken by stimulated emission. Proc Natl Acad Sci U S A 97:8206–8210

18. Hofmann M, Eggeling C, Jakobs S, Hell SW (2005) Breaking the diffraction barrier in fluorescence microscopy at low light intensities by using reversibly photoswitchable proteins. Proc Natl Acad Sci U S A 102:17565–17569

19. Gustafsson MG (2000) Surpassing the lateral resolution limit by a factor of two using structured illumination microscopy. J Microsc 198:82–87

20. Schermelleh L, Carlton PM, Haase S, Shao L, Winoto L, Kner P, Burke B, Cardoso MC, Agard DA, Gustafsson MG, Leonhardt H, Sedat JW (2008) Subdiffraction multicolor imaging of the nuclear periphery with 3D structured illumination microscopy. Science 320:1332–1336

21. Markaki Y, Gunkel M, Schermelleh L, Beichmanis S, Neumann J, Heidemann M, Leonhardt H, Eick D, Cremer C, Cremer T (2010) Functional nuclear organization of transcription and DNA replication: a topographical marriage between chromatin domains and the interchromatin compartment. Cold Spring Harb Symp Quant Biol 75:475–492

22. Rust MJ, Bates M, Zhuang X (2006) Subdiffraction-limit imaging by stochastic optical reconstruction microscopy (STORM). Nat Methods 3:793–795

23. Betzig E, Patterson GH, Sougrat R, Lindwasser OW, Olenych S, Bonifacino JS, Davidson MW, Lippincott-Schwartz J, Hess HF (2006) Imaging intracellular fluorescent proteins at nanometer resolution. Science 313: 1642–1645

24. Schoen I, Ries J, Klotzsch E, Ewers H, Vogel V (2011) Binding-activated localization microscopy of DNA structures. Nano Lett 11:4008–4011

25. Abbe E (1873) Beiträge zur theorie des mikroskops und der mikroskopischen wahrnehmung. Arch Microsc Anat 9:413–468

26. Speil J, Baumgart E, Siebrasse JP, Veith R, Vinkemeier U, Kubitscheck U (2011) Activated STAT1 transcription factors conduct distinct saltatory movements in the cell nucleus. Biophys J 101:2592–2600

27. Mazza D, Abernathy A, Golob N, Morisaki T, McNally JG (2012) A benchmark for chromatin binding measurements in live cells. Nucleic Acids Res 40, e119

28. Gebhardt JC, Suter DM, Roy R, Zhao ZW, Chapman AR, Basu S, Maniatis T, Xie XS (2013) Single-molecule imaging of transcription factor binding to DNA in live mammalian cells. Nat Methods 10:421–426

29. Izeddin I, Récamier V, Bosanac L, Cissé II, Boudarene L, Dugast-Darzacq C, Proux F, Bénichou O, Voituriez R, Bensaude O, Dahan M, Darzacq X (2014) Single-molecule tracking in live cells reveals distinct target-search strategies of transcription factors in the nucleus. eLife 3:PMID: 24925319

30. Chen J, Zhang Z, Li L, Chen BC, Revyakin A, Hajj B, Legant W, Dahan M, Lionnet T, Betzig E, Tjian R, Liu Z (2014) Single-molecule dynamics of enhanceosome assembly in embryonic stem cells. Cell 156:1274–1285

31. Etheridge TJ, Boulineau RL, Herbert A, Watson AT, Daigaku Y, Tucker J, George S, Jönsson P, Palayret M, Lando D, Laue E, Osborne MA, Klenerman D, Lee SF, Carr AM (2014) Quantification of DNA-associated proteins inside eukaryotic cells using single-molecule localization microscopy. Nucleic Acids Res 42, e146

32. Wombacher R, Heidbreder M, van de Linde S, Sheetz MP, Heilemann M, Cornish VW, Sauer M (2010) Live-cell super-resolution imaging with trimethoprim conjugates. Nat Methods 7:717–719

33. Cisse II, Izeddin I, Causse SZ, Boudarene L, Senecal A, Muresan L, Dugast-Darzacq C, Hajj B, Dahan M, Darzacq X (2013) Real-time dynamics of RNA polymerase II clustering in live human cells. Science 341:664–667

34. Hu Y, Zhu Q, Elkins K, Tse K, Li Y, Fitzpatrick J, Verma I, Cang H (2013) Light-sheet

Bayesian microscopy enables deep-cell super-resolution imaging of heterochromatin in live human embryonic stem cells. Opt Nanosc 2:7

35. Palayret M, Armes H, Basu S, Watson AT, Herbert A, Lando D, Etheridge TJ, Endesfelder U, Heilemann M, Laue E, Carr AM, Klenerman D, Lee SF (2015) Virtual-'light-sheet' single-molecule localization microscopy enables quantitative optical sectioning for super-resolution imaging. PLoS One 10, e0125438

36. Tokunaga M, Imamoto N, Sakata-Sogawa K (2008) Highly inclined thin illumination enables clear single-molecule imaging in cells. Nat Methods 5:159–161

37. Galland R, Grenci G, Aravind A, Viasnoff V, Studer V, Sibarita JB (2015) 3D high- and super-resolution imaging using single-objective SPIM. Nat Methods 12:641–644

38. Planchon TA, Gao L, Milkie DE, Davidson MW, Galbraith JA, Galbraith CG, Betzig E (2011) Rapid three-dimensional isotropic imaging of living cells using Bessel beam plane illumination. Nat Methods 8:417–423

39. Michalet X, Colyer RA, Scalia G, Ingargiola A, Lin R, Millaud JE, Weiss S, Siegmund OH, Tremsin AS, Vallerga JV, Cheng A, Levi M, Aharoni D, Arisaka K, Villa F, Guerrieri F, Panzeri F, Rech I, Gulinatti A, Zappa F, Ghioni M, Cova S (2013) Development of new photon-counting detectors for single-molecule fluorescence microscopy. Philos Trans R Soc Lond B Biol Sci 368:20120035

40. Huang B, Wang W, Bates M, Zhuang X (2008) Three-dimensional super-resolution imaging by stochastic optical reconstruction microscopy. Science 319:810–813

41. Pavani SR, Thompson MA, Biteen JS, Lord SJ, Liu N, Twieg RJ, Piestun R, Moerner WE (2009) Three-dimensional, single-molecule fluorescence imaging beyond the diffraction limit by using a double-helix point spread function. Proc Natl Acad Sci U S A 106:2995–2999

42. Juette MF, Gould TJ, Lessard MD, Mlodzianoski MJ, Nagpure BS, Bennett BT, Hess ST, Bewersdorf J (2008) Three-dimensional sub-100 nm resolution fluorescence microscopy of thick samples. Nat Methods 5:527–529

43. Abrahamsson S, Chen J, Hajj B, Stallinga S, Katsov AY, Wisniewski J, Mizuguchi G, Soule P, Mueller F, Dugast Darzacq C, Darzacq X, Wu C, Bargmann CI, Agard DA, Dahan M, Gustafsson MG (2013) Fast multicolor 3D imaging using aberration-corrected multifocus microscopy. Nat Methods 10:60–63

44. Shtengel G, Galbraith JA, Galbraith CG, Lippincott-Schwartz J, Gillette JM, Manley S, Sougrat R, Waterman CM, Kanchanawong P, Davidson MW, Fetter RD, Hess HF (2009) Interferometric fluorescent super-resolution microscopy resolves 3D cellular ultrastructure. Proc Natl Acad Sci U S A 106:3125–3130

45. Shtengel G, Wang Y, Zhang Z, Goh WI, Hess HF, Kanchanawong P (2014) Imaging cellular ultrastructure by PALM, iPALM, and correlative iPALM-EM. Methods Cell Biol 123:273–294

46. Deschamps J, Mund M, Ries J (2014) 3D superresolution microscopy by supercritical angle detection. Opt Express 22: 29081–29091

47. Wang S, Moffitt JR, Dempsey GT, Xie XS, Zhuang X (2014) Characterization and development of photoactivatable fluorescent proteins for single-molecule-based superresolution imaging. Proc Natl Acad Sci U S A 111:8452–8457

48. Dempsey GT, Vaughan JC, Chen KH, Bates M, Zhuang X (2011) Evaluation of fluorophores for optimal performance in localization-based super-resolution imaging. Nat Methods 8:1027–1036

49. Shaner NC, Steinbach PA, Tsien RY (2005) A guide to choosing fluorescent proteins. Nat Methods 2:905–909

50. Nguyen AW, Daugherty PS (2005) Evolutionary optimization of fluorescent proteins for intracellular FRET. Nat Biotechnol 23:355–360

51. Merzlyak EM, Goedhart J, Shcherbo D, Bulina ME, Shcheglov AS, Fradkov AF, Gaintzeva A, Lukyanov KA, Lukyanov S, Gadella TW, Chudakov DM (2007) Bright monomeric red fluorescent protein with an extended fluorescence lifetime. Nat Methods 4:555–557

52. Zhou XX, Lin MZ (2013) Photoswitchable fluorescent proteins: ten years of colorful chemistry and exciting applications. Curr Opin Chem Biol 17:682–690

53. Patterson GH, Lippincott-Schwartz J (2002) A photoactivatable GFP for selective photolabeling of proteins and cells. Science 297:1873–1877

54. Subach FV, Patterson GH, Manley S, Gillette JM, Lippincott-Schwartz J, Verkhusha VV (2009) Photoactivatable mCherry for high-resolution two-color fluorescence microscopy. Nat Methods 6:153–159

55. McKinney SA, Murphy CS, Hazelwood KL, Davidson MW, Looger LL (2009) A bright

and photostable photoconvertible fluorescent protein. Nat Methods 6:131–133

56. Zhang M, Chang H, Zhang Y, Yu J, Wu L, Ji W, Chen J, Liu B, Lu J, Liu Y, Zhang J, Xu P, Xu T (2012) Rational design of true monomeric and bright photoactivatable fluorescent proteins. Nat Methods 9:727–729

57. Gurskaya NG, Verkhusha VV, Shcheglov AS, Staroverov DB, Chepurnykh TV, Fradkov AF, Lukyanov S, Lukyanov KA (2006) Engineering of a monomeric green-to-red photoactivatable fluorescent protein induced by blue light. Nat Biotechnol 24:461–465

58. Wilmes S, Staufenbiel M, Lisse D, Richter CP, Beutel O, Busch KB, Hess ST, Piehler J (2012) Triple-color super-resolution imaging of live cells: resolving submicroscopic receptor organization in the plasma membrane. Angew Chem Int Ed Engl 51:4868–4871

59. Grimm JB, English BP, Chen J, Slaughter JP, Zhang Z, Revyakin A, Patel R, Macklin JJ, Normanno D, Singer RH, Lionnet T, Lavis LD (2015) A general method to improve fluorophores for live-cell and single-molecule microscopy. Nat Methods 12:244-50

60. Nikić I, Plass T, Schraidt O, Szymański J, Briggs JA, Schultz C, Lemke EA (2014) Minimal tags for rapid dual-color live-cell labeling and super-resolution microscopy. Angew Chem Int Ed Engl 53:2245–2249

61. Di Matteo M, Mátrai J, Belay E, Firdissa T, Vandendriessche T, Chuah MK (2012) PiggyBac toolbox. Methods Mol Biol 859:241–254

62. Sander JD, Joung JK (2014) CRISPR-Cas systems for editing, regulating and targeting genomes. Nat Biotechnol 32:347-55

63. Mao G, Marotta F, Yu J, Zhou L, Yu Y, Wang L, Chui D (2008) DNA context and promoter activity affect gene expression in lentiviral vectors. Acta Biomed 79:192–196

64. Huang F, Hartwich TM, Rivera-Molina FE, Lin Y, Duim WC, Long JJ, Uchil PD, Myers JR, Baird MA, Mothes W, Davidson MW, Toomre D, Bewersdorf J (2013) Video-rate nanoscopy using sCMOS camera-specific single-molecule localization algorithms. Nat Methods 10:653–658

65. Endesfelder U, Van De Linde S, Wolter S, Sauer M, Heilemann M (2010) Subdiffraction-resolution fluorescence microscopy of myosin-actin motility. Chemphyschem 11:836–840

66. Wolter S, Löschberger A, Holm T, Aufmkolk S, Dabauvalle MC, van de Linde S, Sauer M (2012) rapidSTORM: accurate, fast open-source software for localization microscopy. Nat Methods 9:1040–1041

67. Sage D, Kirshner H, Pengo T, Stuurman N, Min J, Manley S, Unser M (2015) Quantitative evaluation of software packages for single-molecule localization microscopy. Nat Methods 12(8):717–724

68. Weimann L, Ganzinger KA, McColl J, Irvine KL, Davis SJ, Gay NJ, Bryant CE, Klenerman D (2013) A quantitative comparison of single-dye tracking analysis tools using Monte Carlo simulations. PLoS One 8, e64287

69. Deschout H, Shivanandan A, Annibale P, Scarselli M, Radenovic A (2014) Progress in quantitative single-molecule localization microscopy. Histochem Cell Biol 142:5–17

70. Annibale P, Scarselli M, Kodiyan A, Radenovic A (2010) Photoactivatable fluorescent protein mEos2 displays repeated photoactivation after a long-lived dark state in the red photoconverted form. J Phys Chem Lett 1:1506–1510

71. Ulbrich MH, Isacoff EY (2007) Subunit counting in membrane-bound proteins. Nat Methods 4:319–321

72. Lando D, Endesfelder U, Berger H, Subramanian L, Dunne PD, McColl J, Klenerman D, Carr AM, Sauer M, Allshire RC, Heilemann M, Laue ED (2012) Quantitative single-molecule microscopy reveals that CENP-A(Cnp1) deposition occurs during G2 in fission yeast. Open Biol 2:120078

73. Annibale P, Vanni S, Scarselli M, Rothlisberger U, Radenovic A (2011) Identification of clustering artifacts in photoactivated localization microscopy. Nat Methods 8:527–528

74. Sengupta P, Jovanovic-Talisman T, Lippincott-Schwartz J (2013) Quantifying spatial organization in point-localization superresolution images using pair correlation analysis. Nat Protoc 8:345–354

75. Ester M, Kriegel H-P, Sander J, Xu X (1996) A density-based algorithm for discovering clusters in large spatial databases with noise. Proceedings of the second international conference on knowledge discovery and data mining (KDD-96). AAAI-Press, Palo Alto, CA, pp 226–231

76. Nan X, Collisson EA, Lewis S, Huang J, Tamgüney TM, Liphardt JT, McCormick F, Gray JW, Chu S (2013) Single-molecule superresolution imaging allows quantitative analysis of RAF multimer formation and signaling. Proc Natl Acad Sci U S A 110: 18519–18524

77. Endesfelder U, Finan K, Holden SJ, Cook PR, Kapanidis AN, Heilemann M (2013) Multiscale spatial organization of RNA polymerase in Escherichia coli. Biophys J 105:172–181

78. Saxton MJ, Jacobson K (1997) Single-particle tracking: applications to membrane dynamics. Annu Rev Biophys Biomol Struct 26:373–399

79. Saxton MJ (1997) Single-particle tracking: the distribution of diffusion coefficients. Biophys J 72:1744–1753

80. Savin T, Doyle PS (2005) Static and dynamic errors in particle tracking microrheology. Biophys J 88:623–638

81. Backlund MP, Joyner R, Moerner WE (2015) Chromosomal locus tracking with proper accounting of static and dynamic errors. Phys Rev E Stat Nonlin Soft Matter Phys 91:062716

82. Levi V, Ruan Q, Plutz M, Belmont AS, Gratton E (2005) Chromatin dynamics in interphase cells revealed by tracking in a two-photon excitation microscope. Biophys J 89:4275–4285

83. Persson F, Lindén M, Unoson C, Elf J (2013) Extracting intracellular diffusive states and transition rates from single-molecule tracking data. Nat Methods 10:265–269

84. Huang F, Schwartz SL, Byars JM, Lidke KA (2011) Simultaneous multiple-emitter fitting for single molecule super-resolution imaging. Biomed Opt Express 2:1377–1393

85. Holden SJ, Uphoff S, Kapanidis AN (2011) DAOSTORM: an algorithm for high-density super-resolution microscopy. Nat Methods 8:279–280

86. Mukamel EA, Babcock H, Zhuang X (2012) Statistical deconvolution for superresolution fluorescence microscopy. Biophys J 102:2391–2400

87. Zhu L, Zhang W, Elnatan D, Huang B (2012) Faster STORM using compressed sensing. Nat Methods 9:721–723

88. Cox S, Rosten E, Monypenny J, Jovanovic-Talisman T, Burnette DT, Lippincott-Schwartz J, Jones GE, Heintzmann R (2012) Bayesian localization microscopy reveals nanoscale podosome dynamics. Nat Methods 9:195–200

Chapter 18

Intra-Nuclear Single-Particle Tracking (I-SPT) to Reveal the Functional Architecture of Chromosomes

Vincent Récamier

Abstract

Chromosome architecture needs to be investigated in relation with the chemical function of DNA. The kinetics of gene expression, DNA replication, and repair are driven by the mechanisms by which a functional nuclear protein finds its substrate in the nucleus. Single-particle tracking (SPT) is a method to quantify fluorescent molecules dynamics from the tracks of the single molecules recorded by high-resolution microscopes. SPT offers direct observation of the movement and single-molecule resolution. Usually SPT is performed on membranes because of higher contrast. Here, we introduce a novel method to record the trajectories of weakly fluorescent molecules in the nucleus of living cells. I-SPT uses some specific detection and analysis tools to enable the computation of reliable statistics on nuclear particle movement.

Key words Chromatin functional architecture, Single-particle tracking, Photoactivatable proteins, Molecule diffusion

1 Introduction

Chromatin architecture has been studied using recent imaging technique showing that the organization is not random, displaying, for instance, chromosome territories [1]. However, little is known about how this organization influences the biological function of nuclear DNA. Here we introduce a method called I-SPT [2] (intra-nuclear single-particle tracking) to follow functional proteins at the single-molecule level in relation with the functional architecture of chromosomes. The method can be applied to any nuclear protein, provided that it can be tagged with a photo-activated dye with no alteration of its functional properties.

Single-particle tracking (SPT) is a general term for any assay that combines imaging and image analysis to record trajectories of single objects, i.e. their position in space and time. In fluorescent microscopy, SPT can be performed if the concentration of fluorescent emitters is low enough and the signal to noise ratio high enough to reach single-molecule accuracy [3]. Until recently, SPT

Mark C. Leake (ed.), *Chromosome Architecture: Methods and Protocols*, Methods in Molecular Biology, vol. 1431,
DOI 10.1007/978-1-4939-3631-1_18, © Springer Science+Business Media New York 2016

265

inside live cells has been mostly restricted to membranes [4] but numerous efforts have developed to extend the analysis deeper in the nucleoplasm. On the recorded trajectories, it is possible to compute the statistical descriptors of the movement, which remain an intense subject of investigation in the scientific community [5]. Alternative experiments to SPT to recover the movement characteristics of fluorescent objects are bulk techniques such as florescence recovery after photo-bleaching (FRAP) [6] and fluorescent correlation spectroscopy (FCS) [7]. As opposed to FRAP and FCS which record ensemble average movement, SPT offers a direct observation of the trajectories, possibly revealing the heterogeneity of the fluorescent-labeled molecule population. Therefore, SPT data can theoretically be explained with weaker assumption compared to bulk techniques and enables direct measurement of chemical interactions. The spatial resolution of SPT can also break the fundamental resolution limit of microscopy imposed by diffraction, leading to nanometer precision [8]. For that reasons, cellular live single-particle assays have been a significant breakthrough in the measurement of in vivo reaction kinetics, like transcription factor target search of DNA sequence [9].

In the present protocol, we describe I-SPT is a versatile technique to image, follow, and quantitatively describe single-fluorescent proteins dynamics based on the tagging of functional nuclear proteins by photo-activatable dyes. By stochastic photo-activation of the tag with very low activation, a few, maybe only one protein emits light in the imaging wavelength. Tuning the photo-activation to a suitable regime where the number of emitter is low enough so that we can accurately detect their position but still get robust statistics is the challenge of this technique. The novelty of our approach is to include the photophysics of the fluorophore to compute the tracking reliability, the probability of good connection.

2   Materials

1. Cells: Any cell that grows on coverslip can be used for I-SPT. We used U2OS cells because of their large nucleus. Grow U2OS cells in Dulbecco's Modified Eagle Medium (DMEM) with 10% fetal bovine serum. Prior to imaging, we replaced the imaging medium by a transparent imaging medium.

2. Plasmids. The plasmid of a molecule of interest shall be fused to a sequence of a photo-activatable protein [10]. Several photo-activatable proteins are available that need to be excited and activated in specific wavelengths. We chose the photo-activatable protein Dendra2 [11]. Dendra2 has maximum excitation at 490 nm and emission at 507 nm in the pre-converted

form. In its converted form, Dendra2 has maximum excitation at 553 nm and emission at 573 nm.

3. ISPT is to be performed on an inverted microscope, with a heated stage. The microscope shall be equipped with a high numerical aperture objective (1.49 NA) and 100× magnification. In the light path, place a motorized mirror (TIRFF) to induce a small angle between 0° and 30°, typically to reduce background from out of focus emitters.

4. Sample excitation: Pre-converted form of Dendra2: a mercury lamp with 480/20 excitation filter. Activation-conversion: 405 nm argon-ion LASER. Converted form: 561 yellow green LASER. The illumination sequence is created using imaging software-driven electro acoustic filter (AOTF). The emission signal passes through two bands emission filters: $561-25 \times 36$ in the red channel and $490-25 \times 36$ in the green channel.

5. Image acquisition. EMCCD camera in read-out mode 10 MHz at 16 bits. Do not allow pixel binning. Use camera with pixel size lower than 120 μm.

6. Coverslips: Use 25 nm coverslips cleaned with plasma cleaner and coated with collagen.

3 Methods

To reach single-molecule accuracy, it is necessary to select cells with low level of expression, and then activate dyes at low power to dilute by several orders of magnitude the number of active emitters. To estimate the bleaching time of the dye under the same imaging conditions, on the contrary, it is necessary to select cells with high level of expression and to pulse-activate significantly to have a measurable bulk fluorescence decay. Since the molecule is moving during acquisition, the resulting motion blur does not display a peak that can be fitted to a Gaussian curve and detection based on filtering and segmentation is required. The tracking step is simple nearest neighbor algorithm, up to a maximum distance R, including a quality check process that assigns a good assignment probability to any computed connection according to the dye-bleaching time. The good assignment probability is then integrated in standard single-particle tracking statistics for the investigation of diffusion, the Mean Squared Displacement (MSD), and the translocation histogram.

3.1 Sample Preparation

1. Forty-eight hours prior to the imaging, clean and sterilize 25 nm coverslips with plasma cleaner (2 min with air).

2. Dilute collagen I solution 1:10, then 1:50 with 30% ethanol and spread over the surface of the coverslips in a cell culture hood. Let it dry under the hood.

3. Seed cells at 30–40% confluence on plasma-cleaned and collagen-coated coverslips.

4. Twenty-four hours before imaging, transfect the cells with the plasmid of the functional protein tagged with photo-activatable protein (100 ng/25 mm coverslip) using a non-lipidic transfection reagent and applying the protocol of the provider.

3.2 Single-Molecule Microscopy

1. In the pre-converted channel: Select one cell with low plasmid expression, as judge by low fluorescence intensity and select a focal plane inside the nucleus of the cell.

2. In the converted channel: Shine a pulse of activation and tune the TIRFF angle to 0–30° to reach maximum signal to noise ratio (*see* **Note 1**).

3. In the pre-converted channel: Take a 1-s exposure image of the pre-converted form of the ensemble fluorescence.

4. In the pre-converted channel: select a small region of interest (ROI) to image a large cross section within the nucleus of a single cell.

5. In the converted channel: Allow acquisition rates as fast as 100 Hz (inter-frame $\Delta t = 10\text{ms}$) and set the illumination sequence as in Fig. 1, panel a.

   - *Activation laser (405 nm)* needs to illuminate the sample with very low power between frames so that a fluorescent molecule does not appear during acquisition.

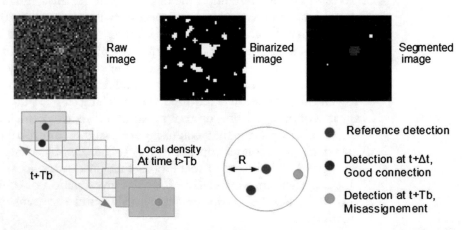

Fig. 1 *Upper panel*: the illumination sequence of an I-SPT experiment: the typical exposure time is 10 ms, the excitation LASER is shut off between frames to avoid unnecessary bleaching and the activation is done in the lag time between frames to avoid molecule appearance during acquisition. *Lower panel*: time montage of a diffusing single molecule. For visualization, the inter-frame is three times the actual exposure time (10 ms) plus lag time (0.5 ms)

- *Illumination laser (561 nm)* needs to illuminate the sample with very high power during frame acquisition for high signal to noise ratio and switched off between frames to avoid bleaching.

6. A typical acquisition is $N = 10,000$ frames (~2 min). Repeat acquisition up to five times per cell and take one image of the nucleus in the pre-converted channel between acquisitions. The cell nucleus shall keep its shape over the experiment and no fluorescence shall be seen outside the cell. Stop acquisition if the cell does not match this criterion.

7. Check visually the acquisition of single-molecule trajectories as shown in Fig. 1.

3.3 Estimation of the Bleaching Time Decay

1. In the pre-converted channel: Select one cell with high expression, as judge by high fluorescence intensity.

2. In the converted channel: Shine a 2–10-s pulse of activation (405) and monitor the fluorescent intensity increasing. Stop activation before reaching pixel saturation.

3. Record the fluorescence decay on the whole cell using the illumination sequence in Fig. 1, panel a *without activation*.

4. Repeat the acquisition of the fluorescence decay on different cells (~10 cells). Align and sum the decays. Compute the bleaching time T_b in situ by fitting the summed fluorescence decay to an exponential function. T_b shall be between 10 s and 1000 s.

$$Ae^{-\frac{t}{T_b}}$$

3.4 Detection (Image Processing)

1. To reduce noise, filter the raw images in 2D (Fig. 2) using a Gaussian mask with standard deviation of $\sigma = \lambda / 2$, where λ is the emission wavelength.

2. Make the image binary using a percentile threshold, which is the rescaled brightest pixel value that can be considered as a detection (Fig. 2). Set the percentile threshold to a value around quantile 10–20% estimated on the whole movie.

3. Aggregate detections that are less than 200 nm apart to merge detections that belong to molecules going in and out of the focal plane during acquisition.

4. For every binary area, estimate the motion blur size (Fig. 2), which is the maximum, and minimum size for a detection to be accepted. A low-percentile threshold shall be compensated by a high-motion blur size. Set the motion blur size to a value between 0.1 and 2 μm^2.

5. Multiply the binary image with the original image. For every detection estimate the signal to noise ratio (SNR), which is the

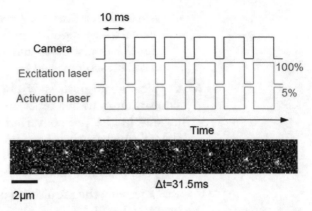

Fig. 2 *Upper panel*: A raw image of a single-molecule detection, followed by the same image after binarization and then a detection as judged as the over the noise area. *Lower panel*: definition of a connection and misassignment. A connection can occur when two detections are within a tracking distance R on consecutive frames. The number of misassignments can be estimated by connecting two detections within a tracking distance R on frame which a time lag higher than the bleaching time Tb

overall signal to noise ratio estimated of the particle. This is defined by the formula:

$$\frac{-\sum_i \mathrm{Value}_i - \mathrm{noise}_i}{\sum_i \mathrm{Variance}_i}$$

The sum is computed over the pixels of the detection. The noise and variance are, respectively, the time median and variance of the one-dimensional time series pixel without detections. Keep detection with SNR ratio higher than 0.1

6. Detection is performed by selecting the other-the-noise pixels and setting the *center of mass* as their position. The final output of the detection step is a table file with *x*, *y*, and time.

3.5 Tracking (Post Processing)

Tacking is performed by setting a maximum tracking radius R. When a detection at time $t + \Delta t$ is found at distance lower than R to a reference detection at time t, then a connection is computed and the reference and the successive detection are linked in a trajectory (*see* **Note 2**).

1. On the detection coordinate file, estimate the number of possible connections between two consecutive frames as a function of the maximum distance R with an increment $dR = 10$ nm. This results in an ever increasing function $C(R)$.

2. If any ambiguity occurs in the tracking such as two detections are found at distance lower than R of a reference detection in the next frame, remove the connections.

3. Duplicate the detections coordinate file and change the time clock t', so that two successive detections at times t' and $t' + \Delta t$ are distant by at least the bleaching time T_b, in absolute value (Fig. 2). This can be done by setting the times t' to:

$$t' = [t / T_b] \times \Delta t + (t - [t / T_b]) \times [N / T_b]$$

where [] is the integer part and N is the total length of the acquisition.

4. On the reshuffled detection coordinate file, estimate also the number of possible connections between two consecutive frames as a function of the maximum distance R. This results in misassignments ever increasing function $M(R)$.

5. The number of good connections as a function of the distance R can be estimated by estimating $C(R) - M(R)$. We observed that under our condition of illumination, this function reaches a maximum at $R_{max} \approx 2\mu m$ approximately. This value can be assigned as the maximum radius tracking parameter.

6. Assign $Rmax$ as the maximum tracking radius. The final output of the tracking step is a table file with x, y, and time and trajectory number (Fig. 2, panel d).

7. Estimate the probability of good connection $P(R)$ as a function of the radius using the formula:

$$P(R) = 1 - \frac{M(R + dR) - M(R)}{C(R + dR) - C(R)}$$

3.6 The Step-Displacement Histograms and the Mean Square Displacements (MSD) (Statistics)

1. Displacements are computed distances within a trajectory between two detections, and step displacements are displacements computed between successive detections.

2. For step displacements i, assign a probability Pi using the following convention: if the displacement does not reach the beginning or the end of the trajectory, then $P_i = 1$. If the displacement reaches the beginning or the end of the trajectory, then the probability is equal to the probability of good connection $P(Ri)$, as a function of the distance Ri of i.

3. Compute the step displacements Ri histogram (Fig. 3, upper panel) for 1, Δt counted with weights Pi, using an appropriate binning (5 nm) (*see* **Note 3**).

4. For displacements j computed between detections that are not successive, but distant in time by $n\Delta t$, assign a probability Pj,n by averaging the probability Pi of the step displacements i, it is composed of Fig. 3, lower panel.

5. Compute the step displacement histograms for $n\Delta t$ as the distribution of $n\Delta t$ displacements Rj, counted with weights Pj,n,

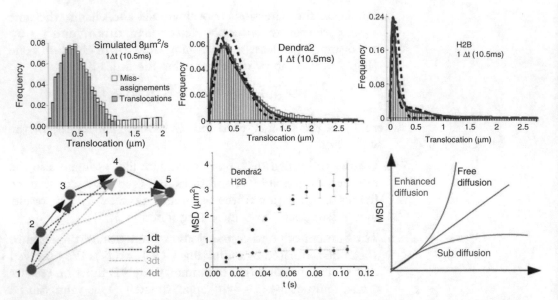

Fig. 3 *Upper panel*: The step-displacement histogram represents the distribution of one-step displacement within the recorded trajectories, together with the estimated misconnections. Here, we display the step displacement histogram of a simulated movement of mole diffusion at 8 µm²/s, of the free fluorophore Dendra2 and the chromatin bound nucleosomal protein H2B in U2OS cells. The histogram displays free diffusion for Dendra2 and restricted diffusion for H2B. *Lower panel*: Considering the displacement for different lag times dt inside trajectories, we can estimate the mean square displacement curve as shown for H2B in Dendra2. MSD curves can be interpreted in the diffusion framework in terms of free diffusion, sub-diffusion, or enhanced diffusion.

     using an appropriate binning (5 nm). I SPT can reliably estimate the step displacement histogram up to $10\Delta t$.

6. For every time step $n\Delta t$, compute the time and ensemble average means square displacement $MSD(n)$ [12]. $MSD(n)$ is the mean of all the computed square displacements, Rj^2 counted with weights Pj,n, and average over all the computed trajectories.

7. Plot the mean square displacement as a function of $n\Delta t$ (Fig. 3, lower panel) (*see* **Note 4**).

---

4   Notes

1. An angle in the illumination path increases significantly the signal to noise ratio of single fluorophores and therefore the focal depth of the experiment [13]. With a larger focal depth, the detected trajectories of single molecule will be longer. The input LASER power is given as an indication and shall vary from one setup to another. A typical activation and illumination power is 10 W/cm²

2. To estimate misassignment probability, we make the following assumptions: (a) Molecules are permanently bleached after a given bleaching time T_b. (b) The density of detections does not vary rapidly along the experiment. Under those assumptions, connections performed with inter-frame larger than T_b is a misassignment: I-SPT therefore estimates tracking misassignment by computing the local density around each detection at time labs larger than T_b.

3. Step displacements histograms can be used to probe different sorts of movements of the nucleus. Here, as a benchmark, in Fig. 3 we show the step displacement histogram of the free fluorophore Dendra2 and of the chromatin-bound molecule H2B in the nucleus of U2OS cells. Displacement histograms determine the number of populations diffusing at different speed, or diffusion coefficient in the sample [14]. Note however that I-SPT has a bias toward slow-moving molecules.

4. MSD is the standard statistic to investigate diffusion. By plotting the average square displacement as a function of the time lag, we have an indication of the type of diffusion. In the case of free diffusion, the slope of the MSD is equal to the diffusion coefficient D. The shape of the MSD can also indicate if the movement is restricted in the framework of anomalous diffusion [15] (Fig. 3).

Acknowledgments

The author would like to thank Ignacio Izeddin and Xavier Darzacq who co-designed this protocol, Mark Leake and Roman Sedlak for critical reading of the manuscript. This research was supported by the Fondartion pour la Recherche Médicale (FRM) and Marie Curie Action.

References

1. Berger AB, Cabal GG, Fabre E et al (2008) High-resolution statistical mapping reveals gene territories in live yeast. Nat Methods 5:1031–1037

2. Izeddin I, Récamier V, Bosanac L et al (2014) Single-molecule tracking in live cells reveals distinct target-search strategies of transcription factors in the nucleus. eLife 3:e02230

3. Lippincott-Schwartz J, Altan-Bonnet N, Patterson GH (2003) Photobleaching and photoactivation: following protein dynamics in living cells. Nat Cell Biol Suppl:S7–S14

4. Alcor D, Gouzer G, Triller A (2009) Single-particle tracking methods for the study of membrane receptors dynamics. Eur J Neurosci 30:987–997

5. Ruthardt N, Lamb DC, Bräuchle C (2011) Single-particle tracking as a quantitative microscopy-based approach to unravel cell entry mechanisms of viruses and pharmaceutical nanoparticles. Mol Ther 19: 1199–1211

6. Mueller F, Mazza D, Stasevich TJ et al (2010) FRAP and kinetic modeling in the analysis of nuclear protein dynamics: what do we really know? Curr Opin Cell Biol 22:403–411

7. Brock R, Jovin TM (2001) Fluorescence correlation microscopy (FCM): fluorescence cor-

relation spectroscopy (FCS) in cell biology. In: Fluorescence correlation spectroscopy. Springer, Berlin, pp 132–161

8. Mazza D, Abernathy A, Golob N et al (2012) A benchmark for chromatin binding measurements in live cells. Nucleic Acids Res 40, e119

9. Normanno D, Boudarène L, Dugast-Darzacq C et al (2015) Probing the target search of DNA-binding proteins in mammalian cells using TetR as model searcher. Nat Commun 6:7357

10. Lippincott-Schwartz J, Patterson GH (2008) Fluorescent proteins for photoactivation experiments. Methods Cell Biol 85:45–61

11. Gurskaya NG, Verkhusha VV, Shcheglov AS et al (2006) Engineering of a monomeric green-to-red photoactivatable fluorescent protein induced by blue light. Nat Biotechnol 24:461–465

12. Michalet X (2010) Mean square displacement analysis of single-particle trajectories with localization error: Brownian motion in an isotropic medium. Phys Rev E Stat Nonlin Soft Matter Phys 82:041914

13. Tokunaga M, Imamoto N, Sakata-Sogawa K (2008) Highly inclined thin illumination enables clear single-molecule imaging in cells. Nat Methods 5:159–161

14. Schütz GJ, Schindler H, Schmidt T (1997) Single-molecule microscopy on model membranes reveals anomalous diffusion. Biophys J 73:1073–1080

15. Metzler R, Klafter J (2000) The random walk's guide to anomalous diffusion: a fractional dynamics approach. Phys Rep 339: 1–77

Chapter 19

Visualizing *Bacillus subtilis* During Vegetative Growth and Spore Formation

Xindan Wang and Paula Montero Llopis

Abstract

Bacillus subtilis is the most commonly used Gram-positive bacterium to study cellular processes because of its genetic tractability. In addition, during nutrient limitation, *B. subtilis* undergoes the development process of spore formation, which is among the simplest examples of cellular differentiation. Many aspects of these processes have benefited from fluorescence microscopy. Here, we describe basic wide-field fluorescence microscopy techniques to visualize *B. subtilis* during vegetative growth, and the developmental process of sporulation.

Key words *Bacillus subtilis*, Vegetative growth, Sporulation, Fluorescence microscopy, Time-lapse microscopy

1 Introduction

Bacillus subtilis is a rod-shaped soil bacterium that grows and divides through binary fission. When nutrients become limited, it undergoes a developmental process that results in the formation of a dormant spore [1]. The highly resistant spore allows the bacteria to survive extreme environmental conditions including heat, desiccation, UV and γ-radiation, and presence of antibiotics and other toxic chemicals [2]. When nutrients become available, the spores can germinate and resume exponential growth [3]. This double life-style and the ease with which genetic, biochemical, and cytological analysis can be carried out in this organism make *B. subtilis* an ideal system to study a variety of cellular processes, such as gene regulation, chromosome dynamics, morphogenesis, and cell fate determination.

The application of fluorescence microscopy to the study of prokaryotes has revealed that bacteria possess a highly organized internal architecture [4]. Even at a time in which super-resolution imaging [5] and microfluidic technologies are becoming more and more common [6–8], wide-field fluorescence microscopy using

Mark C. Leake (ed.), *Chromosome Architecture: Methods and Protocols*, Methods in Molecular Biology, vol. 1431, DOI 10.1007/978-1-4939-3631-1_19, © Springer Science+Business Media New York 2016

simple glass slides still remains a powerful tool and workhorse in the field. In this chapter, we describe how we routinely grow *B. subtilis* in liquid culture, and how we prepare slides for snapshot and time-lapse imaging in a very simple experimental setup. Although it is a popular model organism, compared to other model bacteria like *Escherichia coli* and *Caulobacter crescentus*, *B. subtilis* appears to require more oxygen for growth and most importantly, for microscopy. In this chapter, we specifically emphasize the importance of aeration of liquid cultures and the use of open agarose pads for time-lapse microscopy to maintain adequate oxygen for balanced growth of *B. subtilis* in liquid and on slides. Additionally, we have observed that photobleaching and phototoxicity seem to be a bigger challenge when imaging *B. subtilis*, perhaps related to its requirement for oxygen. Therefore, the use of a low-fluorescence background growth medium and a systematic image acquisition optimization are especially important when visualizing *B. subtilis*.

2   Materials

Media components are prepared in Milli-Q water (ddH$_2$O) unless otherwise stated. Where indicated, liquid media are sterilized by autoclaving for 30 min in liquid cycle, or by filtering through a 0.22-µm syringe-driven filter or a bottle-top filter. Glassware is sterilized by autoclaving for 30 min in dry cycle. Sterile media components and glassware are stored at room temperature unless otherwise specified.

2.1   Media and Equipment for the Growth of B. subtilis

1. Make regular LB agar plates, or plates containing one of the following antibiotics if needed: 5 µg/ml chloramphenicol; 1 µg/ml erythromycin plus 25 µg/ml lincomycin (MLS); 10 µg/ml kanamycin; 0.4 µg/ml phleomycin; 100 µg/ml spectinomycin; 10 µg/ml tetracycline (*see* **Note 1**).

2. Defined rich casein hydrolysate medium (CH medium) [9] component CHI + II: 10 mg/ml casein hydrolysate (Neogen #7229A), 4.7 mg/ml l-glutamate sodium salt monohydrate, 3.2 mg/ml l-asparagine monohydrate, 2.5 mg/ml l-alanine, 2.72 mg/ml potassium phosphate monobasic anhydrous (KH$_2$PO4), 2.68 mg/ml ammonium chloride (NH$_4$Cl), 1.1 mg/ml sodium sulfate (Na$_2$SO$_4$), 1 mg/ml ammonium nitrate (NH$_4$NO$_3$), and 0.01 mg/ml ferric chloride 6-hydrate (FeCl$_3$·6H$_2$O); autoclaved.

3. CH medium component CHIII: 0.66 mg/ml calcium chloride dehydrate (CaCl$_2$·2H$_2$O), and 1.21 mg/ml magnesium sulfate anhydrous (MgSO$_4$); autoclaved.

4. CH medium component CHIV: 1.67 mg/ml manganese sulfate monohydrate ($MnSO_4 \cdot H_2O$); autoclaved.

5. CH medium component CHV: 2 mg/ml l-Tryptophan; filtered and distributed in 10 ml aliquots in 15 ml conical tubes. Store at 4 °C.

6. S750 minimal medium [10] component deionized water (dH_2O); autoclaved (*see* **Note 2**).

7. S750 minimal medium component 10× S750 salt: 104.7 mg/ml 4-morpholinepropanesulfonic acid (MOPS free acid), 13.2 mg/ml ammonium sulfate [$(NH_4)_2SO_4$], and 6.8 mg/ml potassium phosphate monobasic (KH_2PO_4); autoclaved.

8. S750 minimal medium component 100× metals: 200 mM $MgCl_2$, 70 mM $CaCl_2$, 5 mM $MnCl_2$, 0.1 mM $ZnCl_2$, 0.1 mg/ml thiamine HCl, 0.002 N HCl, 0.5 mM $FeCl_3$; filtered and distributed in 10 ml aliquots in 15 ml conical tubes. Wrap tubes in foil and store at 4 °C.

9. S750 minimal medium component 1 M glutamic acid potassium salt: adjust to pH 7.0 using potassium hydroximate (KOH); filtered.

10. S750 minimal medium component 50 % glucose; filtered. If a slower growth rate is needed, 50 % sorbitol can be used instead of glucose.

11. Glass culture tubes (18 × 150 mm, VWR 47729-583), autoclaved; and roller drum in 22 °C incubator. Similar tubes or rolling/shaking systems can be used to grow 5 ml of liquid culture with aeration.

12. 250 ml baffled flasks, autoclaved.

13. Temperature-controlled shaking waterbath that can accommodate 250 ml flasks. Alternatively, temperature controlled air-shakers can be used.

14. Spectrophotometer to monitor optical density (OD_{600}).

2.2 Components for Snapshot Imaging

1. Standard glass slides, and cover slips (glass thickness 0.17 mm/No.1.5).

2. (Optional) Red membrane stain FM4-64 (*N*-(3-triethylammoniumpropyl)-4-(6-(4 (diethylamino) phenyl) hexatrienyl) pyridinium dibromide) (Life Technologies T-3166) (100×): 0.15 mg/ml in ddH_2O; protect from light and store at 4 °C. This dye can be visualized using Chroma's ET 49008 single band filter set (*see* **Note 3**).

3. (Optional) Blue DNA stain DAPI (4′,6-diamidino-2-phenylindole) (Life Technologies D-1306) (100×): 0.2 mg/ml in ddH_2O; protect from light and store at 4 °C. This dye

can be visualized using Chroma's ET 49000 single band filter set (*see* **Note 3**).

4. (Optional) Blue membrane stain TMA-DPH (1-(4-trimethylammoniumphenyl)-6-phenyl-1,3,5-hexatriene *p*-toluenesulfonate) (Life Technologies, T-204) (100×): 5 mM in DMSO; protect from light and store at 4 °C. This dye can be visualized using Chroma's ET 49000 single band filter set (*see* **Note 3**).

5. Molecular grade agarose.

6. Microwave oven.

7. Kimwipes.

8. Ethanol in squirt bottle.

9. Nikon Ti microscope equipped with a Plan Apo 100×/1.4 N.A., phase-contrast oil objective, a CoolSnapHQ^2 camera, Nikon Ti-S-ER motorized stage, filter cubes for GFP (Chroma 49002), YFP (Chroma 49003), CFP (Chroma 49001), DAPI (Chroma 49000), Texas Red (Chroma 49008), and a Lumencor Spectra X light engine. Similar microscopes can be used.

2.3 Components for Time-Lapse Imaging

1. Molecular grade agarose.

2. Microwave oven.

3. 60 × 15 mm petri dish (Becton Dickinson Labware 351007).

4. Scalpel.

5. Glass bottom dish (Willco Wells 50/40 mm Glass Thickness 0.17 mm/No.1.5 HBSt-5040).

6. Humidified stage-top incubator (TC-MIS; Bioscience Tools) and objective heater (Bioptechs). Other humidified, temperature-controlled environmental chambers for microscopes can be used.

7. Microscope (*see* **item 9** in Subheading 2.2) with a Well Plate Holder stage (TI-SH-W; Nikon) for stage-top incubator. Other inverted microscopes can be used.

2.4 Components for Visualizing Sporulating Cells

1. Sporulation resuspension medium [9] component ddH$_2$O, autoclaved.

2. Sporulation resuspension medium component Solution A: 0.089 mg/ml ferric chloride 6-hydrate (FeCl$_3$·6H$_2$O), 0.83 mg/ml magnesium chloride hexahydrate (MgCl$_2$·6H$_2$O), 1.98 mg/ml manganese chloride tetrahydrate (MnCl$_2$·4H$_2$O); filtered and dispensed into 10 ml aliquots in 15 ml conical tubes. Wrap with foil and store at 4 °C.

3. Sporulation resuspension medium component Solution B: 13.4 mg/ml ammonium chloride (NH$_4$Cl), 2.65 mg/ml sodium sulfate (Na$_2$SO$_4$), 1.7 mg/ml ammonium nitrate

(NH_4NO_3), 2.43 mg/ml potassium phosphate monobasic anhydrous (KH_2PO_4); Dissolve in 80 % volume, adjust to pH 7.0 using 1 N NaOH, add ddH_2O to final volume; autoclaved.

4. Sporulation resuspension medium component Solution C: 63.6 mg/ml l-glutamic acid sodium salt monohydrate, which represents 5 % l-glutamic acid; autoclaved.

5. Sporulation resuspension medium component Solution D: 3.68 mg/ml calcium chloride dehydrate ($CaCl_2 \cdot 2H_2O$); autoclaved.

6. Sporulation resuspension medium component Solution E: 120.4 mg/ml magnesium sulfate anhydrous ($MgSO_4$); autoclaved.

7. Bench top centrifuge for spinning 50 ml conical tubes.

8. Components for snapshot imaging, same as **items 1–9** in Subheading 2.2.

3   Methods

3.1   Exponential Growth of Cells

1. Streak out the *B. subtilis* strain of interest on an LB agar plate containing the appropriate antibiotics and incubate at 37 °C overnight (*see* **Note 4**). Use a different temperature if the strain has a specific requirement.

2. If the colonies are visible the next morning, take the plate out and leave at room temperature during the day to prevent over growth (*see* **Note 5**).

3. In the evening, prepare 100 ml of complete CH medium using the individual components. The doubling time for wild-type PY79 strain growing in CH is ~35 min (*see* **Note 6**). For complete CH medium, combine 94 ml of CHI + II, 4 ml of CHIII, 1 ml of CH IV, and 1 ml of CHV in a sterile bottle. If minimal medium is used instead of CH medium, make 100 ml of S750 medium by combining 86 ml of autoclaved dH_2O, 10 ml of 10× S750 salt, 1 ml of 100× metals, 2 ml of 1 M glutamic acid potassium salt, and 2 ml of 50 % glucose or sorbitol in a sterile bottle. The doubling time for wild type PY79 strain growing in S750 glucose is ~48 min and in S750 sorbitol is 80–100 min.

4. Set up a starter culture by inoculating a single colony into 5 ml of growth medium (complete CH medium or S750 minimal medium), vortex gently to disperse the colony (*see* **Note 7**). Make a 1–5 dilution of the inoculum by transferring 1 ml of the inoculum into 4 ml of fresh medium. Put both tubes in roller drum and roll overnight at 22 °C (*see* **Note 8**).

5. In the next morning, measure the optical density (OD_{600}) of both cultures and use the starter culture that is between 0.2 and 0.6. Dilute the culture in 25 ml of fresh growth medium prepared the previous day (*see* **step 3**) in a 250 ml baffled flask to an OD_{600} of 0.02 (*see* **Note 9**).

6. Put the flask in the shaking waterbath and shake at 250 rpm at 37 °C (or other desired temperature). Other temperature-controlled air-shaker can be used.

7. Monitor the OD_{600} and harvest cells at the density specified by different applications (see below).

3.2 Visualize B. subtilis Using Snapshot Microscopy

1. If cell membrane and DNA are going to be visualized, prepare the fluorescent dyes before the culture is ready: add 1 μl of 100× FM4-64 stock and 1 μl of 100× DAPI stock into 100 μl of growth medium (same medium used for growth, *see* **step 3** in Subheading 3.1). Protect from light.

2. While the cells are growing, prepare 2% agarose solution in growth media for making agarose pads: dissolve 0.6 g of molecular grade agarose in 30 ml of growth medium. Microwave until homogenous. Keep at 65 °C (*see* **Note 10**).

3. Prepare the agarose pads (Fig. 1) (*see* **Note 11**). Prepare two spacers by putting three layers of lab tape on a glass slide (*see*

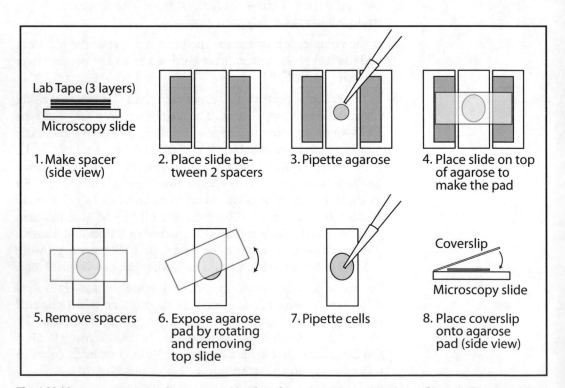

Fig. 1 Making an agarose pad for snapshot imaging. *Steps 1* and *8* are side views. *Steps 2–7* are top views

Note 12). Clean two microscopy slides per sample by wiping them with a kimwipe wetted with ethanol using a squirt bottle. Place one of the slides between the two spacers and add 100 μl of the 2 % agarose solution to the center of the slide (*see* **Note 13**). Immediately after, gently drop a second slide over the agarose droplet. This will make a thin agarose pad "sandwiched" in between the two glass slides (Fig. 1) (*see* **Note 14**). Leave on the bench for 2–5 min to allow the agarose to solidify. Carefully remove the spacers from the agarose sandwich and remove one of the slides to expose the agarose pad (*see* **Note 15**).

4. Harvest cells when OD_{600} is between 0.2 and 0.4. Take 1 ml of culture and spin at $3300 \times g$ for 30 s. Remove 900 μl of supernatant by pipetting or aspiration. Repeat centrifugation and remove supernatant completely using a P200 tip (*see* **Note 16**).

5. Resuspend the cell pellet using 10 μl of medium containing FM4-64 and DAPI from **step 1**. Pipette to mix and spot 1 μl of cells on an agarose pad prepared at **step 3**. Place a coverslip over the pad and visualize using the microscope (Fig. 2) (*see* **Note 17**).

3.3 Visualize B. subtilis Using Time-Lapse Microscopy

1. Grow the cells in CH or S750 minimal medium as in Subheading 3.1 to an OD_{600} of 0.2–0.4.

2. Prepare the stage top incubator for imaging. Carefully fill the water reservoir to maintain high humidity in the incubator (*see* **Note 18**). Turn on the stage top incubator and objective heater and allow them to reach and stabilize at the required temperature, which takes about 30 min. If other environmental chamber is used instead, set it up beforehand to let the temperature stabilize.

CH, τ=35 min   S750 glucose, τ=48 min   S750 sorbitol, τ=98 min

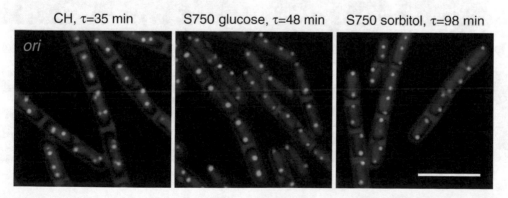

Fig. 2 Snapshot micrographs of cells growing in CH medium, or S750 minimal medium supplemented with glucose or sorbitol [11]. Membranes (*red*) were stained with FM4-64, nucleoids (*blue*) were stained with DAPI, origins (*green*) were labeled using *tetO48*/TetR-CFP. τ, doubling time. Bar, 4 μm

3. Prepare 2 % agarose solution in growth medium as in **step 2** in Subheading 3.2.

4. Pour 6 ml of the 2 % agarose solution into a 60×15 mm petri dish and leave on the bench for 15–20 min (Fig. 3) (*see* **Note 19**).

5. Using a scalpel, cut 0.5×1.5 mm strips of agarose from the petri dish.

6. Take 1 ml of culture and spin at $3300 \times g$ for 30 s. Remove 900 µl of supernatant by pipetting or aspiration. Resuspend the cell pellet using the remaining medium. Gently pipette up and down to mix (*see* **Note 20**).

7. Spot 1–2 µl of cells on a glass bottom dish, which will be used as a cover glass for the microscope. Lay a strip of agarose pad on top of cells using the scalpel (*see* **Note 21**).

8. Put the glass bottom dish containing cells and agarose pads in the stage top incubator. Close the lid of the incubator. Incubate for 15–30 min before imaging to stabilize the temperature in the pads and in the incubator (*see* **Note 22**).

9. To reduce image drift due to evaporation, chose a field of view that is not too close to the edge of the agarose strip. Optimize image acquisition to reduce photobleaching and phototoxicity (*see* **Note 23**). Take images at desired time intervals (Fig. 4).

3.4 Visualize B. subtilis During Sporulation

1. Grow the cells in CH medium as in Subheading 3.1.

2. While the cells are growing, prepare 100 ml of sporulation resuspension medium in a sterile bottle by combining 84 ml of

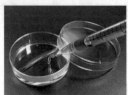

1. Pour 6 ml of molten agarose

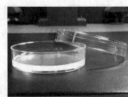

2. Incubate 15 min to solidify

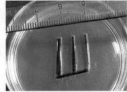

3. Cut 0.5x1.5 cm agarose strips

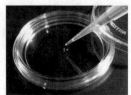

4. Pipette cells onto glass-bottom dish

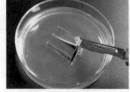

5. Collect an agarose strip

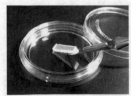

6. Place the agarose strip on top of cells

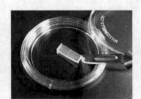

7. Slowly lower agarose strip to prevent bubbles

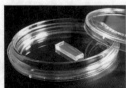

8. Ready to image

Fig. 3 Set up a slide for time-lapse microscopy using a glass bottom dish. During imaging, the agarose pad is fully exposed in the humidified temperature-controlled incubator

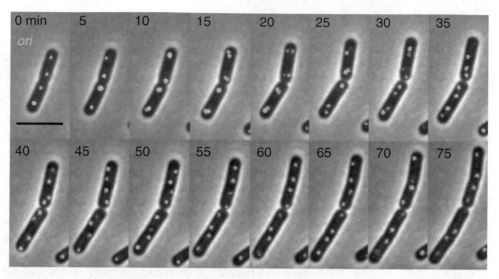

Fig. 4 A time-lapse progression (5-min intervals) of cells growing in S750 sorbitol minimal medium [11]. Nucleoids (*red*) were visualized using HbsU-GFP, origins (*green*) were labeled using *tetO48*/TetR-CFP. Bar, 4 μm

ddH$_2$O, 100 μl of Solution A, 4 ml each of Solutions B, C, D, and E.

3. Prepare the fluorescent dyes in sporulation resuspension medium as in **step 1** in Subheading 3.2 (*see* **Notes 3**).

4. Prepare a 2% agarose solution in sporulation resuspension medium as in **step 2** in Subheading 3.2. Prepare agarose pad right before use as in **step 3** in Subheading 3.2.

5. When the culture reaches an OD$_{600}$ of 0.5, transfer all the cells from the flask (about 20–25 ml) into a 50 ml conical tube by pouring. Save the empty flask for **step 7**.

6. Spin the tube in a bench-top centrifuge at 5000×*g* for 5 min. Remove the supernatant by aspiration (*see* **Note 24**).

7. Add 20 ml of resuspension medium (from **step 2**) to the cell pellet. Pipette to resuspend and transfer the cells back to the original flask (from **step 5**). This is the time 0. Take a sample for microscopy if needed.

8. Put the flask back to the shaking waterbath and take samples at required time points to examine the progression of sporulation.

9. At each time point, take 200 μl of cells, spin at 3300×*g* for 30 s, remove and discard the supernatant, and resuspend the cells in 10 μl of sporulation resuspension medium containing dye from **step 3**.

10. Prepare the slide as in **step 3** in Subheading 3.2 (Fig. 1) and visualize using a microscope (Fig. 5).

4   Notes

1. Plates can be stored at 4 °C for up to 3 months. Tetracycline plates should be protected from light.

2. Use deionized water (dH₂O) here, which contains trace amount of minerals.

3. FM4-64 and DAPI can be used at the same time. FM4-64 is not compatible with fluorescent fusions to mCherry. If membrane needs to be visualized together with an mCherry fusion, the blue membrane stain TMA-DPH can be used. In this case, to visualize the DNA, a GFP fusion to the nucleoid-associated protein HbsU (HbsU-GFP) [11] can be used instead of DAPI, which uses the same filter set as TMA-DPH. For sporulation, if a later time point is needed, TMA-DPH a preferred membrane dye because it is semi-permeable to cell membrane and the spore membrane can be visualized even after the spore is fully engulfed by the mother cell, while FM4-64 is impermeable to membrane and cannot stain the spore membrane once it is fully engulfed (Fig. 5).

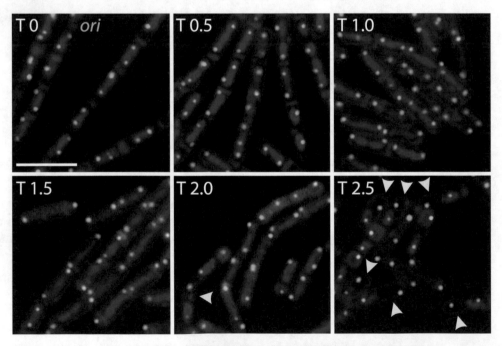

Fig. 5 Sporulation time course. Membranes (*red*) were stained with FM4-64, nucleoids (*blue*) were stained with DAPI, origins (*green*) were labeled using *tetO48*/TetR-CFP. Time (in hours) after the initiation of sporulation is indicated. Bar, 4 μm. *Yellow carets* indicate the fully engulfed spores, the membrane of which cannot be stained using FM4-64 (*see* **Note 3**)

4. Streak out strains freshly for every experiment.

5. Do not leave the plates at 4 °C. *B. subtilis* cells on the plates die at 4 °C.

6. CH medium has lower background fluorescence compared to LB medium.

7. *B. subtilis* tends to clump in the colony. Vortex gently for 5 s to make a homogenous inoculum.

8. This is to make sure that one of these two cultures will be in mid-exponential phase in the next morning.

9. To ensure adequate aeration, the volume of the medium used should not be more than 1/10th of the volume of the flask.

10. To prevent agarose from boiling over, heat the agarose solution in the microwave at 5 s pulses and gently swirl the bottle to mix thoroughly between pulses, until the agarose is fully melted. Use caution to prevent burns.

11. Prepare the agarose pads 2–5 min before harvesting the cells. Pads can be made 1–2 h in advance but need to be stored in a humid chamber to prevent them from drying off.

12. Spacers can be reused.

13. To prevent formation of bubbles, pipette the agarose solution using a pipette tip with its tip cut off.

14. Position the second slide over the agarose droplet and let it drop. This prevents the agarose pad from being slanted, which will produce uneven focal planes in the field of view while imaging.

15. To expose the agarose pad, carefully slide one of the microscopy slides over the other one. The agarose pad will remain adhered to one of the slides. Do not pull the slides apart because it can distort the agarose pad. Pads made this way are even in thickness. The slide that is removed can be reused.

16. *B. subtilis* grows in filaments. Higher speed of spinning could potentially shear the cells and affect protein localization. Cell pellet is loose so aspirate or pipette with care to prevent losing too many cells.

17. To prevent bubbles forming between the agarose pad and the coverslip, put the coverslip at an angle over the pad and gently lower it until it touches the agarose. To prevent depletion of oxygen from the cells, do not let cells sit in the agarose pad for longer than 10 min before imaging.

18. This is to prevent the agarose pad from drying out.

19. Do not over-dry the agarose pad.

20. We do not use dyes for time-lapse imaging because they may affect cell viability over time. If DNA needs to be visualized, a

fluorescent fusion to the nucleoid-associated protein HbsU, such as HbsU-GFP [11], can be used.

21. As with the coverslips, angle the agarose strip and slowly lower it onto the cells, to prevent bubbles. If the microscope stage allows multi-position acquisition, multiple strains can be visualized simultaneously on the same dish by putting cells and agarose strips in parallel, each for a different strain.

22. The agarose pad is fully exposed to oxygen to help growth of *B. subtilis* cells on the slide.

23. Optimize image acquisition by introducing Neutral Density (ND) filters in the light path and adjusting exposure times and time intervals. It is less damaging to the cell to introduce an ND filter and increase the exposure time than to only reduce the exposure time. This optimization is especially important when imaging *B. subtilis*. Phototoxicity causes the chromosome to expand and fill the entire cell compartment and it stalls cell growth and affects the dynamic behavior of many cell wall related proteins.

24. The cell pellet is not tight. Try to remove as much medium as possible without losing cells.

Acknowledgment

Support for this work comes from National Institutes of Health Grants GM086466 and GM073831 (to David Z. Rudner). X.W. was a long-term fellow of the Human Frontier Science Program. P.M.L. is a Helen Hay Whitney postdoctoral fellow.

References

1. Tan IS, Ramamurthi KS (2014) Spore formation in Bacillus subtilis. Environ Microbiol Rep 6(3):212–225. doi:10.1111/1758-2229.12130

2. Setlow P (2014) Spore resistance properties. Microbiol Spectr 2(5):PMID: 26104355. doi:10.1128/microbiolspec.TBS-0003-2012

3. Paredes-Sabja D, Setlow P, Sarker MR (2011) Germination of spores of Bacillales and Clostridiales species: mechanisms and proteins involved. Trends Microbiol 19(2):85–94. doi:10.1016/j.tim.2010.10.004

4. Rudner DZ, Losick R (2010) Protein subcellular localization in bacteria. Cold Spring Harb

Perspect Biol 2(4):a000307. doi:10.1101/cshperspect.a000307

5. Fornasiero EF, Opazo F (2015) Super-resolution imaging for cell biologists: concepts, applications, current challenges and developments. Bioessays 37(4):436–451. doi:10.1002/bies.201400170

6. Norman TM, Lord ND, Paulsson J, Losick R (2013) Memory and modularity in cell-fate decision making. Nature 503(7477):481–486. doi:10.1038/nature12804

7. Wang P, Robert L, Pelletier J, Dang WL, Taddei F, Wright A, Jun S (2010) Robust growth of

Escherichia coli. Curr Biol 20(12):1099–1103. doi:10.1016/j.cub.2010.04.045

8. Balaban NQ, Merrin J, Chait R, Kowalik L, Leibler S (2004) Bacterial persistence as a phenotypic switch. Science 305(5690):1622–1625. doi:10.1126/science.1099390

9. Harwood CR, Cutting SM (1990) Molecular biological methods for Bacillus. Wiley, New York, NY

10. Grossman AD, Losick R (1988) Extracellular control of spore formation in Bacillus subtilis. Proc Natl Acad Sci U S A 85(12):4369–4373

11. Wang X, Montero Llopis P, Rudner DZ (2014) Bacillus subtilis chromosome organization oscillates between two distinct patterns. Proc Natl Acad Sci U S A 111:12877–12882. doi:10.1073/pnas.1407461111

INDEX

Mark C. Leake (ed.), *Chromosome Architecture: Methods and Protocols*, Methods in Molecular Biology, vol. 1431,
DOI 10.1007/978-1-4939-3631-1, © Springer Science+Business Media New York 2016